WITHDRAWN
UTSA LIBRARIES
P9-DUH-604

THE COSMETIC FORMULARY

The
COSMETIC FORMULARY

HOW TO MAKE COSMETICS, PERFUMES, SOAPS, AND ALLIED PRODUCTS

By

H. BENNETT

Fellow American Institute of Chemists
Editor-in-Chief The Chemical Formulary
Practical Everyday Chemistry
More For Your Money

CHEMICAL PUBLISHING CO. of N. Y. INC.

148 Lafayette St. New York

1937

PRINTED IN U.S.A.

PREFACE

COSMETICS are no longer considered luxuries. Most women consider them necessities. The cosmetic industry comes next to the food and clothing industries in volume of business done. Like all important industries, it is continually changing, as well as growing. Cosmetic products, their packages and sales appeals must be closely attuned with the times. What was a popular product a year ago may soon be passed by another product and eventually may be forgotten entirely.

Just as the industry is growing, so is the literature on this subject growing. For any individual, especially the non-chemist or lay-worker, it is almost a hopeless task to keep up with new developments.

The purpose of this book is to correlate the most practical, up-to-date information and formulae in the cosmetic and allied fields. Since our knowledge in this field is mainly empirical, theories and opinions should be taken with the proverbial "grain of salt." No two chemists or manufacturers will agree exactly on any formula. It is manifestly impossible to suit everyone. A formula is useful as a starting point or to give one an idea.

The manufacture of cosmetics in general is often an elaborate procedure. The technique is more manual than creative and most of the products that fall under this classification are within the reach of the average person provided with a formula and common sense. The creation of new formulas and new products is, of course, restricted to the specialist. Anyone, given a satisfactory formula, can produce successfully a batch of cold cream, but to alter that cream, to modify its properties in conformity with certain desired ends, requires knowledge and experience. If the procedure results in disappointment, it may be assumed that the trouble is due to improper technique, incorrect or impure materials or quantities, lack of knowledge of the specific properties of certain ingredients or perhaps the non-realization of product conforming to specific and not general requirements.

The "whys and wherefores" of cosmetic formulation are founded on tradition and based on "rule-of-thumb" experiments with little "rhyme or reason." The number of chemists employed in the cosmetic industry is steadily increasing. More and more are cosmetic manufacturers beginning to realize the value of the chemist to this industry. Those who cannot engage a full time chemist are turning to consultants. In this way they are enabled to turn out uniform products, with a lesser tendency to deteriorate, and they are in a position to keep up with new developments.

Schools and colleges which, in the past, have not considered this industry are now aware of its importance. Many high schools are giving simple courses in making cosmetics in connection with their domestic science courses. Colleges, too, are awakening and are preparing students to take their places in this tremendous industry.

It is hoped that this text will prove a starting point for education in the field of cosmetic manufacture. The editors will appreciate suggestions and criticisms from readers of this work with a view to extending its usefulness in future editions.

It is a sincere pleasure to acknowledge the valuable assistance of the members of the board of editors and others who have so willingly given of their time, effort and knowledge in contributing special, private data to this volume.

H. Bennett

CONTENTS

	PAGE
Preface	vii
Contents	ix
Introduction	xi
Figuring	xii
Apparatus	xiv
Methods	xv

CHAPTER		
I.	Creams	1
II.	Lotions	47
III.	Skin Treatments, Special	65
IV.	Depilatories and Deodorants	75
V.	Sunburn Preparations	79
VI.	Lipsticks and Rouges	86
VII.	Eye Preparations	92
VIII.	Soaps and Cleaners	96
IX.	Bath Preparations	104
X.	Hair Preparations	112
XI.	Manicure Preparations	143
XII.	Face Powders and Talcs	150
XIII.	Perfumes and Toilet Waters	161
XIV.	Shaving Preparations	194
XV.	Dentifrices	211
XVI.	Miscellaneous	225
XVII.	Tables	235

References	246
Where to Buy	
Raw Materials	247
Equipment	257
Containers	258
Index	263

INTRODUCTION

THE contents of this section are written in a simple way so that anyone, regardless of technical education or experience, can start making simple products without any complicated or expensive machinery. For commercial productions, however, suitable equipment is necessary.

Cosmetics en masse are composed of oils, greases, fats, waxes, emulsifying agents, water, chemicals of great diversity, dyestuffs, and perfumes. To assemble some of these with some of the others requires certain definite and well-studied procedure, any departure from which will inevitably result in failure. The successful steps are given with the formulas. Follow them explicitly. If the directions require that A should be added to B, carry this out literally, and not in reverse fashion. In making an emulsion (and many cosmetics, particularly creams, are emulsions), the job is often quite as tricky as the making of mayonnaise. In making mayonnaise, you add the oil to the egg, *slowly,* with constant and even and regular stirring. If you do it correctly, you get mayonnaise. If you depart from any of these details: if you add the egg to the oil, or pour the oil in too quickly, or fail to stir regularly, the result is a complete disappointment. The same disappointment might be expected if the prescribed procedure of a cosmetic formula is violated.

The next point in importance is the scrupulous use of the proper ingredients. Substitutions are sure to result in inferior quality, if not in complete failure. Use what the formula calls for. If a cheaper product is desired, do not obtain it by substituting a cheaper material for the one prescribed: resort to a different formula. Not infrequently a formula will call for some ingredient which is difficult to obtain: in such cases, either reject the formula or substitute a similar material only after preliminary experiment demonstrates its usability. There is a limit to which this rule may reasonably be extended. In some instances the substitution of an equivalent ingredient may legitimately be made. For example: when the formula calls for *white wax* (beeswax), yellow wax can be used, if the color of the finished product is a matter of secondary importance. Yellow beeswax will replace white beeswax, making due allowance for color: but paraffin will *not* replace beeswax, even though its light color recommends it above yellow beeswax.

And this leads to the third point: the use of good quality ingredients, and ingredients of the correct quality. Ordinary lanolin is not the same thing as *anhydrous* lanolin: the replacement of one for the other, weight for weight, will give discouragingly different results. Use exactly what the formula calls for: if you are unacquainted with the material and a doubt arises as to just what is meant, discard the formula and use one that you understand. Buy your materials from reliable sources. Many of the ingredients in cosmetics are obtainable in a number of different grades: if the formula does not designate the grade, it is understood that the best grade is to be used. Remember that a formula and the directions can tell you only a part of the story. Some skill is often required to attain success. Practice with a small batch in such cases until you are sure of your technique. Many instances can be cited. If the formula calls for steeping quince seed for 30 minutes in cold water, your duplication of this procedure may produce a mucilage of too thin a consistency. The originator of the formula may have used a fresher grade of seed, or his conception of what "cold" water means may be different from yours. You should have a feeling for the right degree of mucilaginousness, and if steeping the seed for 30 minutes fails to produce it, steep them longer until you get the right kind of mucilage. If you do not know what the right kind is, you will have to experiment until you find out. Hence the recommendation to make small experimental batches until successful results are arrived at. Another case is the use of dyestuffs for coloring lotions, and the like. Dyes vary in strength: they are all very powerful in tinting value: it is not always easy to state in quantitative terms how much to use. You must establish the quantity by carefully adding minute quantities until you have the desired tint. Gum tragacanth is one of those products which can give much trouble. It varies widely in solubility and bodying power: the quantity prescribed in the formula may be entirely unsuitable for *your* grade of tragacanth. Hence a correction is necessary, which can only be made after experiments to determine *how much* to correct.

In short, if you are completely inexperienced, you can profit greatly by gaining some experience through recourse to experiment. Such products as mouth washes, hair tonics, astringent lotions, need little or no experience, because they are as a rule merely mixtures of simple liquid and solid ingredients, the latter dissolving without difficulty and the whole being a clear solution that is ready for use when mixed. On the other hand, face creams, tooth pastes, shaving creams, which require relatively elaborate procedure and which depend for their usability on a definite final viscosity, must be made with the exercise of some skill, and not infrequently some experience.

Figuring

Some prefer proportions expressed by weight, volume or in terms of percentages. In different industries and foreign countries various systems of weights and measures are used. For this reason no one set of units could be satisfactory for everyone. Thus divers formulae appear with different units in accordance with their sources of origin. In some cases, parts instead of percentages or weight or volume is designated. On the pages preceding the index, tables of weights and measures are given. These are of use in changing from one system to another. The following examples illustrate typical units:

Example No. 1

Permanent Wave Lotion

Ammonium Sulphite	50
Water	1000
Glycerin	30
Turkey Red Oil	5

Here no units are mentioned. When such is the case it is standard practice to use parts by weight, using the same system throughout. Thus here we may use ounces or grams as desired. But if ounces are used for one item then ounces must be the unit for all the other items in the particular formula.

Example No. 2

Cream Rouge

Stearic Acid	25 %
Water	61½%
Glycerin	10 %
Potassium Hydroxide	1 %
Oil Soluble Dye	2½%
Perfume	to suit %

Where no units of weight or volume but percentages are given then forget the percentages and use the same instructions as given under Example No. 1.

Example No. 3

Antiseptic Ointment

Petrolatum	16 parts
Coconut Oil	12 parts
Salicylic Acid	1 part
Benzoic Acid	1 part
Chlorthymol	1 part

The same instructions as given under Example No. 1 apply to Example No. 3.

It is not wise in many cases to make up too large a quantity of material until one has first made a number of small batches to first master the necessary technique and also to see whether it is suitable for the particular outlet for which it is intended. Since, in many cases, a formula may be given in proportions as made up on a commercial factory scale, it is advisable to reduce the proportions accordingly. Thus, taking the following formula:

Example No. 4

Neutral Cleansing Cream

Mineral Oil	80 lb.
Spermaceti	30 lb.
Glyceryl Monostearate	24 lb.
Water	90 lb.
Glycerin	10 lb.
Perfume	to suit

Here, instead of pounds, grams may be used. Thus this formula would then read:

Mineral Oil	80 g.
Spermaceti	30 g.
Glyceryl Monostearate	24 g.
Water	90 g.
Glycerin	10 g.
Perfume	to suit

Reduction in bulk may also be obtained by taking the same fractional part or portion of each ingredient in a formula. Thus in the following formula:

Example No. 5

Vinegar Face Lotion

Acetic Acid (80%)	20
Glycerin	20
Perfume	20
Alcohol	440
Water	500

We can divide each amount by ten and the finished bulk is only $\frac{1}{10}$th of the original formula. Thus it becomes:

Acetic Acid (80%)	2
Glycerin	2
Perfume	2
Alcohol	44
Water	50

Apparatus

For most preparations pots, pans, china and glassware, such as is used in every household, will be satisfactory. For making fine mixtures and emulsions a "malted-milk" mixer or egg-beater is necessary. For weighing, a small, low priced scale should be purchased from a laboratory supply house. For measuring of fluids, glass graduates or measuring glasses may be purchased from your local druggist. Where a thermometer is necessary a chemical thermometer should be obtained from a druggist or chemical supply house.

Methods

To better understand the products which you intend making, it is advisable that you read the complete section covering such products. Very often an important idea is thus gotten. You may learn different methods that may be used and also avoid errors which many beginners are prone to make.

Containers for Compounding

Where discoloration or contamination is to be avoided (as in light colored, or food and drug products) it is best to use enamelled or earthenware vessels. Aluminum as well, is highly desirable in such cases but it should not be used with alkalies as the latter dissolve and corrode this metal.

Heating

To avoid overheating, it is advisable to use a double boiler when temperatures below 212°F (temperature of boiling water) will suffice. If a double boiler is not at hand, any pot may be filled with water and the vessel containing the ingredients to be heated is placed therein. The pot may then be heated by any flame without fear of overheating. The water in the pot, however, should be replenished from time to time as necessary—it must not be allowed to "go dry." To get uniform higher temperatures, oil, grease or wax is used in the outer container in place of water. Here of course care must be taken to stop heating when thick fumes are given off as these are inflammable. When higher uniform temperatures are necessary, molten lead may be used as a heating medium. Of course, where materials melt uniformly and stirring is possible, direct heating over an open flame is possible.

Where instructions indicate working at a certain temperature, it is important that the proper temperature be attained—not by guess work, but by the use of a thermometer. Deviations from indicated temperatures will usually result in spoiled preparations.

Temperature Measurements

In Great Britain and the United States, the Fahrenheit scale of temperature measurement is used. The temperature of boiling water is 212° Fahrenheit (212°F); the temperature of melting ice is 32 degrees Fahrenheit (32°F).

In scientific work and in most foreign countries the Centigrade scale is used. On this scale of temperature measurement, the temperature of boiling water is 100 degrees Centigrade (100°C) and the temperature of melting ice is 0 degrees Centigrade (0°C).

The temperature of liquids is measured by a glass thermometer. The latter is inserted as deeply as possible in the liquid and is moved about until the temperature remains steady. It takes a little time for the glass of the thermometer to come to the temperatures of the liquid. The thermometer should not be placed against the bottom or side of the container, but near the center of the liquid in the vessel. Since the glass of the bulb of the thermometer is very thin, it can be broken easily by striking it against any hard surface. A cold thermometer should be warmed gradually (by holding over the surface of a hot liquid) before immersion. Similarly the hot thermometer when taken out should not be put into cold water suddenly. A sharp change in temperature will often crack the glass.

Mixing and Dissolving

Ordinary solution (e.g. sugar in water) is hastened by stirring and warming. Where the ingredients are not corrosive, a clean stick, bone or composition fork or spoon is used as a mixing device. These may also be used for mixing thick creams or pastes. In cases where most efficient stirring is necessary (as in making mayonnaise, milky polishes, etc.) an egg beater or a malted milk mixer is necessary.

Filtering and Clarification

When dirt or undissolved particles are present in a liquid, they are removed by settling or filtering. In the former the solution is allowed to stand and if the particles are heavier than the liquid they will gradually sink to the bottom. The upper liquid may be poured or siphoned off carefully and in some cases is then of sufficient clarity to be used. If, however, the particles do not settle out then they must be filtered off. If the particles are coarse they may be filtered or strained through muslin or other cloth. If they are very small particles then filter paper is used. Filter papers may be obtained in various degrees of fineness. Coarse filter paper filters rapidly but will not, of course, take out extremely fine particles. For the latter, it is necessary to use a very fine grade of filter paper. In extreme cases even this paper may not be fine enough. Here it will be necessary to add to the liquid ⅓% of infusorial earth or magnesium carbonate. The latter clog up the pores of the filter paper and thus reduce their size and hold back undissolved material of extreme fineness. In all such filtering, it is advisable to take the first portions of the filtered liquid and pour them through the filter again as they may develop cloudiness in standing.

Decolorizing

The most commonly used decolorizer is decolorizing carbon. The latter is added to the liquid to the extent of 1/5% and heated with stirring for 1/2 hour to as high a temperature as is feasible. It is then allowed to stand for a while and filtered. In some cases bleaching must be resorted to. Examples of this are given in this book.

Pulverizing and Grinding

Large masses or lumps are first broken up by wrapping in a clean cloth and placing between two boards and pounding with a hammer. The smaller pieces are then pounded again to reduce their size. Finer grinding is done in a mortar with a pestle.

Spoilage and Loss

All containers should be closed when not in use to prevent evaporation or contamination by dust; also because, in some cases, air affects the material adversely. Many materials attack or corrode the metal containers in which they are received. This is particularly true of liquids. The latter, therefore, should be transferred to glass bottles which should be as full as possible. Corks should be covered with aluminum foil (or dipped in melted paraffin wax when alkalies are present).

Materials such as glue, gums, olive oil or other vegetable or animal products may ferment or become rancid. This produces discoloration or unpleasant odors. To avoid this, suitable antiseptics or preservatives must be used. Too great stress cannot be placed on cleanliness. All containers must be cleaned thoroughly before use to avoid various complications.

Weighing and Measuring

Since, in most cases, small quantities are to be weighed, it is necessary to get a light scale. Heavy scales should not be used for weighing small amounts as they are not accurate for this type of weighing.

For measuring volume (liquids) measuring glasses or cylinders (graduates) should be used. Since this glassware cracks when heated or cooled suddenly it should not be subjected to sudden changes of temperature.

Caution

Some chemicals are corrosive and poisonous. In many cases they are labeled as such. As a precautionary measure, it is advised not to smell bottles directly, but only to sniff a few inches from the cork or stopper. Always work in a well ventilated room when handling poisonous or unknown chemicals. If anything is spilled, it should be wiped off and washed away at once.

Where to Buy Chemicals and Apparatus

Many chemicals and most glassware can be purchased from your druggist. Notices of suppliers of all products will be found at the end of this book.

Advice

This book is the result of co-operation of many chemists and engineers who have given freely of their time and knowledge. It is their business to act as consultants and, for a fee, to give advice on technical matters. As publishers, we do not maintain a laboratory or consulting service to compete with them.

Please, therefore, do not ask us for advice or opinions, but confer with a chemist in your vicinity.

CALCULATING COSTS

WHEN materials are bought in small quantities their cost is necessarily higher than when bought in large quantities. Commercial prices are based on purchases in barrels or bags and prices on such units should be obtained from manufacturers or their sales representatives. For example, a pound of shellac may cost 60 cents or more but in bags it may be gotten for about 23 cents per pound.

Typical Commercial Costing Calculation

Water Shellac

Ammonium Hydroxide—	8 pounds	@	$ .04 per lb.—	$ 0.32
Water	100 "		—	—
Glycerine (Yellow)	— 2 "	@	.16 " "	0.32
Shellac, Bleached	— 20 "	@	.32 " "	6.40
Total	130 pounds		Total	$7.04

If 130 pounds cost $7.04, 1 pound will cost $7.04 divided by 130 or about $5\frac{4}{10}$c per pound.

Always weigh up the amount of finished product and use this weight for calculating costs as some part may be lost in the process or will stick to the vessel, mixer, etc. Costs of making sample lots will necessarily be high and should not be used as a basis but the excess should be charged to development expense.

Extra Reading

It is strongly urged that if at all possible that the following magazines be gotten and read regularly. Only in this way will it be possible to keep up with new materials, equipment and finished products.

Cosmetic Magazines Recommended

Drug and Cosmetic Industry, New York, N. Y.
American Perfumer, New York, N. Y.
Soap and Perfumery Review, London, England.

CHAPTER I

CREAMS

Cold Cream

COLD creams are the most basic and still the most important creams that are sold. Cold creams are usually formulated using mineral oil as a softening and cleansing agent, and emulsifying with water by the action of borax on beeswax.

Cold creams are emulsions of water in oil (oil + wax). They are oily or greasy to the touch and produce a cooling effect on the skin as the water slowly evaporates.

Countless variations in formulation have been and are being made to try to obtain special effects or to conform with various theories.

In the manufacture of cold creams it is necessary to use raw materials of the lightest color and avoid discolorations that may be introduced through attack or corrosion of vessels and mixers used. Dirt and foreign matter must be scrupulously excluded.

Mixing vessels and all other materials with which the cream comes in contact should be made of aluminum, monel, special stainless steel or high grade enamel. They should be steam jacketed or of the double boiler type to avoid over heating. Mixers should be so pitched and regulated to avoid beating in excessive amounts of air.

When creams are poured into jars, while warm, they should not be capped until cool; otherwise water will condense and separate on the surface of the cream.

Procedure:

The beeswax is chipped and melted, not allowing the temperature to go over 70° C. The borax and water are placed in the kettle on the opposite side of the mixing tank. Start to warm gently when the beeswax is melted and at the time start to add the rest of the mineral oil. Bring the temperature of the wax and oil mixture to 72° C. Now quickly bring the temperature of the borax solution to the same temperature 72° C.

These temperatures must be the same, but the closer they are the better the cream will be.

Warm the mixing tank a little; strain the wax and oil mixture into it. Now start the mixer and run in the borax solution, not too quickly, but with a fairly moderate speed. Add perfume when the temperature is about 50° C.

A cream made with these precautions will have a fine texture and yield a good surface. It may be run through a colloid mill but it is not necessary.

Run cream to the storage tank above the filling machine.

Formula No. 1

Beeswax, White	14 oz.
Mineral Oil	52 oz.
Borax	1 oz.
Water	33 oz.

Formula No. 2

Mineral Oil	1 gal.
Beeswax, White	2 lb.
Water (Distilled)	½ gal.
Powdered Borax (Bolted)	2 oz.

Mix beeswax and oil in one container. Bring to 150° F. then reduce to 120° F. Dissolve borax in water. Bring to 120° F. Pour borax and water solution slowly into wax and oil solution stirring constantly but not rapidly. At 115° F., perfume and pour into containers.

Formula No. 3

Beeswax	540 g.
Spermaceti	300 g.
Mineral Oil	1730 g.
Stearin	430 g.
Water	720 cc.
Borax	100 g.
Sodium Benzoate	10 g.
Perfume	

The fat bases should be melted with mineral oil. The borax and benzoate of soda dissolved in water and brought to the boil and stirred while still hot into the molten fats. Allow to cool with slow agitation. Add perfume.

Formula No. 4

Beeswax	8.5 g.
Spermaceti	8.5 g.
Cholesterin	1.0 g.
Ozokerite	3.5 g.
Olive, Peanut, or Mineral Oil	50.5 g.
Water, Distilled	30.0 g.

Emulsify and homogenize at lowest possible temperature.

Formula No. 5

White Mineral Oil	73.5 g.
White Beeswax	16.5 g.
Paraffin Wax	5.0 g.
Ozokerite	5.0 g.

The above should be heated to a temperature slightly above its melting point. The proper type of perfume is then added.

In a separate container, 1½ g. borax is dissolved in water. The amount of water can vary from 26 to 36 g. per 100 g. of finished cold cream.

The borax dissolved in the water and heated almost to the boiling point (approximately 200° F.) is then added all at one time to the above mixture. Stir during the addition of the borax water and continue stirring until a complete emulsion has been formed. The cream should be filled into the jars while still warm; not hot but just warm enough to pour easily so that it will have a perfectly smooth and even appearance at normal temperature.

Caution: If the water is not hot enough when added to the base, the cream will separate drops of water upon standing. If the stirring is not properly done or not continued long enough, the cream will likewise separate water.

Formula No. 6

White Mineral Oil	45.0 g.
White Beeswax U.S.P.	13.0 g.
Spermaceti	6.0 g.

Heat all together until liquid; then add under stirring

Powdered Borax	1.0 g.
Water	35.0 g.

which has been heated previously to about 200° F. In the summer time or warm weather, it is advisable to increase percentage of beeswax and decrease percentage of spermaceti, reducing the amount of water slightly.

Formula No. 7

Stearic Acid	120 g.
Lanolin (Anhydrous)	24 g.
Beeswax (White)	20 g.
Mineral Oil (White)	42 g.
Olive Oil	90 g.
Paraffin	12 g.
Triethanolamine	15.2 g.
"Carbitol"	64 g.
Water	380 g.

Melt the first six constituents and heat to about 70° C. Heat the triethanolamine and water to boiling, and stir vigorously into the hot solution of waxes. Add perfume and stir into the above cream after it has cooled somewhat. Stir the mixture until it is homogeneous and pour into jars while still warm.

Formula No. 8

Stearic Acid	30 g.
Lanolin	6 g.
Paraffin Wax	16 g.
Paraffin Oil (White)	50 g.
Triethanolamine	7 g.

"Carbitol"	15 g.
Water (Distilled)	200 g.
Perfume Oil	

Melt together the stearic acid, lanolin, paraffin, and paraffin oil. Add this mixture to the triethanolamine and water, which have been mixed and heated to the boiling point, stirring constantly. As the cream begins to thicken, add the "Carbitol" and perfume, continuing the stirring until a smooth cream is obtained.

Formula No. 9

Olive Oil (Benzoinated)	10 g.
Beeswax	35 g.
White Petroleum Jelly	35 g.
Paraffin Wax	10 g.
Liquid Paraffin Oil	80 g.
Water	60 g.
Borax	1 g.

Melt the fats and wax. Boil the water and add the borax, cool a little and mix.

Formula No. 10

The old standard cold cream is an emulsion of water in an oil wax mixture. The emulsifying agent is borax and the body is supplied by the waxes. A combination of "Ceraflux" and Ozokerite has been found to give the best results at a moderate cost. This is illustrated by the following formula:

Mineral (Paraffin Oil), Light or Medium Viscosity	2 gal.
White Beeswax	2 lb.
White Ozokerite	1 lb.
"Ceraflux"	2 lb.

Heat the above to 170° F. and add to it slowly while stirring thoroughly a solution of:

Borax	3 oz.
Water	1 gal.

which has been heated to 175° F. The cream is stirred and allowed to cool to 150° F., when 2 ounces of perfume are added. The cream is poured at 130° F.

If all of the cream is not packed at once, it may be stored in bulk. When it is desired to pack it, it should be reheated to 130° F. on a water or steam bath with slow stirring and then poured into jars. If desired the water in this formula may be replaced by rose water.

The body of these creams may be varied by changing the amounts of "Ceraflux" and Ozokerite. Part of the mineral oil may be replaced by petrolatum. For special needs part of the mineral oil may be replaced by olive, almond, cherry, turtle, peanut or other oils. Where a non-mineral oil is used an amount of Moldex equal to 1% of the oil used should be dissolved in the water to prevent rancidity.

Formula No. 11

Cold Cream, Modern

Paraffin Wax	1 lb.
Cetamin	2 lb.
Petrolatum, White	1½ lb.
Mineral Oil, White	3 pt.

Heat to 180° F. and to it add with stirring

Water (Boiling)	1 gal.

When at 150° F., while mixing, add 1 dram perfume and mix till thick. Pack cold.

Lavender Cream

As above except using water soluble lavender color and lavender perfume.

Violet Cream

Follow cold cream formula using water soluble violet color and violet perfume.

Tangerine Cream

Follow cold cream formula using water soluble orange color and tangerine perfume.

Mint Cream

Follow cold cream formula using water soluble green color and peppermint perfume.

Wild Cherry Cream

Follow cold cream formula using water soluble cherry color and wild cherry perfume.

Formula No. 12

Cetyl Alcohol	10 g.
Paraffin, Liquid	10 g.
Vaseline, White	80 g.
Water	60 g.

A transparent, soft, white cream.

Formula No. 13

Cetyl Alcohol	10 g.
Paraffin, Liquid	40 g.

Vaseline, White	50 g.
Water	60 g.

Formula No. 14

Cetyl Alcohol	10 g.
Paraffin, Liquid	40 g.
Vaseline, White	15 g.
Water	35 g.

Formula No. 15

Cetyl Alcohol	20 g.
Paraffin, Liquid	20 g.
Vaseline, White	60 g.
Water	60 g.

In place of the liquid paraffin there can be used a good vegetable oil. The maximum water-content (37.5%) can be increased by adding 10% wool fat.

Procedure: Melt the fatty materials together and stir, then run in boiling water, a little at a time, not adding additional water until previous amount is absorbed.

Formula No. 16

White Beeswax	12 g.
White Petroleum Jelly	12 g.
Peach Kernel Oil	50 g.
Rose Water	25 g.
Borax	1 g.
Perfume	to suit

Formula No. 17

1. Diglycol Stearate	14	lb.
2. Paraffin Wax	2	lb.
3. Mineral Oil	3¾	gal.
4. Petrolatum (White)	6	lb.
5. Water	6	gal.
6. Perfume Oil	5½	fl. oz.

Method of Manufacture:

a. Melt Nos. 1, 2, 3 and 4 at 170° F.

b. Heat 5 to 180°F.

c. Add *b* to *a* while mixing. Allow mixer to run until batch is completely emulsified.

d. Allow batch to cool to 125° F. and add 6 and mix at low speed.

e. Batch should be allowed to cool without stirring to 105° F. at which temperature it is poured into jars.

Formula No. 18

A rather soft but exceptionally smooth cream is made as follows:

Mineral Oil	1 gal.
Beeswax	1¾ lb.

Heat the above to 160° F. Dissolve 1½ oz. of borax in 5 pints of water, heat to 160° F. and add this solution to the oil and wax with rapid stirring. When the temperature drops to 140°, add 1 oz. of perfume oil and pour the cream at about 120°.

This basic formula may be modified by replacing up to half of the beeswax with paraffin, ceresin, ozokerite or spermaceti.

The oil may be replaced in part by petrolatum or by the vegetable oils. If vegetable oils are used, a preservative should be employed.

Materials such as lanolin and absorption base may be introduced in small quantities.

Formula No. 19

Diglycol Stearate	10.2 g.
Petrolatum, White	7 g.
Paraffin, 52° C.	5.6 g.
Mineral Oil, White	14.9 g.
Water, Distilled	60 g.
Borax	1.4 g.
Sodium Benzoate	0.9 g.

Emulsify at 75° C., perfume at 55° C. Pack in collapsible tubes or jars.

Formula No. 20

Stearic Acid	30	lb.
Lanolin (Anhydrous)	20	lb.
Beeswax (White)	16	lb.
Mineral Oil (White)	33	lb.
Triethanolamine	3.8	lb.
"Carbitol"	16	lb.
Water	95	lb.

Preparation

Melt the stearic acid, lanolin and beeswax in the mineral oil and heat to about 70° C. Prepare in a separate kettle a boiling solution of the Triethanolamine and water, and add to this the hot solution of waxes. Stir vigorously until a creamy emulsion is obtained and add the "Carbitol" to which the perfume has been added. Continue stirring until homogeneous and the product has reached the proper consistency. Pour into jars while still warm.

Properties

Cold creams are somewhat similar to cleansing creams in composition. They contain less oil and usually a mixture of fats and waxes of a type absorbed by the skin. Since cold creams usually remain in contact with the skin for several hours, they should contain the proper skin conditioners and the maximum absorbability of the fatty matter. The given cream is of good texture, is white and stable, and soothing in its action. It is also a washable cream.

Variations

The given formula should serve as a starting point for making up a cream to suit the individual preference and should not be considered as necessarily the best product obtainable. Great variation in the wax and oil constituents is allowable with little change in the basic ingredients. For example, vegetable and animal oils or fats may be substituted for all or a part of the mineral oil which is used only in the cheaper creams. Specific attention should be paid to the choice of perfumes, for some tend to discolor cosmetic creams after standing for a time. Neither Triethanolamine nor Carbitol, however, will have a deteriorating effect on perfumes properly chosen.

Formula No. 21

Mineral Oil	54.0 g.
White Wax	18.0 g.
Absorption Base (Parachol)	5.5 g.
Borax	1.0 g.
Water	21.0 g.
Perfume	.5 g.

Melt the white wax, add the mineral oil. Dissolve borax in part of water with heat. Add to melted fats. Heat rest of water, stir in absorption base until smooth and mix with fats. Agitate thoroughly and when just above solidifying point, add perfume.

Formula No. 22

Theatrical (Inexpensive)

Spermaceti	125 g.
White Wax	120 g.
Liquid Petrolatum	560 g.
Borax	5 g.
Distilled Water	190 g.
Oil of Rose, Synthetic	to suit

Melt the wax and spermaceti on the water bath and add the liquid petrolatum. Heat the distilled water and in it dissolve the borax. Add this warm solution to the melted mixture while both are warm and at about the same temperature. Beat rapidly; as soon as it begins to congeal add the oil of rose and beat until congealed. Dispense preferably in pure tin tubes.

Formula No. 23

Cold Cream (Low Cost)

Glycosterin	20 g.
Paraffin Wax	30 g.
Petrolatum White	18 g.
Mineral Oil	8 g.
Water	200 g.
Perfume	to suit

Formula No. 24

(Cleansing Type)

White Wax	10 oz.
Paraffin Wax	9 oz.
Ceresin	2 oz.
White Petrolatum	8 oz.
Liquid Petrolatum	3 lb.
Borax	1 oz.
Water, Distilled	1 pt., 4 fl. oz.

Formula No. 25

Cold Cream

Stearic Acid	15 g.
Paraffin Wax	25 g.
Paraffin Oil	25 g.
Triethanolamine	5 g.
"Carbitol"	5 g.
Water	45 cc.

Directions: Melt acid, wax and oil together and pour into a mixture of the triethanolamine, "Carbitol" and water. After suitable mixing and when partially cooled, add perfume to suit.

Formula No. 26

Beeswax, White	8.7 g.
Spermaceti	8.6 g.
Mineral Oil, White	51.8 g.
Ozokerite, White	2.2 g.
Paraffin, 52° C	3.2 g.
Water, Distilled	24.25 g.
Borax, or Potassium Biborate	1.25 g.
Perfume	up to 0.5 g.

Melt the waxes in the oil, heat to 60° C. Heat the borax-water to 60° C. Pour water-to-oil with slow, continued stirring. Perfume at 55–50° C. Pour at 45° C.

Formula No. 27

Beeswax, White	8.7 g.
Spermaceti	8.6 g.
Ozokerite, White	2.4 g.
Paraffin Wax, (52° C)	2.0 g.
Cholesterol	1.0 g.
Mineral Oil, White	40.8 g.

Sperm Oil, Deodorized	0.6 g.
Olive Oil, Preserved	5.25 g.
Water, Distilled	24.0 g.
Borax	0.75 g.
Perfume	0.5 g.

Emulsify at 60° C, add water-to-oil. Stir slowly until cooled, or pour at 45° C.

Cold Cream with High Content of Water

Cholesterol	2.0 g.
Beeswax, White	9.0 g.
Spermaceti	11.0 g.
Petrolatum, White	7.0 g.
Peanut Oil	68.0 g.
Water	143.0 g.

Important: in cholesterol creams, perfume additions should be made to the oils *before* adding the water. The water should be at 25–30° C, and should be added at a temperature slightly higher than room-temperature.

It is best to add only ½ of the water, the other ½ being added the following day after slightly warming the cream until manageable.

Night Cream (Greasy)

a.	Paraffin Oil, White	2500 g.
	Wax, Scale	500 g.
	Beeswax, Bleached	500 g.
	Adeps Lanae, Anhydrous	500 g.
b.	Distilled Water	3000 cc.
	Triethanolamine	75 g.
	Borax	35 g.

Melt *a* together at 75° C.; add *b* which is at same temperature, to *a*. Stir until cold.

Lanolin—Cold Cream

Beeswax, White	42 g.
Spermaceti	48 g.
Petrolatum, White	360 g.
Woolfat, Anhydrous	200 g.
Water	350 g.
Rose Perfume	10 g.

Vegetable Cold Cream

Sweet Almond Oil	48 g.
Olive Oil	5 g.
Beeswax	14 g.
Diglycol Laurate	1 g.
Borax	1 g.
Perfume	½ g.
Water	28 cc.

Cocoa Butter Cold Cream

Spermaceti	8.5 g.
Beeswax, White	8.5 g.
Cocoa Butter	12.0 g.
Mineral Oil	45.0 g.
Water, Distilled	24.75 g.
Borax	1.25 g.

Glycerin Cold Cream

a.	Wax, White	80 g.
	Spermaceti	80 g.
	Peanut Oil	300 g.
	Vaseline	300 g.
	Melt.	
b.	Glycerin	120 g.
	Water	120 g.
	Borax	10 g.

Warm up to 90°; pour into melted *a*. Add when cool:

Perfume Composition, Fresh Odor 20 g.

Cold Cream with Wool Wax

Beeswax	7.0 g.
Spermaceti	7.0 g.
Woolwax, Bleached (Woolfat Alcohols)	3.0 g.
Ceresin, White	2.5 g.
Paraffin	1.5 g.
Mineral Oil	37.5 g.
Olive or Peanut Oil, or Mineral Oil	12.5 g.
Water, Distilled	28.5 g.
Borax	0.5 g.
Perfume	

Emulsify at 60° C. (add water-to-oil). Stir slowly until cooled.

Washable Cold Cream

This is a cold cream which washes off readily with water.

Stearic Acid	20 g.
Triethanolamine	4 g.
"Carbitol"	1 g.
White Petrolatum	65 g.
Water	10 cc.

Two Purpose Cold Cream

Mineral Oil	22 g.
Glycosterin	10 g.
Paraffin Wax	6 g.

Heat to 65° C. and stir until uniform. To this add

Water (Boiling) 62 cc.

Mix well and when thickening begins add

Perfume	¼ cc.

Cold Cream with Cetyl Alcohol

Beeswax, White	8.5 g.
Spermaceti	8.5 g.
Ozokerite	2.0 g.
Cetyl Alcohol, Pure	4.0 g.
Paraffin Oil	51.3 g.
Water, Distilled	24.45 g.
Borax	1.24 g.

Emulsify at 60° C.

Cold Cream Base (Ointment)

Cetyl Alcohol	4 oz.
Wool Fat, Anhydrous	10 oz.
White Soft Paraffin	86 oz.

Melt on a steam-bath, mix well and allow to cool.

Cetyl ointment has the consistency and the glassy sheen of soft paraffin. When an equal weight of water is worked in a creamy, almost white ointment is produced, which is of the modern vanishing toilet-cream type, and which can be made into a greasy cream by the addition of olive oil, and this, perfumed with rose oil, gives the cold cream of the Swiss pharmacopœia, the formula of which is:—

Cetyl Alcohol	50 g.
Olive Oil	4 g.
Rose Water	46 g.
Rose Oil	2 drops

The mixture of cetyl alcohol and olive oil warmed at gentle heat is mixed carefully with the lukewarm rosewater, and the whole is stirred until cold, when the rose oil is added.

From the cold cream of other pharmacopœias it is readily distinguished, and resembles the now widely-used new skin creams. It has the advantage of plasticity, spreading power, freedom from rancidity, and a permanently "fast" water content. There is also a considerable saving in cost in the use of 4 per cent. olive oil instead of 60 per cent. almond oil. This cold cream, made with a basis of soft paraffin as a lubricant, is clearly an ointment which has only a minimum absorption, unlike the older cold creams made with easily-absorbed vegetable oils. That has naturally been the intention, and it is to be regarded as a step in advance.

Non-Greasy Cold Creams

(Almost Non-Greasy)

Formula No. 1

Beeswax	5 g.
Spermaceti	5 g.
Stearic Acid	15 g.
Mineral Oil, White	16 g.
Ammonia (0.910)	0.5 g.
Borax	2 g.
Water, Distilled	54.5 g.

Formula No. 2

Glycosterin	22 lb.
Petrolatum (Vaseline)	16 lb.
Paraffin Wax	12 lb.
Mineral Oil	30 lb.
Water	100 lb.

Heat first four ingredients to 170° F. and stir together. Then slowly with stirring pour in the water which has been heated to the same temperature. Stir thoroughly and then allow to stand (hot) until air bubbles are gone. Add perfume and stir and pour at 110–130° F. Cover jars as soon as possible.

Formula No. 3

Stearic Acid	16 oz.
Glycerin	48 oz.
Mineral Oil	12 oz.
Paraffin Wax	2 oz.
Stronger Ammonia Water	4 oz.
Water	64 oz.
Perfume	.75 oz.

Formula No. 4

A very low priced light bodied but stable cream is made as follows:

1.	Glycosterin	22 lb.
	Petrolatum White	16 lb.
	Paraffin Wax	12 lb.
	Mineral Oil	32 lb.
2.	Water	128 lb.
	Borax	3 lb.
	Potassium Carbonate	2 lb.

Heat above separately to 80° C. and pour (2) into (1) slowly while stirring. Add perfume at 55° C. stir and pack. If cold packed a high gloss is given to surface by passing a flame lightly over surface in each jar.

Cold Cream Base—Greaseless

White Petrolatum	5.25 g.
Beeswax	11.25 g.
White Mineral Oil	2.50 g.

Diglycol Stearate	6.00 g.
Water	75.00 cc.
Perfume, Color, Etc.	to suit

Liquid Greaseless Cream

Stearic Acid	32 oz.
Trihydroxyethyleneamine Stearate	8 oz.
Distilled Water	176 oz.
"Carbitol"	16 oz.
Zinc Sulphocarbolate	1 oz.
Alcohol	12 oz.
Perfume to suit	

Directions: #1. Melt stearic acid and trihydroxyethyleneamine stearate together.

#2. Dissolve the zinc sulphocarbolate in 76 parts of distilled water by heating, then add the balance of distilled water and carbolate and bring to a boil.

#3. Mix perfume oil with alcohol. Add #1 to #2 and agitate well. Then continue stirring slowly during the cooling process. When temperature has reached 50° C. add perfume.

Stearate Cold Cream

Formula No. 1

Stearic Acid	12.5 g.
Spermaceti Best, or Cetyl Alcohol	0.5 g.
Paraffin Oil (0.850)	2 g.
Corn (Maíze) Starch	2.5 g.
Water, Distilled	2.5 g.
Glycerin, 28° Bé	25 g.
Water, Distilled	20 g.
Caustic Potash or Ammonia Water	35 g.

Melt up the three first ingredients to 80–85° C., mix well. Separately make a paste of the starch with the same amount of water; the homogeneous starch paste is thinned with the glycerin water (100° C.) keep the hot starch dispersion at 70° C. for 1–2 hours, until it is a jelly.

Dissolve, in the meantime, the alkali (enough for a 30% saponification) in the remaining water, heat to 85° C., and add the oils to it with stirring. Keep temperature constant for 20 minutes with agitation, let cool to 70° C., and add the starch mucilage, always stirring.

Cool.

Formula No. 2

Stearic Acid, Triple Pressed	12.5 g.
Caustic Soda 30° Bé	2.1 g.
Glycerin	20.0 g.
Gelatine	0.8 g.
<or Tragacanth	0.5> g.
Water, Distilled	64.2 g.
Perfume	0.4 g.

Ammonia-Stearate Creams

Cold Cream Type "Elcaya"

Stearic Acid	11.0 g.
Spermaceti, Deodorized	2.0 g.
Ammonia (sp.g. 0.910)	0.8 g.
Glycerin	10.0 g.
Paraffin Oil	3.0 g.
Sodium Hydroxide	0.1 g.
Borax	0.3 g.
Corn Starch	1.5 g.
Perfume	1.0 g.
Water, Distilled	69.3 g.

Heat stearic acid and spermaceti and paraffin oil to 85° C. Dissolve caustic soda and borax in ⅔ of the water, heat up to 85° C. Mix starch and glycerin, and add the last ⅓ of water to it while boiling. Keep the mucilage hot.

Now pour the stearin-spermaceti mixture into the borax solution (to which, shortly before, the ammonia is added,) rather quickly with slow stirring. Boil the emulsion gently to free of unreacted ammonia. Cool, stir. At 70° C., the starch mucilage is added. Stir until cold. Perfume at 40° C.

Determine the loss of water, and replace some of it (less 8%).

Lemon Cream

The basic Cold Cream A formula is used with a little Tartrazine dissolved in the water used. "Lemenone" or citral is used as the perfume.

Strawberry Cream

The basic Cold Cream A formula with a little erythrosine dissolved in the water is used. Aldehyde C16 is used as the perfume.

Peaches and Cream

The basic Cold Cream A formula is used along with a small amount of Aldehyde C14 as the perfume.

Almond Cream

The basic Cold Cream A formula is used with a little benzaldehyde as the perfume.

Menthol (Cooling) Cream

The basic Cold Cream A formula is used along with 1 oz. of menthol as a perfume and cooling agent. These creams may be converted to tissue creams by incorporating some lanolin as in the Tissue Cream formula.

Cucumber Cream

The basic Cold Cream A is used and a little green dye is dissolved in the water used and cucumber juice replaces the usual perfume.

Acid Cream

(Patented in Germany)

Formula No. 1

Diglycol Stearate	14	g.
Stearyl-Sapamin Phosphate, 100%	0.8	g.
Citric Acid	2.2	g.
(or Lactic Acid, Buffered	1	g.)
Glycerin	5	g.
Mineral Oil	3	g.
Ceresin	1	g.
Beeswax, White	1	g.
Water, Distilled	73	g.

Formula No. 2

(Patented in Germany)

Diglycol Stearate	14	g.
Mineral Oil	3	g.
Beeswax, White	2	g.
Ceresine	1	g.
Lanolin	1	g.
Sodium Lauryl-Sulphonate	1	g.
Pectin, Citrus	0.5	g.
Perfume, Lemon Type *	0.5	g.
Citric Acid, Phosphoric Acid	2	g.
Glycerin	6	g.
Water, Distilled	69	g.

* *Lemon Perfume*

Lemon Oil	5	g.
Citral	1	g.
Benzyl Salicylate, C.P.	24	g.

Liquid Cold Cream

According to the *Pharmaceutical Journal*, nearly all of the existing liquid cold creams on the market have serious faults. They are either soap emulsions, which are alkaline and tend to remove the last bit of grease left in the skin, or acacia emulsions which leave the skin sticky and uncomfortable. In addition, they usually separate. A preparation has been devised in England which possesses none of these disadvantages. It has the following formula:

Formula No. 1

Liquid Paraffin	36	oz.
Trihydroxyethylamine Stearate	7¼	oz.
Warm Water	70	fl. oz.
Glycerin	10	fl. oz.
Perfume		to suit

Heat the oil and stearate together until just melted, add the warm water, stirring until a good emulsion is formed. Transfer to a bottle, add the perfume, and allow to stand until the next day. Shake for a few minutes and bottle. The cream can be made more viscous if desired by reducing the quantity of water.

To thicken the cream, vegetable oil may be used instead of liquid paraffin, up to 5% of white beeswax, spermaceti or lanolin, or a mixture of these may be used.

Formula No. 2

Triethanolamine	0.8	g.
Stearic Acid	4.0	g.
Cetyl Alcohol	2.0	g.
Glycerin	2.0	g.
Sodium Benzoate	0.5	g.
Borax	0.75	g.
Perfume		to suit
Water, Distilled to make	100.0	g.

Formula No. 3

Paraffin Oil	29	g.
Triethanolamine Stearate	4	g.
Triethanolamine Oleate	2	g.
+Distilled Water	65	g.
Perfume	0.5	g.

Melt up the first three ingredients at lowest possible temperature, and stir in the water which has been slightly warmed.

Formula No. 4

Paraffin Oil	300	g.
Stearic Acid	40	g.
Triethanolamine	30	g.
Water, Distilled	700	g.

Alcohol—Perfume (20%) 10 g.

Melt up paraffin and stearic acid (60–70° C). Stir this into the solution of triethanolamine in water of equal temperature.

Cool, and add perfume drop by drop.

Formula No. 5

1. Mineral Oil	72	lb.
2. Trihydroxyethylamine Stearate	14½	lb.
3. Water (Warm)	160	lb.
4. Perfume	1½	lb.

Heat (1) and (2) until just melted together, and stir. Next add (3) slowly with thorough stirring and continue until the batch is homogeneous. Allow to stand one night and stir for 15 minutes before packing.

This cream washes off easily with cold water. The consistency can be changed by varying the amount of water in this formula.

Emollient Cream

Very soft emollient creams, containing glycerin, can be made by the aid of vanishing cream. The method of production is very simple. All that is necessary is to thoroughly mix the vanishing cream with glycerite of starch with which a little zinc oxide has been previously incorporated. If zinc oxide is objected to because of the possibility of its reacting with the free stearic acid present, it may be advantageously replaced by titanium dioxide; and the following new formula for a cream of the type in question is suggested, which is based on a vanishing cream:

Glycerite of Starch	40 g.
Titanium Dioxide (Pure)	2 g.
Vanishing Cream	58 g.

To prepare this cream, first triturate the titanium dioxide with the glycerin of starch thoroughly in a mortar. Then work in the vanishing cream, a little at a time. The product is a beautifully white very soft emollient cream, excellent for the hands in cold weather. As the glycerite of starch exercises a softening effect on the vanishing cream, this should not be itself too soft in texture. The method may, indeed, be employed for using up vanishing cream which has become somewhat hardened by evaporation. The vanishing cream should itself be perfumed before use, and a larger proportion than that indicated may be incorporated if desired.

Hand Cream

Glyceryl Monostearate	10 g.
Cocoa Butter	2 g.
Glycerin	5 g.
Anhydrous Lanolin	2 g.
Stearic Acid	1 g.
Water	80 cc.

Add the ingredients to the water, turn on the heat and bring to the boiling point with constant stirring. When all the ingredients are melted and a clear emulsion is formed, shut off the heat and continue the mixing until the product is cold.

Cream Hand Cleaner

A cream for removing dirt from the hands without the use of water contains casein 9 g., lime water 16 g., ammonia 0.5, g., soda 1 g., oxycellulose or hydrocellulose 9 g., perfume 0.5 and water 64 g.

Liquid Hand Cream

Cetyl Alcohol	3.0 g.
Lanolin	1.0 g.
Lactic Acid	1.0 g.
Peanut Oil	2.0 g.
Sulfated Fatty Alcohol	0.5 g.
Water	92.5 g.
Perfume	0.5 g.

Melt the cetyl alcohol, lanolin and peanut oil at 50–60°C. and mix thoroughly with the sulfated fatty alcohol dissolved in half the water at the same temperature. Stir very thoroughly, avoiding the incorporation of air as much as possible. When the mixture has cooled somewhat but is still warm, stir in the lactic acid dissolved in the rest of the water. Homogenization is advantageous. The sulfated fatty alcohol is the emulsifier here and is used here in preference to one of the soaps because it retains its emulsifying power in the presence of free acid. The acid is added to neutralize alkaline residues left after dishwashing. Lanolin and peanut oil are emollients while the cetyl alcohol is present both as an emollient and to act as an auxiliary. The product has been shelf tested for over six months and has showed no signs of separation or other deterioration.

White Powder for Creams

Titanium Dioxide, 100%	10 kg.
Colloidal Clay	20 kg.
Zinc Stearate	10 kg.
Talcum, Best Quality	60 kg.

Zinc Stearate Creams

Formula No. 1

Zinc stearate cream may be prepared with 150 grams glycerin, 100 grams water, 80 grams zinc stearate. The stearate is first triturated with glycerin and water is gradually added. This cream is very soft, white and absolutely homogeneous. Sometimes ingredients of this cream separate after long standing. This can be corrected by addition of about 5% of medicinal pulverized soap which ensures permanent cohesion of various ingredients in a uniform mixture.

Formula No. 2

Five parts zinc stearate may be easily mixed with 50 parts petrolatum and is useful for many purposes, particularly in healing cuts.

Formula No. 3

Lanolin salve is made with 325 parts lanolin, 35 parts ceresin wax, 150 parts mineral oil and 150 parts water. Ceresin wax is melted in heated mineral oil and then lanolin is added and mixture allowed to cool. Mass is triturated into soft salve and water and perfume are worked in gradually. Five to 10% of zinc stearate is added to obtain preparation suitable for dry skin.

Vanishing Cream

This type of cream is essentially a stearic acid soap with excess suspended stearic acid dispersed in water. Pearliness is the optical effect produced by crystalline stearic acid in suspension.

The stearic acid used should be of the triple pressed grade having a melting point not lower than 56° C. Cheaper grades of stearic acids give softer, darker and malodorous creams. The glycerin used should be chemically pure, water-white and free from any objectionable odor. Some "white" glycerines are really yellow but appear "white" because a small amount of blue dye has been added. Such glycerin will give off-colored creams.

The alkalies used, too, should be colorless. When alkali carbonates such as potassium or sodium carbonates are used to saponify the stearic acid, they liberate large volumes of gaseous carbon dioxide. This gas is dissipated at high temperatures. At lower temperatures the cream will retain some of this gas. For this reason stirring should be continued intermittently for a number of days. Even then, the cream should be allowed to age in the mixing kettle for a few days, to settle. Before packing it should be stirred again working the crust into the mixture thoroughly so as to avoid any lumps.

Soft creams are produced by potassium carbonate or potassium hydroxide. Hard creams are produced by sodium carbonate or sodium hydroxide. Mixtures of the above sodium and potassium compounds produce creams intermediate in consistency. When ammonium hydroxide is used as the saponifying alkali a slightly darker cream is formed. This color deepens on aging. To avoid this anhydrous ammonium stearate is now being used to replace the mixture of ammonium hydroxide and stearic acid.

Certain bacteria thrive on stearic acid and water dispersible stearates. One never knows when they will be present and cause mold growth. It is best to be on the safe side by incorporating an efficient preservative. For this purpose moldex (a special p-hydroxy benzoic acid ester is used; 18 oz. of this preservative is used per 100 gal. of finished product).

Two kettles, preferably steam heated, are necessary for making vanishing creams. In one the stearic acid is melted; in the other the glycerin, ⅓ of the water and alkali are heated. Both of the above mixtures are heated to about 212° F and the water mixture is run into the melted stearic acid while mixing vigorously. Stirring should be continued until emulsification is complete. The balance of the water, heated to 212° F, is then added while mixing well. Then turn off the heat and continue mixing until the batch has cooled to 110–116° F and add the perfume while mixing. Continue mixing for ½ hour and then allow to age. If a finer textured and more stable product is desired the batch should be run through a colloid mill or homogenizer as soon as all the water has been introduced. The perfume is incorporated at 110–116° F.

Cetyl Alcohol is being used in some of the newer vanishing creams to give smoother and more penetrating products. Butyl stearate and diglycol laurate is replacing glycerin in vanishing creams to eliminate irritations to sensitive skins and prevent stickiness on humid days.

Formula No. 1

Vanishing Cream

Stearic Acid	50	lb.
Lanolin (Anhydrous)	9	lb.
Triethanolamine	2.5	lb.
"Carbitol"	18	lb.
Water	120	lb.

Preparation

In one container melt the stearic acid carefully and add the lanolin. Heat the Triethanolamine and water separately to boiling and then add the melted fatty acid to it with constant stirring. When a smooth mixture is obtained, stir in the "Carbitol" to which has been added the perfume. Continue with even stirring while cooling until a heavy, smooth cream is obtained, and then stir occasionally until cold. The cream will become thinner as it cools and the acid crystallizes.

Properties

A vanishing cream should be completely absorbed without leaving a greasy residue. It should have no tendency to flake or roll and should impart a feeling of softness and smoothness to the skin. It should afford some protection against wind and sun and also act as a powder base. The given product gives these desired properties to the fullest extent, and is free from irritating effect.

Variations

An excellent suntan or sunburn cream can be made with the above formula using 40 lb. stearic acid and 20 lb. lanolin.

Stearic acid is the essential ingredient of a vanishing cream since it produces the desired "dryness" and pearliness. It should be a very pure product if no rancidity or discoloration is to develop. The grade of acid has some effect upon the consistency of a vanishing cream, and if it is very hard and waxy, more water will have to be added to give the proper body. As a rule, by variations in the amount of this ingredient, any desired consistency can be obtained. The speed of stirring also has an effect upon the body of the cream. During the cooling, as soon as a stiff smooth emulsion is obtained, stirring should be reduced until just sufficient to prevent crusting on top. Rapid stirring after this point has been reached will usually cause aeration and yield a thin cream.

Formula No. 2

Five g. of cocoa butter is melted with 25 to 30 g. of pure stearin on a water bath at not above 100° C. A warm solution (at 60° C.) of 100 g. water, seven g. potash, eight g. borax, 16 g. glycerin, 12 g. alcohol and 3 g. ammonia, is added to 30 g. of molten waxes. Much carbon dioxide gas is liberated, which necessitates a large kettle for operation. Vigorous agitation is required. After most of carbon dioxide has escaped, a hot-filtered solution of 0.5 g. agar-agar in 20 g. water is added and the mixture stirred until cool. Perfume is added shortly before the mass congeals. The cream is filled into containers after standing 1 to 2 days.

Formula No. 3

Stearic Acid	35	lb.
Witch Hazel	6	gal.
Distilled Water	10	gal.
Glycerin	50	lb.
Castor Oil	8	oz.
Sodium Borate	8	oz.
Ammonia (28%)	56½	oz.
Perfume		

Melt stearic acid and castor oil in one container and in another heat Witch Hazel and water in which has been dissolved the sodium borate. When at about 190° F, add ammonia to water solution and instantly introduce into this solution the stearic acid. Agitate cream for 12 hours until every trace of ammonia gas has passed off. Agitate again the next day for two hours. Add perfume.

Formula No. 4

Stearic Acid	16	lb.
Water	74	lb.
Glycerin	10	lb.
Borax	1½	lb.
Potassium Carbonate	½	lb.
When finished add		
Glycerin	5	lb.
Perfume		

Melt stearic acid and glycerin on water bath, keeping at 70° C. Dissolve potassium carbonate and borax in water at 70° C. Add this solution very slowly constantly stirring to stearic acid and glycerin having turned off the heat. After all water is added, keep on stirring until cream forms. Then turn on the heat again and stir until whole mass is practically liquid. Turn off heat and stir till cold. Shortly before getting cool, add 5 lbs. glycerin.

Formula No. 5

Stearic Acid	18 lb.
Glycerin	6 pt.
Ammonia Water (26° Bé)	1 pt. 2 oz.
Water	11 gal.
Perfume	

Melt stearic acid at low heat. Mix glycerin with ammonia and 11 gal. of water. Add to stearic acid in several portions, heating and stirring until smooth and liquid. When all water has been added remove from fire. Add perfume. Stir occasionally until mass is cold. Strain cold through cheese cloth.

Formula No. 5

To make a quart.

Stearic Acid	1920 g.
Glycerin	960 g.
Soda Ash	60 g.
Borax	840 g.

Distilled water to make 32 fl. oz.

Melt stearic in glycerin and one-half the water. Dissolve soda ash and borax in other half. Mix the two with stirring until cream is cooled sufficiently. Perfume to suit.

Formula No. 6

For a soft type vanishing cream, triethanolamine is used as a saponifying agent.

Stearic Acid (heated to 170° F.)	24 lb.

Heat the following to 170° F.:

Triethanolamine	1 lb.
Glycerin	8 lb.
Water	8 gal.

and add to the melted stearic acid slowly, while stirring rapidly for a few minutes until emulsification is completed.

When the temperature falls to 135° F. add 4 oz. perfume oil and stir intermittently at slow speed until cold.

Allow to stand for a few days stirring slowly at least once a day for a few minutes.

For harder products, potassium carbonate or hydrate is used as a saponification agent. For example:

Stearic Acid (heat to 170° F.)	24 lb.

Then heat, also to 170° F., the following:

Potassium Carbonate	5 oz.
Glycerin	8 lb.
Water	12 gal.

and add to the melted stearic acid. The procedure is the same as above. Use 5 oz. of perfume.

Formula No. 7

Vanishing Creams made with Glycomine (a real forward step in cosmetics) enable anyone to produce perfect products, noteworthy because—

1. The use of caustic soda, potash and ammonia is eliminated.
2. No glycerin is necessary.
3. A most beautiful pearly finish results.
4. Closed jars will not dry or shrink.
5. It may be poured in jars when cold.
6. The batch is complete in 24 hours.

Formula

1.	Stearic Acid	20 lb.
2.	Glycomine	11 lb.
	Water	50 lb.
3.	Perfume	12 oz.

Heat No. 2 to 200° F. and add No. 1 (previously heated to 200° F.) to it slowly with stirring in an emulsifier or whipper. Continue stirring until mass is homogeneous. Allow to stand overnight. Add No. 3 and mix for 20 minutes. This cream is softer than the old-fashioned creams but typifies the highest grade modern vanishing cream. The pearliness in this cream increases with age and is helped by stirring cold the next day.

A softer cream can be produced by increasing the amount of water.

A harder cream is made by pouring hot or by increasing the amount of stearic acid; and also if stirring is very slow.

Formula No. 8

Vanishing Cream

(Also Makes a Good Brushless Shaving Cream)

Lime Water	79 pt.	8 fl. oz.		
Gelatin		8 oz.		
Glycerin	4 pt.			
Stearic Acid		12 oz.		
Coconut Oil	8 pt.			
Boric Acid *and*		8 oz.		
Stearic Acid, Powdered		8 oz.		
Ammonia Water (26%)	1 pt.	12 fl. oz.		
Borax		1 oz.	363 gr.	
Potassium Carbonate		1 oz.	363 gr.	
Eucalyptol				120 min.
Menthol			163 gr.	
Camphor			80 gr.	
Carbolic Acid		6 oz.		
(Perfume)		10 oz.		

Makes 96 lb.

Formula No. 9

Vanishing Cream Base

(Also Brushless Shave, Medicated Creams, Etc.)

Stearic Acid	24.75 g.
Triethanolamine	13.75 g.
Borax	0.05 g.
Water	61.45 g.
Perfume, Color, Medicaments, Etc.	to suit

The development of a new synthetic chemical has changed entirely the type of vanishing cream now in favor. With this, uniform, non-irritating, stable products are produced very easily. This new chemical is called Deramin.

Deramin permits of the production of a soft, silky non-irritating cream free from fixed alkalies. It avoids the necessity of using glycerin, which is irritating to some tender skins.

If a harder type of cream is desired Trikalin is used as the emulsifier. To make this type of cream smooth some Polycol is incorporated. Combinations of Deramin and Trikalin give an intermediate or medium texture cream. All of these creams develop a pearly texture. They are made as follows:

Formula No. 10

Soft Vanishing Cream

Stearic Acid	6 lb.
Heat to 170° F	
Deramin	1½ lb.
Water	15 pt.

Heat the Deramin and water to 170° F and add to the melted stearic acid slowly, while stirring rapidly for a few minutes, until emulsification is complete. Allow to cool slowly while stirring slowly. When the temperature has fallen to 130° F add 1½ ounces perfume oil and stir intermittently at slow speed until cold. Allow to stand for a few days, stirring slowly at least once a day. Pack in air-tight jars.

Formula No. 11

Medium Vanishing Cream

A.	Stearic Acid	6 lb.
	Heat to 170° F	
B.	Deramin	12 oz.
	Trikalin	9 oz.
	Polycol	15 oz.
	Water	2 gal. 1 pt.

B is heated to 170° F. and added to the melted stearic acid. The procedure is as above using 2 oz. perfume oil.

Formula No. 12

Hard Vanishing Cream

A.	Stearic Acid	24 lb.
	Heat to 170° F	
B.	Trikalin	4 lb. 7 oz.
	Polycol	5 lb. 1 oz.
	Water	96 lb.

Heat B to 170° F. and add to the melted stearic acid. The procedure is as above using about 10 ounces perfume.

In the above formulae where Polycol is specified and a lower quality, lower priced cream is warranted it may be replaced by glycerin.

These creams may be modified as follows:

Part of the stearic acid (up to 15%) may be replaced by Glycosterin to get a smoother and less pearly cream. Polycol or glycerin may be used to replace part of the water.

To produce a "nourishing" effect, a small part of the stearic acid may be replaced by Parachol. If 1% of titanium dioxide is ground into the cream (it is best to grind this into a small amount of the finished cream and then grind this into the balance of the cream) a whitening effect is produced on dark skins.

Formula No. 13

U. S. Patent 1,979,385

Stearic Acid	220 g.
Lanolin (Anhydrous)	40 g.
Triethanolamine	12.5 g.
"Carbitol"	75 g.
Water	500 g.

The cream is prepared by melting the acid and lanolin and adding them with constant stirring to the remaining ingredients, which are heated to 95° C. An emulsion forms at once which thickens upon cooling. Efficient agitation of the mixture is essential to obtain a smooth product. The solid content, i.e., in No. 13, the lanolin and stearic acid, of a cream of this type may vary from 15% to 35% depending upon the ingredients used and the type of product desired.

Formula No. 14

Glyceryl Monostearate	10.0 g.
Glycerin	3.0 g.
Petrolatum	3.0 g.
Spermaceti	5.0 g.
Mineral Oil	2.0 g.
Stearic Acid	2.0 g.
Caustic Potash	0.1 g.
Titanium Oxide	1.0 g.
Water	73.9 cc.

Formula No. 15

Pearly Type

Glyceryl Monostearate	2.5 g.
Stearic Acid	10.5 g.
Glycerin	4.5 g.
Ammonia (0.91)	2.5 g.
Water	80.0 cc.

Formula No. 16

Moderately Fatty Cream

Glyceryl Monostearate	12 g.
Petrolatum	6 g.
Lanolin	4 g.
Mineral Oil	6 g.
Almond Oil	6 g.
Glycerin	3 g.
Water	63 cc.

Formula No. 17

This cream is non-beading as it is free from glycerin.

Deramin	4 lb.
Water	5 gal.

Heat to 180° F. and pour into

Stearic Acid	16 lb.

previously heated to 180° F. while stirring, not too quickly. Add 4 oz. perfume when cream thickens and stir until cold. Allow to stand overnight and pack. The pearly finish becomes more pronounced with age.

This cream is noteworthy because it is free from ammonia, soda, potash and glycerin and therefore will not affect tender skins.

Formula No. 18

Stearic Acid	24 lb.
Triethanolamine	1 lb.
Water	8 gal.
Ethylene Glycol	12 lb.
Water	8 gal.
Perfume	8 oz.

In separate vessels heat stearic acid and all other ingredients except perfume to 180° F. Add one to the other and stir until uniform. Mix in perfume at about 105° F.

Formula No. 19

A.	Stearic Acid	4 lb.
	Lanolin	1 lb.
B.	Water	2 gal.
	Glycerin	2 lb.
	Potassium Carbonate	2 oz.
C.	Perfume Oil	2 oz.

In separate aluminum or enamel pots heat A and B to 180° F. Add B to A slowly with stirring until uniform. Stir in C at 110° F.

The above makes an excellent sunburn cream with or without the addition of 1% Quinine Ricinoleate.

Formula No. 20

Aminostearin	5 g.
Stearic Acid	25 g.
"Carbitol"	10 g.
Water	60 g.

Melt the Aminostearin and Stearic Acid and add to the "Carbitol," water solution at 70° C with rapid agitation. When completely emulsified stir slowly. Add perfume at 60° C, stir and pour at 50–55° C.

Formula No. 21

Stearic Acid	25 g.
Potassium Hydroxide,	1 g.
Water	75 cc.
Glycerin	8 g.
Perfume	to suit

Melt stearic acid and heat to 80° C., dissolve the potassium hydroxide in half of the water and heat to the same temperature and add to the acid while stirring. Mix the glycerin with the remainder of the water and heat to 80° C. and add to the mixture. If the process is carried on slowly and in small quantities, water will have to be added because of evaporation. While warm ordinary hydrogen peroxide may be added and a peroxide cream produced. This is a beautiful pearly cream. The pearliness is due to stearic acid. The glycerin prevents drying out of the skin that is so common for vanishing creams. Without perfume this makes an excellent brushless shaving cream by increasing potassium hydroxide to 2 parts.

Formula No. 22

Stearic Acid	40 lb.
Water	22 gal.
Glycerin	3 gal. 1 pt.
Borax	3 lb. 12 oz.
Potassium Carbonate	18 oz.
Mineral Oil	1 pt.

Use 20 gal. water in kettle with Stearic Acid and melt. Stir well. Add potassium carbonate and borax dissolved in 2 gal. hot water. Beat until smooth. Stir constantly. Add mineral oil in about 15 minutes, gradually add glycerin. Heat all for ½ hour. Stir constantly until cool. Add perfume.

Formula No. 23

Stearic Acid	30	oz.
Cocoa Butter	2½	oz.
Water	12	pt.
Add		
Borax	2½	oz.
Water	9	pt.
Add		
Sodium Carbonate	2	oz.
Water	4	oz.
Glycerin	15	oz.
Peroxide of Hydrogen	15	oz.
Ammonia Water	2.6	lb.
Perfume		

Formula No. 24

Stearic Acid	4	oz.
Paraffin Wax	½	oz.
Glycerin	12	oz.
Add Ammonia (26°)	½	oz.

When there is a perfect saponification, add 16 oz. warm distilled water in which must be dissolved 15 grams powdered borax.

Formula No. 25

Stearic Acid	4 lb. 12	oz.
Glycerin	8 lb. 8	oz.
Water	14	pt.
Ammonia Water	4¼	oz.

Heat 2 lb. glycerin with 12 pints water into the ammonia. Then melt Stearic Acid. Add first mixture and balance of glycerin and water. Heat to 80° C.

Formula No. 26

Stearic Acid	14	oz.
Glycerin	12	oz.
Potash	4	oz.
Water	8	oz.
Borax	1	oz.
Perfume	to suit	

Formula No. 27 (Pearly)

Stearic Acid	169.9	g.	6	oz.
Castor Oil U.S.P.	28.32	g.	1	oz.
Glycerin	113.28	g.	4	oz.
Ammonia (26°)	14.16	g.	½	oz.
Water	906	cc.	2	pt.

Melt stearic acid and castor oil, then add glycerin and heat to 180° F., and at the last moment, before adding the stearic mixture, add the ammonia to the water, then mix in the stearic mixture with the ammonia and water, stirring slowly, not too briskly. Too brisk stirring will destroy the pearly effect.

Formula No. 28

Stearic Acid	40	g.
Triethanolamine	2	g.
"Carbitol"	2	g.
Water	56	cc.

Formula No. 29

Stearic Acid	2½	lb.
Potassium Carbonate	21.24	g.
Sodium Carbonate	16.19	g.
Borax Powdered	1	oz.
Glycerin	1¼	pt.
Lanolin (Anhydrous)	1	oz.
Water (Distilled)	1½	gal.
Perfume	1	oz.

Directions: Dissolve Potassium and Sodium Carbonate in the water, add Glycerin, then heat solution to boiling. To this solution add slowly, with constant stirring, the Stearic Acid and Lanolin, which has been previously melted together to a temperature of 150° F. The vessel used should be large, to take care of effervescence, continuing the stirring until cold, adding perfume toward the end of the operation.

Vanishing Cream without Glycerin

1. Stearic Acid	36	lb.
Water	6	gal.
Cocoa Butter	2	lb.

Melt together.

2. Caustic Potash	22	oz.
Caustic Soda	5	oz.
Water	10	gal.
3. Mineral Oil	1	gal.
Perfume	to suit	

Melt together No. 1, dissolve No. 2 in hot water, and add cautiously to No. 1, stirring constantly. When nearly cold, add No. 3 slowly and stir in.

Non-Greasy Creams

Formula No. 1

a.	Stearic Acid	230	g.
	Wax, Scale	40	g.
	Adeps Lanae, Anhydrous	10	g.
b.	Glycerin	140	g.
	Triethanolamine	13	g.
	Borax	5	g.
	Distilled Water	562	cc.

Melt *a* and warm up *b* in another container. Mix both (*a* and *b* should be 65° C. boiling) pouring *b* into *a* in thin jet. Stir until cold.

Formula No. 2

a.	Stearic Acid	170	g.
	Adeps Lanae, Anhydrous	13	g.
	Wax, Scale	13	g.
	Spermaceti	5	g.
	Cetyl Alcohol	4	g.
b.	Glycerin (28° Bé.)	80	g.
	Triethanolamine	13	g.
	Borax	5	g.
	Distilled Water	697	cc.

Melt up waxes (65–70°), add *b* hot (boils) in thin jet, stirring thoroughly.

Optionally, 100 water may be substituted by witch hazel (1:1). Stir until cold.

Formula No. 3

Liquid Cream

a.	Stearic Acid	50 g.
	Adeps Lanae, Anhydrous	4 g.
	Cetyl Alcohol	1 g.
	Beeswax	1 g.
b.	Glycerin	20 g.
	Triethanolamine	2 g.
	Borax	2 g.
	Witch Hazel (1:1)	75 g.
	Distilled Water	625 cc.

Melt up together *a* at 60–70° C. Heat *b* to boiling, then add in thin jet, stirring vigorously, to *a*. Stir until cold.

To all above-mentioned creams, perfume should be added during cooling (0.5–0.7%). The perfume components should be colorless, and should not irritate the skin. No alcoholic compositions should be used.

Formula No. 4

Stearic Acid	120.0 g.
Cocoa Butter	45.0 g.
Sodium Biborate	2.5 g.
Potassium Carbonate	1.25 g.
Monohydrated Sodium Carbonate	1.25 g.
Glycerin	110.0 g.
Distilled Water	560.0 cc.
Rose Oil	4.0 cc.

Melt acid and cocoa-butter together. Decant carefully into a dish having a capacity of about 2000 cc. Add the borax and carbonates dissolved in 80 cc. of hot water and boil for one minute. Next add the glycerin and the remainder of the water (480 cc.) which has been heated to boiling. Mix the whole and just bring to a boil. Withdraw the heat and stir rapidly and continuously until a perfect emulsion is formed and the cream is cold. The perfume should be incorporated as the cream becomes cool.

Ammonia Vanishing Creams

(Free from Ammonia Odor)

The production of anhydrous ammonium stearate permits of the manufacture of ammonia vanishing and brushless shaving creams free from an undesirable ammonia odor.

The ammonium stearate should be powdered or ground to small pieces for best results. In working with this new material it is necessary to use powerful mixing as the emulsions stiffen suddenly. This cream is packed cold.

Formula No. 1

A	Ammonium Stearate (Anhydrous) Powdered	5 oz.
	Stearic Acid	13 oz.
B	Glycerin	10 oz.
	Water	72–78 oz.
	Perfume	to suit

A is melted at lowest possible temperature; B is warmed to 70–72° C. and is poured slowly into A with good mixing. Add perfume at 66° C.

Formula No. 2

A	Stearic Acid	15 oz.
	Ammonium Stearate (Anhydrous)	5 oz.
	Coconut Oil, Cochin	5 oz.
B	Glycerin	5 oz.
	Water	70 oz.

Method as above.

Ethylene Diamine Cream

Stearic Acid	14 g.
Ethylene Diamine 100%	1 g.
Glycerin or Glycol	10 g.
Water, Distilled	75 g.

Warm together and mix with a high speed mixer until smooth.

Zinc Stearate Vanishing Cream

Glycerin	150 g.
Water, Distilled	100 g.
Zinc Stearate	80 g.

Grind stearate and glycerin, add water.

To stabilize, use about 5% of Castile Soap, powdered.

Cosmetic Stearate Cream

(Potash Cream)

Stearic Acid	20 g.
Distilled Water	76 g.
Alcohol	4 g.
Potash Hydroxide sticks	1.4 g.

The alcohol should be added to the cooled cream at 30° C. together with the perfume.

Stearate Cream

Stearic Acid	16	g.
Glycerin	5	g.
Wheat Starch	0.5	g.
Spermaceti	1	g.
Potassium Hydroxide	1.5	g.
Distilled Water	76	g.

Prepare the cream at 85° C. A part of the water is used, together with the glycerin to prepare the starch mucilage which is added to the cooling cream at 70° C.

Stearate Creams by "Combined Saponification"

Formula No. 1

Stearic Acid	16.3	g.
Lanolin, Deodorized	0.5	g.
Paraffin Oil	4.3	g.
Glycerin	5.7	g.
Sodium-Potassium Carbonate C.P.	0.8–0.9	g.
Borax	0.4	g.
Perfume to suit	0.4	g.
Water, Distilled	70.6	g.

Formula No. 2

Stearic Acid	15	g.
Coconut Oil, Cochin	1.2	g.
Lanolin	0.5	g.
Paraffin Oil	4	g.
Glycerin	2	g.
Borax	0.4	g.
Potassium-Sodium Carbonate C.P.	0.8	g.
Distilled Water, or Witch Hazel	75.6	g.
Perfume	0.4	g.

Formula No. 3

Stearic Acid	12.5	g.
Potassium-Sodium Carbonate	0.53	g.
Cocoa Butter	0.5	g.
Glycerin	10.5	g.
Perfume	0.5	g.
Distilled Water	75.5	g.

Formula No. 4

Stearic Acid	14	g.
Potassium-Sodium Carbonate	0.6	g.
Tallow Fatty Acid, 100%	1	g.
Borax	0.5	g.
Glycerin	10	g.
Starch	1	g.
Distilled Water	72.6	g.

Melt the fats and fatty acids to 85° C., and pour them into the alkali-solution of the same temperature. Keep at 95° C. for 15 minutes, until free of carbon dioxide. Stir until cooled.

Starch is wetted with a part of the water and the glycerin and added at about 70° C.

Stearate Cream—Concentrate

Stearic Acid	33.2	g.
Ammonia (0.88)	1.8	g.
Wheat or Rice Starch	4.0	g.
Glycerin, 28° Bé	31.0	g.
Water, Distilled	30.0	g.
Preservative		

Heat the stearic acid to 85° C. Heat the ammonia and ⅓ of the water to the same temperature. Make a glycerin-starch paste, and thin with ⅔ of the water. Heat to 70° C.

Add the melted stearin to the aqueous ammonia with stirring, keep hot to complete saponification, cool to 70° C. with agitation, add the starch mucilage, cool and stir.

This concentrate can be used as follows:

Concentrate, heated to 50° C.	38	g.
Water, Distilled, 55° C.	61.5	g.
Perfume (add at 35° C.)	0.5	g.

Cream Using Anhydrous Ammonium Stearate

Stearic Acid	7.5	g.
Ammonium Stearate Anhydrous	7.5	g.
Glycerin	15	g.
Borax	0.3	g.
Distilled Water	69.2	g.

Melt stearic acid, glycerin and ammonium stearate together, and emulsify with the water (and borax) of 80° C. Take up to a boil, stir until cold. Perfume (0.5%) add to it at 35–40° C. This cream does not smell of ammonia when cooled.

Stearate Creams

Formula No. 1

Stearic Acid	15	g.
Glycerin	15	g.
Sodium Carbonate, Crystallized C.P.	1	g.
Ammonia (0.88)	0.4	g.
Alcohol	2.6	g.
Water, Distilled	65	g.

Formula No. 2

Stearic Acid	19.5 kg.
Sweet Almond Oil	0.5 kg.
Potassium Hydroxide	375 g.
Ammonia (0.88)	1 kg.
Borax	1 kg.
Water, Distilled, and Glycerin	80 kg.

Mix at 82° C., boil, stir down to 70° C., let stand. After 12 hours, warm to 38–43° C. Cool.

Formula No. 3

Stearic Acid	15 g.
Glycerin	25 g.
Sodium Bicarbonate	1.2 g.
Ammonium Carbonate, Crystals	1.2 g.
Perfume	0.5 g.
Witch Hazel	30 g.
Water, Distilled	27 g.

Cream with Glyceryl Mono Stearate

Glyceryl Mono Stearate	2.5 g.
Stearic Acid	10.5 g.
Glycerin	5 g.
Ammonia, Dilute	2.5 g.
Water, Distilled	79.0 g.
Perfume	0.5 g.

Powder Base Cream

Formula No. 1

Stearic Acid	10 g.
Zinc Oxide	6 g.
Rice or Wheat Starch	11 g.
Glycerin	39 g.
Witch Hazel	15 g.
Water, Distilled	15 g.
Quillaja Bark Tincture (1:50)	1 g.
Benzoin Tincture (1:50)	1 g.
Solution of Gomme Liatrix, 2%	1 g.
Caustic Potash	0.8 g.
Borax	0.2 g.
Chlorophyll	sufficient to color

Make up a mucilage from glycerin and starch; separately prepare a paste from zinc oxide and the soap bark solution. Mix these two together and add to the hot (70° C.) stearate cream (which is prepared before in the usual manner.) Add the benzoin, perfume. Homogenize.

The cream can also be a make-up cream (grease paint) when suitable pigments are incorporated.

Formula No. 2

A mixture of about 500 g. distilled water, 20 g. potassium carbonate and 125 g. glycerin is heated almost to the boiling point in a capacious vessel constructed of well enamelled material. Two hundred g. stearic acid melted in another vessel are cautiously introduced, a little at a time, into the hot potassium carbonate solution. Violent carbon dioxide evolution ensues and continues until the last portion of stearic acid has been added. When gas development ceases, indicating completion of the reaction, heating is discontinued and the batch transferred to another vessel fitted with stirring gear. An additional 1000 g. water and 125 g. glycerin are added and the mix stirred until cold and viscous. Cold-stirring is important for securing a fine, uniform emulsion and for preventing settlement of stearic acid particles. Certain variations in preparation can be practiced, such as replacement of glycerin by white liquid paraffin or addition of 125 g. groundnut oil to facilitate emulsification.

Formula No. 3

Stearic Acid	1.0 g.
Cetyl Alcohol	1.0 g.
Potassium Hydroxide	0.1 g.
Water	91.9 g.

All Weather Cream

a.	Stearic Acid	210 g.
	Adeps Lanae, Anhydrous	50 g.
b.	Glycerin	133 g.
	Triethanolamine	20 g.
	Borax	5 g.
	Distilled Water	582 cc.

Melt up *a* to about 65° C., add *b* boiling hot, in thin jet, stirring thoroughly until cold.

Tinted Creams

An effective color will be developed by mixing one to two per cent. of pigment into the liquid cream batch. The dry color mixture may be made in the following proportions: Peach, 59% precipitated chalk, 40% golden ochre and 1% of brilliant pink lake; rachel, 75% precipitated chalk, 25% golden ochre; flesh, precipitated chalk 90%, golden ochre 9.5% and brilliant pink lake .5%; naturelle, precipitated chalk 75%, golden ochre 24%, brilliant pink lake 1%; ochre, 54% precipitated chalk, 3% brilliant pink lake, 43% golden ochre; suntan, 36% precipitated chalk, 58% golden ochre, 6% brilliant pink lake. To make the cream, melt 22 g. stearic acid with 2 g. cetyl alcohol. Dissolve 1 g. of potassium hydroxide in 64 cc. water, add 10.5 g. glycerin and heat to 70° C. Slowly add the aqueous solution to the melted stearic acid, stirring thoroughly. When the mixture is completely emulsified, add one or more parts of any of the above pigment mixtures, according to the shade desired. Continue stirring until quite thick. Add .5 g. of perfume at 40° C.

Benzoin and Almond Cream

Stearic Acid	20 g.
Potassium Hydroxide	1 g.
Curd Soap	3 g.
Water	150 cc.
Almond Oil	2 g.
Tincture of Benzoin	2 g.

Dissolve the soap in 40 cc. of water (hot); form a vanishing cream with the remainder of the formula, using 80 cc. water; mix the two and heat again, adding the remainder of the water when cold. A better sheen would no doubt result if the almond oil were omitted. Two or three days will elapse before the sheen appears.

Cleansing Cream

A cleansing cream is one containing little or no water. It should not be too viscous or pasty so as to spread easily and liquefy at the body temperature. It should enter into the pores of the skin and clean them. It must soften and smooth the skin and refreshen it. Unfortunately most cleansing creams do not meet all of the above specifications.

Cleansing Creams

Formula No. 1

Mineral Oil	34.2 g.
Beeswax, White	2.2 g.
Spermaceti	12.3 g.
Triethanolamine Stearate	8.8 g.
Glycerin	1.8 g.
Water, Distilled	40.3 g.
Perfume	0.4 g.

Water and glycerin are added to the melted waxes and oils, both being at about 90–95° C. Keep stirring slowly until the cream thickens. Perfume. Stir until almost cold. Stir again before packing.

Formula No. 2

Spermaceti	12.8 g.
Diglycol Stearate	10.2 g.
Mineral Oil	34.2 g.
Glycerin	4.0 g.
Water, Distilled	38.5 g.
Perfume	0.5 g.

Stir water and glycerin heated to 60° C. into the melted oils and waxes at the same temperature.

Perfume at 40° C. Stir continuously until cold.

Formula No. 3

Stearic Acid	30 g.
Lanolin, Anhydrous	20 g.
Beeswax, White	16 g.
Mineral Oil	33 g.
Polyglycol (Polycol)	16 g.
Triethanolamine	3.8 g.
Water, Distilled	95 g.

Add water-to-oil at 70° C.

Formula No. 4

Glycosterin	120 g.
Mineral Oil	225 cc.
Petrolatum, White	45 g.
Parachol (Absorption Base)	15 g.
Water, Distilled	578 cc.
Triethylene Glycol	17 g.

Emulsify at 70° C., perfume at 40° C. Stir until it cools to 35° C., pour.

Formula No. 5

Flaked White Beeswax	10 g.
Ceresin Wax (Melting Point 138° F.)	5 g.
Mineral Oil (Viscosity 68/75)	65 g.
Water	40 g.
Borax	½ g.
Perfume	to suit

The beeswax, ceresin and a portion of the mineral oil are placed in a steam jacketed kettle and the temperature in melting the waxes should be at no time in excess of 80° C. (The emulsifying power of beeswax is retarded or broken down when the temperature is above 80° C.) When the waxes have melted, the steam should be so regulated (this can be accomplished only by actual experiment on the part of the cream maker) that when the balance of the mineral oil is added cold, the temperature will be approximately 57° C. It will take a little experimenting to gain the knack of properly controlling the kettle temperature in order to speed production.

When the melted waxes and mineral oil are at a temperature of 57° C., the perfume oil should be added and the agitator started. The agitator should have only one propeller at the bottom, causing a complete vortex when agitating the melted waxes and oil, and forming only a slight vortex when all the water and borax have been added.

In another kettle, the water and borax should be kept at exactly the same temperature, 57° C. It is important that agitation be continued while the water and borax are being added and while the curds form until the cream begins to thin down and becomes a homogeneous mass. As soon as this occurs, stirring should be continued for a few minutes only. When the cream must stand before passing into the filling machine, it may be necessary to agitate it to destroy any crust caused by surface cooling.

Formula No. 6

Liquid Cleansing Cream

Glyceryl Monostearate	6.0 g.
Water	75.5 g.
Glycerin	10.0 g.
Stearic Acid	1.0 g.
Oleic Acid	2.0 g.
Mineral Oil	5.0 g.
Perfume	.5 g.

Put all the ingredients into a kettle excepting the perfume and heat until melted and mass is slimy. Agitate continuously until mass is cool. Then perfume.

Formula No. 7

Colorless Liquid Skin Cleanser

Glycerin	22.0 g.
Alcohol	10.0 g.
Water	64.5 g.
Tribasic Sodium Phosphate	3.0 g.
Perfume	.5 g.

Dissolve the phosphate in the water, add the glycerin. Mix the alcohol and perfume and add to the first solution. Mix and filter.

Formula No. 8

Quick Melting, Mineral Jelly

Mineral Oil	50.0 g.
Petrolatum	33.5 g.
Spermaceti	10.0 g.
Stearic Acid	6.0 g.
Perfume	.5 g.

Melt waxes and petrolatum in oil, add perfume when cool.

Formula No. 9

Cold Cream Type

Beeswax	15.0 g.
Petrolatum	14.0 g.
Mineral Oil	50.0 g.
Water	20.0 g.
Borax	.5 g.
Perfume	.5 g.

Melt wax and petrolatum. Add oil. Dissolve borax in hot water. Add to above with stirring. Perfume at 120° F.

Formula No. 10

Quick Melting, Absorption Type

Beeswax	7 g.
Spermaceti	8 g.
Absorption Base	20 g.
Water	50 g.
Mineral Oil	15 g.

Melt the waxes and add the mineral oil. Warm the absorption base to 40° C. and the water likewise; then slowly add the water with steady but not violent agitation. Then add the melted waxes which should be of the same temperature.

Formula No. 11

Quick Melting, Oily Type

Petrolatum	40 g.
Anhydrous Lanolin	10 g.
Mineral Oil	50 g.

Melt the petrolatum, add the lanolin and mineral oil. Mix and perfume.

Formula No. 12

Cleansing Cream

1.	Mineral Oil	76 g.
	White Wax	5 g.
	Spermaceti	26 g.
	Trihydroxyethylamine Stearate	20 g.
2.	Perfume	1 g.
3.	Glycerin	4 g.
	Water	92 g.

Heat Nos. 1 and 3 separately to 200° F.; then add Nos. 1 to 2 slowly, stirring thoroughly. When the cream begins to set, the perfume is added and stirred in. Allow to stand over night. Stir thoroughly the next morning and package. This cream will not sweat oil during hot weather and will maintain its consistency.

Formula No. 13

Neutral

1. Mineral Oil 80 g.
2. Spermaceti 30 g.
3. Glyceryl Monostearate 24 g.
4. Water 90 g.
5. Glycerin 10 g.
6. Perfume to suit

Heat 1, 2 and 3 to 140° F. and stir into it slowly 4 and 5 heated to same temperature. Add perfume, at 105° F., stir slowly until cold; after allowing to stand for 5 minutes stir until smooth and pack.

Formula No. 14

(Semi-Absorbent)

Lanolin	22 g.
White Mineral Oil	25 g.
White Petroleum Jelly	11 g.
Distilled Water	42 g.
Perfume	to suit

Formula No. 15

(Non-Absorbent)

Ceresin	18 g.
White Mineral Oil	81 g.
White Petroleum Jelly	1 g.
Perfume	0.5 g.

Formula No. 16

(Greasy Type)

Spermaceti	23 g.
Petrolatum White	20 g.
Mineral Oil	57 g.
Perfume	to suit

Formula No. 17

White Beeswax	85 gr.
White Soft Paraffin Wax	100 gr.
Liquid Paraffin	240 min.
Hydrous Wool Fat	25 gr.
Water	28 min.
Sulphonated Castor Oil	28 min.
Perfume	to suit

Melt together the beeswax, soft paraffin, liquid paraffin and lanolin, and bring the temperature to 70° C. Mix together the water and the sulphonated oil and heat them to 75° C. Then stir them rapidly into the melted oil, continuing the stirring until the temperature falls to 45° C. before adding the perfume.

Formula No. 18

1. Mineral Oil (White) 54.0 g.
2. Beeswax 18.0 g.
3. Parachol (Absorption Base) 5.5 g.
4. Borax 1.0 g.
5. Water 21.0 g.
6. Perfume 0.5 g.

Melt together 1, 2 and 3. Dissolve 4 in 5 and heat to boiling. Add this to first mixture slowly with stirring; add perfume before solidification begins.

Formula No. 19

(Non-Greasy)

1. Beeswax 1.5 g.
2. Spermaceti 6.5 g.
3. Cherry Kernel Oil 6.0 g.
4. Glycosterin 4.0 g.
5. Water 122.0 g.
6. Alcohol 3.0 g.
7. Galagum 1.0 g.
8. Borax 3.0 g.
9. Perfume 3.0 g.
10. Glycerin 4.0 g.

Melt together 1, 2 and 3. Heat while stirring 4, 5, 7 and 8 together until uniform. Mix these two solutions stirring until uniform. Stir in 6, 9 and 10 and mix until uniform.

Formula No. 20

Cleansing Cream

Ozokerite (M. P. 78° C.)	20 lb.
Mineral Oil, White	80 lb.
Perfume	4 oz.

The procedure should be as follows:

If the volume of production is large a special machine for breaking the ozokerite should be used; if not, the slabs should be chopped into as small pieces as possible with a hatchet, or place the ozokerite in a strong wooden box and chop into pieces with an ordinary ice chopper. The ozokerite after being chopped is placed in one of the melting kettles above the mixing kettle, with about one third of the mineral oil and heated until all of the ozokerite is melted. For best results do not heat over 80° C. for at this temperature the wax will, on cooling, give a nice white cream. Then add the rest of the mineral oil. This is best added a small quantity at a time with some stirring, with a hard wood paddle. The reason for adding the mineral oil in small quantities is that by this method the wax is not chilled and crystallized.

Now strain the melted wax and oil in the mixing kettle and when cooled add the perfume, and if the cream is to be tinted, the color. From here the cream is run into the storage tank above the filling machine and when the temperature has reached the proper degree for filling, that operation is started.

In filling the cream in jars a little experimenting is necessary to find just the correct temperature, as on different days the temperature will vary a little. The cream should never be so hot that on cooling an indentation will show on the surface, or so cold that a lump will be in the middle of the surface of the jar of cream. If the jars have been stored in a cold place it is best to have them warmed to the filling temperature.

Formula No. 21

Stearic Acid	20 g.
Liquid Petrolatum	5 g.
Triethanolamine	5 g.
Coconut Oil Soap	40 g.
Distilled Water	25 g.
Glycerin	5 g.

Heat the stearic acid, liquid petrolatum and triethanolamine to 85° C. in a porcelain or glass container. Heat the distilled water and the glycerin to 85° C. in a separate porcelain or glass container. Maintain the heat at 85° C. and dissolve the coconut oil soap by agitation. Add the aqueous solution to the stearic acid mixture with slow but constant stirring. Remove the mixture from the source of heat and continue stirring until it is cool. Do not beat air into the cream.

The result is a smooth, pleasant mass which does not separate even in summer and which gives a good lather when mixed with water. May be used on sensitive skins and as an adjunct in the treatment of acne vulgaris and acne rosacea. It is applied with a pledget of cotton and removed with lukewarm water.

Formula No. 22

Stearin	4.7 g.
Lanolin, Anhydrous	6.4 g.
Paraffin Oil	10.7 g.
Triethanolamine	1.7 g.
Polycol (Polyglycol)	14.0 g.
Quince Seed Mucilage *	3.5 g.
Water, Distilled	59.0 g.
Perfume to suit	

Melt up the first three ingredients to 70° C, and saponify with the solution of triethanolamine in water. To this add the quince seed mucilage, and the glycol together with the perfume after cooling.

Stir thoroughly all the time.

* The *quince seed mucilage* is made by pouring

water, (80° C)	900 cc.
on quince seed	30 g.

and pressing off the liquid after standing for 5 hours.

Formula No. 23

Stearic Acid	10 g.
Mineral Oil	40 g.
Triethanolamine	4 g.
"Carbitol"	2 g.
Water	44 cc.

Formula No. 24

Cleansing Cream

Mineral Oil	28 g.
Beeswax, White	4.5 g.
Spermaceti	22.5 g.
Triethanolamine Stearate	18.0 g.
Glycerin	4.5 g.
Water	22.5 cc.

Cleansing Cream with Cetyl Alcohol

Cholesterol	1 g.
Spermaceti	7 g.
Cetyl Alcohol	20 g.
Beeswax, White	5 g.
Triethanolamine Stearate	20 g.
Paraffin Oil, Best	78 g.
Glycerin	4 g.

Water, Distilled	92 g.
Perfume	1 g.

Emulsify at 95° C

Liquid Cleansing Creams

The following milky creams are stable and effective cleansers. They will even remove indelible lipstick and rouge from the skin in addition to the usual grime and dirt. They leave the skin clean, fresh and stimulated and serve as perfect powder bases without any harmful effects.

Formula No. 1

Stearic Acid	3 lb.
Mineral Oil	2 gal.
Heat to 170 F.	
Water	3 gal.
Deramin	6 lb.

Heat to 170° F. and add slowly with rapid stirring to the melted stearic acid and mineral oil. Continue stirring until temperature falls to 150° F. when 2 oz. of perfume is added. Stir until cool. A thicker cream is made by replacing part of the mineral oil by petrolatum.

Formula No. 2

Mineral Oil	5 pt. 11 oz.
Savolin	24 oz.
Heat to 160 F. with stirring.	
Water	1½ gal.

Heat to 160° F. and add slowly to the oil mixture with good stirring.

Perfume Oil 1½ oz. is stirred in when cooled to 140° F. Continue stirring slowly until cold. This cream is thinner than the previous one. It is an effective cleanser but will not remove indelible rouge or lipstick.

Formula No. 3

Stearic Acid	25 lb.
Lanolin (Anhydrous)	34 lb.
Mineral Oil (White)	57 lb.
Triethanolamine	9 lb.
Carbitol	75 lb.
Water	315 lb.
Quince Seed Mucilage	19 lb.
Terpineol	0.35 lb.

Preparation

Melt the stearic acid in the mineral oil, add the lanolin and terpineol and bring the temperature of this oil solution to 70° C. Add it to the solution of Triethanolamine and water which has been brought to the boiling point in a separate container. Stir vigorously until a good emulsion is formed and then add the quince seed mucilage, slowly, with continued stirring. Add the perfume to the Carbitol and stir this slowly into the cream. The stirring should be fast enough to keep the cream well mixed but not aerate it. If the stirring is not continued until the cream is cold, it thickens upon standing. The quince seed mucilage is made by adding 9½ ounces of quince seed to 20 pounds of water at 80° C., soaking 5 or 6 hours, and straining through a cloth. Some suitable material should be added to the quince seed mucilage to prevent its molding over a period of time.

Properties

The high percentage of Triethanolamine used in this cream serves to completely emulsify the oil and lanolin, aids their penetration into the pores and forms a cream which is readily removed with water, if desired. Carbitol exerts a soothing action on the skin and facilitates the cleansing action of the cream. Due to the high Carbitol and lanolin contents this cream is soothing and healing to the skin and can be used as a hand lotion as well as a cleansing cream.

Formula No. 4

Stearic Acid Triple Pressed	12 g.
White Mineral Oil	30 g.
Triethanolamine	4 g.
Glycerin	4 g.
Perfume	½ g.
Water	80 g.

Formula No. 5

Trihydroxyethyleneamine Stearate	14½ lb.
Perfume Oil	2 lb.
Mineral Oil	72 lb.
Water	148½ lb.

Directions: Place trihydroxyethyleneamine stearate in a kettle, heat until melted. In another kettle heat mineral oil just enough so that it will not congeal when it is added to the trihydroxyethylene-amine-stearate. Avoid excessive heat. Add perfume and small amount of water, which has been previously heated to same temperature as the oily ingredients. Add just enough water until cream will run smoothly from a paddle and be sure all lumps will be dissolved, adding balance of water. Up to this point the cream should be stirred vigorously and should have a cream consistency. After this the balance of the water should be added slowly and slow mixing continued at the rate of about 50 and 60 revolutions a minute. This will give a fine silky emulsion.

Formula No. 6

Stearic Acid	29	lb.
Lanolin (Anhydrous)	8	lb.
Mineral Oil (White)	50	lb.
Triethanolamine	3.6	lb.
"Carbitol"	10	lb.
Water	100	lb.

Preparation

Melt the stearic acid in the mineral oil, add the lanolin and bring the temperature of this oil solution to 70° C. Then add it to the solution of Triethanolamine and water which has been brought to the boiling point in a separate container. Stir vigorously to obtain a uniform emulsion and add the Carbitol solution of the perfume. Continue with even stirring until a smooth cream is obtained and then occasionally until cold. Too rapid stirring causes an undesirable aeration of the cream.

Properties

Cleansing creams contain a fairly high content of mineral oil and usually a wax base. The latter is not essential in a properly formulated cream although it is frequently used. The mineral oil content is normally quite high as it is this material which dissolves or suspends the dirt particles so that they may be readily removed by a cloth or absorbent paper. The higher percentage of Triethanolamine used in this type of cream than in a vanishing cream serves to completely emulsify the oil, aids in its penetration into the pores, and forms a cream which is readily removed with water. Carbitol exerts a soothing action on the skin and facilitates the cleansing action.

Variations

While various waxes and oils may be used in this type of cream, it is important that the correct proportion of Triethanolamine be used. A deficiency of the base is indicated by a thin emulsion, which is not readily washable, and a surplus by a granular cream which tends to separate on cooling. The water content can be increased or decreased slightly to change the consistency of the cream as desired.

Formula No. 7

U. S. Patent 1,979,385

Stearic Acid	122.5	g.
Lanolin (Anhydrous)	35	g.
White Mineral Oil	210	g.
Triethanolamine	17.5	g.
"Carbitol"	40	g.
Water	420	g.

A cream of this type should have a fairly high content of the ethanolamine in order to completely emulsify the oil so that it may be removed from the skin by washing with water. Various oils and waxes may be used in this type of cream, and the oil content should be fairly high.

Liquefying (Liquifying) Creams

This type of cream is a cleansing cream containing no water. It is composed of approximately 50% mineral oil together with petrolatum to give sufficient viscosity so that when the cream liquefies on the skin, it suspends the dirt which is removed from the pores.

Liquefying Creams

Formula No.	1	2	3	4	5
Paraffin wax	18	5	0	0	15 g.
Ceresin	0	0	0	3	0 g.
Beeswax, White	0	0	5	0	10 g.
Ozokerite	0	0	0	4	0 g.
Petroleum Jelly	18	2	85	0	0 g.
Mineral Oil	64	16	10	48	75 g.
Borax	0	0	0	0	1 g.
Water	0	0	0	0	12 g.

Melt the ingredients at the lowest possible temperature, using a water bath to prevent burning. Add any color or tint desired. Stir well, and allow the mixture to cool slowly. Stir at 5 or 10 r.p.m. to avoid the formation of a crust at the side of the container. After the cream has cooled considerably, add the perfume and stir again. By now the cream is quite cool, and ready to be poured. If the jars are previously warmed to about 37° C. or about 99° F., the cream will form a regular and smooth surface on top. If the cream is poured too hot, a hole will remain down through the center of the jar. If this happens, remelt the cream. Too much wax will make the cream crack away from the side of the jar. Regarding sweating, it can be said that practically all liquefying creams sweat. Formulas 1 and 2 obviate the condition somewhat. This is due to the contraction of the physical jell structure of the set cream, causing the oil to ooze out. If the mass is cooled previous to pouring, the condition can be obviated to a great extent. Use of low melting waxes along with petroleum jelly will help too.

Liquefying cleansing cream can do nothing more than cleanse the skin. Any additional claims are unfounded. A cream of this type can scarcely have multiple purposes. It is not a skin food, nor a powder base. To state on the label that the cream should be removed with soap and water after the usual removal with tissue is another good point. Refrain from using aromatic oils that will burn the skin. Be careful in manipulation and along with the type formulas suggested, little trouble will be experienced. If an extra high gloss finish is desired, pass a jet of cold air over each jar as soon as it is filled.

Formula No. 6

Mineral Oil	7 lb.
Ceraflux	3 lb.
Petrolatum	2 lb.

Melt together at 220° F. and stir at room temperature until cold add perfume; pour into jars while liquid but at lowest possible temperature. This cream will not sweat oil during hot weather.

Formula No. 7

Peanut Oil	5 g.
Ozokerite	20 g.
Mineral Oil	74 g.
Perfume	to suit

Formula No. 8

Soft Translucent

Mineral Oil (Light or Medium)	56 g.
Paraffin Wax	25 g.
Petrolatum (White)	19 g.

Formula No. 9

Medium Translucent

Mineral Oil (light or medium)	50 g.
Paraffin Wax	18 g.
Petrolatum (White)	23 g.
Spermaceti	9 g.

Formula No. 10

Medium Opaque

Mineral Oil (Light or Medium)	50 g.
Paraffin Wax	30 g.
Petrolatum (White)	20 g.

Formula No. 11

Hard Opaque

Mineral Oil (Light or Medium)	45 g.
Paraffin Wax	25 g.
Petrolatum (White)	20 g.
Spermaceti	10 g.

The ingredients are melted and stirred together on a water-bath and 4 oz. of perfume is added per 100 lb. These creams are poured at the lowest possible temperature and allowed to stand undisturbed until solid.

This cream possesses exceptional penetrating powers and is absorbed very readily by the skin.

Formula No. 12

Soft Type

Petrolatum, White	3 lb.
Ceraflux	2 lb.
Petrolatum, Liquid	1 gal.

Melt together and add 1 dram perfume; pour at lowest possible temperature.

Formula No. 13

Medium Type

Spermaceti	5 lb.
Petrolatum, White	8 lb.
Ceraflux	4 lb.
Petrolatum, Liquid	1½ gal.

Melt together and add 1½ drams perfume; pour at lowest possible temperature.

Formula No. 14

Hard Type (for Hot Climates)

Spermaceti	5 lb.
Petrolatum, White	8 lb.
Ozokerite	5 lb.
Petrolatum, Liquid	1½ gal.

Proceed as in Medium Type above.

Lemon Juice Cleansing Creams

Formula No. 1

U. S. Patent 1,990,676

Five oz. oxy-cholesterin and 95 oz. petrolatum are thoroughly mixed to form an absorption base. Twenty oz. petrolatum and three oz. beeswax are melted together, and 30 parts of the base are added with thorough stirring. Fifty oz. natural lemon juice are added to the above mixture while still hot and stirring is continued until the mass is cool.

Formula No. 2

Pure Lemon Juice	70 g.
White Petrolatum	12 g.
Parachol (Absorption Base)	17 g.
Acid proof Lemon Perfume (to perfume)	1 g.

Mix the absorption base with the petrolatum with heat and mix until homogeneous. Allow to cool slightly and then slowly add the lemon juice while mixing rapidly. Add the acid proof lemon and stir until uniform.

Tissue Creams

In spite of the many claims made for tissue and allied creams, they have not been shown to have an effect other than that of lubrication and softening of the skin. In conjunction with massage they do help dry and scaly skins and may temporarily increase circulation. The variety of raw materials which enter these compositions are founded on fancy rather than on fact. If, however, they stimulate or elate the individual, their psychological value should not be underestimated.

Tissue Cream

Formula No. 1

Lanolin	20 kg.
Diglycol Stearate	46 kg.
Olive Oil	20 kg.
Spermaceti	10 kg.
Sweet Almond Oil	30 kg.
Water, Distilled	90 kg.
Sodium Benzoate	0.25 kg.

Emulsify at 65° C., stir. Perfume at 40° C., pour at 35° C.

Formula No. 2

Tissue Cream

(See Cold Cream A)

To the waxes in this formula there are added 2 lb. of lanolin. A slightly greater amount of perfume should be used.

Formula No. 3

Paraffin Wax	1 lb.
Cetamin	2 lb.
Lanolin Anhydrous	1 lb.
Petrolatum, Amber	1 lb.
Mineral Oil	3 pt.

Heat above to 180° F. and while mixing add slowly

Water (Boiling) 1 gal.

Continue stirring and at 150° F. add 1½ drams perfume. This cream is poured into jars at 130–135° C.

Formula No. 4

Spermaceti	4 lb.
Beeswax	6 lb.
Lanolin	4 lb.
Mineral Oil	52 lb.
Borax	1 lb.
Water	33 lb.
Perfume	

Formula No. 5

White Wax	5 oz.
Spermaceti	1 lb.
Petrolatum (Light Amber)	1 lb.
Mineral Oil	1½ pt.
Lanolin (Hydrous)	2 lb.
Borax	⅜ oz.
Water	10 oz.
Benzyl Alcohol	1 dr.
Bitter Almond Oil	1 dr.
Rose Geranium Oil	1½ dr.
Bergamot Oil	2 dr.

Formula No. 6

White Mineral Oil	20 lb.
Boracic Acid	6 lb.
Glycerin	14 lb.
Lanolin	20 lb.
Water	120 lb.

Heat the white mineral oil and lanolin with half of the water to about 190° F.; cool gradually, stirring continuously until mass is smooth and homogeneous. Then add balance of water together with boracic acid and glycerin. Stir cold and add perfume. Use distilled water which has been heated to a temperature of 15 to 20 degrees higher than melted wax.

Formula No. 7

Lanolin	80	oz.
Almond Oil	10	oz.
Glycerin	10	oz.
Benzoic Acid	0.2	oz.
Perfume to suit.		

Melt lanolin on water bath, and add the oils and glycerin. Stir until of uniform consistency. When cool, add perfume.

Formula No. 8

Tissue Cream

Lanolin	11.5	g.
Cocoa Butter	7.0	g.
Beeswax, White	12.0	g.
Cetyl Alcohol	2.0	g.
Mineral Oil, White	47.7	g.
Cholesterin	2.5	g.
Borax	1.5	g.
Water	15.0	cc.
Sodium Benzoate	0.3	g.
Perfume	1.0	g.

Tissue Cream with Lecithin

Lanolin, Anhydrous	22	g.
Spermaceti	22	g.
Beeswax, White	40	g.
Cocoa Butter, Odorless	28	g.
Almond Oil (With Preservative)	390	g.
Lecithin	50	g.
Borax	5	g.
Sodium Benzoate	5	g.
Parahydroxybenzoic Acid	2	g.
Water	220	g.

Tissue Cream with Cholesterin

Lanolin	325	g.
Cocoa Butter, Odorless	200	g.
Beeswax, White	300	g.
Spermaceti	55	g.
Oleic Acid	50	g.
Stearic Acid	200	g.
Sesame Oil (With Preservative)	800	g.
Cholesterin (Pure)	65	g.
Borax	50	g.
Water	800	g.
Sodium Benzoate	8	g.

Procedure: Melt the waxes, fats, and oil. Add the cholesterin. Make a hot solution of the borax, sodium benzoate and water and stir into the melted fats after the cholesterin has dissolved. Mix thoroughly and perfume to suit.

Tissue Cream (Soft) with Cholesterin Base

Absorption Base	30	g.
Lanolin	5	g.
Water	55	g.
Beeswax, White	10	g.

Procedure: Melt the wax and lanolin, add the base and stir in the water (warm).

(Note: Consistency in the foregoing formulas can be adjusted by changing the wax content to suit.)

Lanolin Tissue Cream

To Nourishing Cream A formula add

Lanolin Anhydrous	1 lb.

and replace the beeswax, white by yellow beeswax.

Turtle Oil Tissue Cream

Same as Tissue Cream (above) with the addition of turtle oil ½ lb. and ½ oz. Moldex, dissolved in the water.

Tissue Cream with Lecithin and Cholesterin

Lanolin, Anhydrous	220	g.
Cocoa Butter, Odorless	100	g.
Beeswax, White	200	g.
Stearic Acid	100	g.
Olive Oil (with preservative)	1000	g.
Lecithin	22	g.
Cholesterin	44	g.
Water	600	g.
Parahydroxybenzoic Acid	4	g.
Sodium Benzoate	10	g.

Procedure: Melt fats, waxes and oils, add cholesterin and lecithin. Stir in a solution (hot) of the water and sodium benzoate. Dissolve the parahydroxybenzoic acid in a small quantity of alcohol. Mix, perfume, and color.

Tissue Cream with Cholesterol, Lecithin and Turtle Oil

Beeswax, White	220	g.
Stearic Acid	100	g.
Cocoa Butter, Odorless	200	g.
Lanolin	200	g.
Turtle Oil	1000	g.
Almond Oil (with preservative)	1000	g.
Cholesterin	58	g.
Lecithin	120	g.
Water	800	g.
Parahydroxybenzoic Acid	8	g.

Sodium Benzoate	12 g.
Borax	120 g.

Proceed as above.

Tissue Cream (Non-Alkaline)

1.	Spermaceti	10 lb.
	Lanolin	20 lb.
	Glycosterin	46 lb.
	Olive Oil	20 lb.
	Almond Oil	30 lb.
2.	Water	90 lb.
	Sodium Benzoate	¼ lb.
3.	Perfume	to suit

Heat (1) to 150° F. and run into it slowly with stirring (2) which has been heated to the same temperature. Add the perfume at about 105° F. and stir in. Pour at 95–100° F.

Cholesterol-Lecithin Cream

1.	Lanolin, Anhydrous	20 g.
	Stearin	10 g.
	Cacao Butter	20 g.
	White Wax	20 g.
	Sweet Almond Oil, Preserved with Nipagin	200 g.
	Cholesterol	6 g.
	Lecithin	12 g.
	Water	80 g.
	Sodium Benzoate	1.5 g.
	Borax	15 g.
	Moldex or other efficient preservative	0.8 g.

Cholesterol and Lecithin Skin Creams

2.	Lanolin, Anhydrous	30 g.
	White Wax	50 g.
	Spermaceti	10 g.
	Borax	2 g.
	Water	18 g.
	Cholesterol	1.5 g.
	Egg Lecithin	0.5 g.

NOURISHING CREAMS

Formula No. 1

Nourishing Cream A

1.	Beeswax	15 oz.
	Mineral Oil	45 oz.
	Lanolin (Anhydrous)	12 oz.
	"Glyco-Wax A"	15 oz.
2.	Water	25 oz.
	Borax	1¼ oz.
	Benzoate of Soda	½ oz.
3.	Perfume	½ oz.

Heat Nos. 1 and 2 separately to 200° F., then add 1 to 2 slowly with stirring in an emulsifier or beater. When the cream begins to set add the perfume. Allow to stand over-night; stir the next morning and package.

This cream possesses exceptional penetrating powers and is absorbed very readily by the skin.

Formula No. 2

White Beeswax	9 g.
Spermaceti	3 g.
White Petroleum Jelly	35 g.
Benzoinated Lard	18 g.
Lanolin	4 g.
Liquid Paraffin	9 g.
Distilled Water	21 g.
Borax	1 g.

Liquid Nourishing Cream

Lanolin, Anhydrous	16 g.
Stearic Acid	3 g.
Triethanolamine	1 g.
Water, Distilled	80 g.

Formula No. 3

(Skin "Food" Type)

Glycosterin	12 lb.
Petrolatum, White	4 lb.
Lanolin	6 lb.
Mineral Oil	12 lb.
Water	65 lb.

Nourishing Cream, Cholesterol

White Wax	600 g.
Spermaceti	100 g.
Stearin	500 g.
Lanolin, Anhydrous	600 g.
Cacao Butter	400 g.
Sweet Almond Oil (with preservative)	1,800 g.
Cholesterol, Pure	120 g.

After solution of the cholesterol has been effected, stir the following hot solution into the above molten mass until pasty:

Sodium Benzoate	15 g.
Borax	100 g.
Water	1,700 g.

Formula No. 4

Nourishing Cream

Lanolin	20 g.
Peanut Oil	20 g.
Almond Oil	30 g.

Spermaceti	10 g.
Diglycol Stearate	46 g.
Water, Distilled	90 g.
Sodium Benzoate	0.25 g.

Formula No. 5

Nourishing Cream

Stearic Acid	5.0 g.
Mineral Oil	25.0 g.
Triethanolamine	1.0 g.
Water	69.0 g.

A change in viscosity may be made by changing the proportion of water.

Formula No. 6

Absorption Base	30.0 g.
Lanolin	5.0 g.
Lecithin	0.5 g.
Cholesterin	1.0 g.
Cetyl Alcohol	5.0 g.
Deodorized Cocoa Butter	2.5 g.
"Moldex"	0.2 g.
Glycerin	5.0 g.
Water	51.0 g.

The fats, including the cholesterin and lecithin, are melted gradually together, on the water bath, until the cetyl alcohol is dissolved. The water containing the glycerin is raised to the same temperature, and slowly stirred into the fats a little at a time, further water not being added until the previous amount has been entirely absorbed.

This gives a neutral cream, which, despite its water content, will not dry out easily.

Dry Skin Nourishing Cream

Absorption Base	25 g.
Diglycol Stearate	15 g.
Olive Oil	15 g.
Preservative	1.3 g.
Water	75 g.

Melt absorption base, diglycol stearate, and olive oil and add to water which has been heated to same temperature and contains preservative. Mix well and stir slowly till cool. Incorporate perfume and package.

Lecithin Nourishing Cream

Lanolin	15 g.
Beeswax	15 g.
Spermaceti	10 g.
Petrolatum	35 g.
Borax	1 g.
Water	22 g.
Cholesterin	1 g.
Lecithin	1 g.
Perfume	as required

Lanolin Creams

Formula No. 1

Beeswax, White	4.2 g.
Spermaceti	4.8 g.
Peanut Oil or Petrolatum	46.0 g.
Lanolin, Anhydrous	10.0 g.
Water	35.0 g.
Rose Perfume	0.5 g.

Formula No. 2

Beeswax	6.5 g.
Paraffin Wax, (52° C)	2.5 g.
Lanolin, Deodorized	25.6 g.
Mineral Oil, (Viscosity 30)	25.6 g.
Borax	1.2 g.
Water, Distilled	38.6 g.

Melt fats and oil to 55–60° C. Heat borax in water to same temperature, and pour it into the melted oils with slow agitation. Perfume; stir until cooled, or pour at 45° C.

Formula No. 3

Beeswax, White	6.2 g.
Ceresin	3.2 g.
Woolwax, Bleached, or Isocholesterol, Technical	3 g.
Mineral Oil	24.5 g.
Borax	1.0 g.
Lanolin	24.5 g.
Water, Distilled	37.5 g.
Perfume	to suit

Emulsify at 60° C., perfume, and stir until cold, or pour at 45° C.

Formula No. 4

Lanolin	325 g.
Ceresin	35 g.
Petrolatum, White	150 g.
Water, Distilled	150 g.
Perfume	to suit

Melt up the first three ingredients on waterbath, cool, and add slowly the distilled water and the perfume in small portions. Add 5–10% zinc stearate to make it more efficient for dry skin.

Formula No. 5

Lanolin	80 g.
Stearic Acid	15 g.
Triethanolamine	5 g.
Water, Distilled	200 g.

Pourable Lanolin Cream

Beeswax, White	6.2 g.
Paraffin, (52° C)	6.2 g.
Lanolin, Deodorized	24.5 g.
Mineral Oil, White	24.5 g.
Water, Distilled	37.5 g.
Borax	1.1 g.

Mix oils and borax solution at 55–60° C., perfume, and pour at 45° C.

Lanolin Cream, Liquid

Liquid lanolin cream depends upon a suspension of lanolin by means of soap. The following is a satisfactory formula:

Hard Soap	1 dr.
Distilled Water	1 oz.

Dissolve and add

Hydrous Wool Fat	1 oz.
Glycerin	1 oz.

If a more liquid cream is desired the amount of soap may be increased to 1½ drachm, and the glycerin and hydrous wool fat reduced to ½ oz. each.

Lanolin Emulsion

Lanolin	80 lb.
Stearic Acid	15 lb.
Triethanolamine	5 lb.
Water	200 lb.

Preparation

Weigh out the Triethanolamine and stearic acid and add to the whole quantity of water. Heat the mixture in a kettle and, when the stearic acid is melted, stir to a creamy soap solution. Add the lanolin and continue heating without stirring until the lanolin is melted and the mixture is just below the boiling point.

At this point stir the mixture thoroughly until a thick creamy emulsion results. Continue stirring intermittently until the emulsion has cooled to room temperature.

Properties

This emulsion is a very smooth, lightly colored cream of excellent stability, and can be diluted to any desired consistency with water. Such a lanolin emulsion is essentially a water-soluble lanolin and can be used in place of the straight fat whenever washability is advantageous.

Variations

To overcome a slight rancid odor in lanolin it is suggested that one per cent terpineol by weight be added to the lanolin prior to emulsification. Moreover, only the purest anhydrous grade should be used for cosmetic and medicinal preparations. Lanolin, as a readily absorbed and beneficial oil, is recommended for use in many skin creams, and may readily be incorporated in vanishing creams, cold creams and shaving creams.

Uses

Sunburn creams, hand lotions, shaving creams.

Lanolin-Stearate Cream

Stearic Acid	10 g.
Mineral Oil	12 g.
Lanolin	3.5 g.
Ammonia (0.88)	1 g.
Borax	0.5 g.
Water, Distilled	73 g.

Emulsify at 80° C., keep heating for 20 minutes, stir until cold.

Lanolin-Cocoa Butter Cream

Lanolin, Anhydrous	100 g.
Cocoa Butter	100 g.
Peanut or Mineral Oil	50 g.
Rose Perfume	2.5 g.
Water, Distilled	250 g.

"Penetran" Skin Cosmetic

Paraffin Oil	20 cc.
Sperm (Whale) Oil	25 cc.
Parachol (Absorption Base)	5 g.
Cholesterin	0.5 g.
Lecithin	2.5 g.
Fatty Oil, Preserved	47 cc.

Cholesterol Cream

Cholesterol, Pure	0.5 g.
White Beeswax	2.5 g.
Spermaceti	2.5 g.
White Mineral Oil	20.0 g.
White Petrolatum	25.0 g.
Water, Distilled	25.0 g.
Perfume	0.25 g.
Preservative	0.15 g.

Melt waxes on waterbath, add cholesterol and stir until melted. Add preservative (Methylparahydroxy benzoate). Stir until quite thick, add perfume, and add the water to the waxes in small portions, stirring thoroughly.

Cholesterol-Cream Base

Cholesterol	1–2 g.
Paraffin Wax or Ceresin	6 g.
Mineral Oil, (0.875)	43 g.
Petrolatum, White	50 g.

Warm and stir until uniform. Takes up 30–80% of water.

Oxycholesterol—Cream Base

Oxycholesterol	5 g.
Paraffin	5 g.
Mineral Oil, (0.875)	40 g.
Petrolatum, White	50 g.

Warm and stir until uniform.

Cream, Fatty Alcohol

Glyceryl Mono Stearate	11 g.
Sodium Cetyl-Sulfonate, Pure	1.5 g.
Cetyl Alcohol	2 g.
Beeswax, White	0.5 g.
Mineral Oil	3 g.
Glycerin	4 g.
Water, Distilled	78 g.
Ammonia (0.910)	0.1 g.

Cream Base with Woolfat Alcohols

Woolfat Alcohols (Bleached)	5 g.
Lanolin, Deodorized	5 g.
Paraffin Wax, Ceresin, or Cetyl Alcohol	5 g.
Mineral Oil	45 g.
Petrolatum, White	40 g.

Warm and mix until uniform.

Cream Base From Woolfat-Extract

Woolfat Extract (Methanol Extract from Neutral Lanolin)	5 g.
Petrolatum, White	50 g.
Mineral Oil	40 g.
Ceresin, Best Quality	5 g.

"Boro Glycerin Lanolin"

Formula No. 1

Boric Acid	10 g.
Glycerin	40 g.
Water	190 g.
Ceresin	200 g.
Mineral Oil	500 g.
Woolfat, Purified	50 g.
Bergamot Oil	5 g.
Lemon Oil	5 g.

Dissolve the boric acid in the glycerin by warming and stirring and add this to the melted lanolin-ceresin-mineral oil; add the perfume oils and finally the water in portions.

Formula No. 2

Boric Acid	10 g.
Beeswax, White	40 g.
Woolfat, Purified	115 g.
Petrolatum, White	225 g.
Mineral Oil, White	120 g.
Glycerin	185 g.
Water	300 g.
Perfume Composition	5 g.

Dissolve the boric acid in the glycerin, add this to the melted fats and oils, cool, add perfumes, and work in the water in small portions.

Formula No. 3

Boro-Glycerin Lanolin Cream

a.	Boric Acid	10 g.
	Glycerin	40 g.
	Water	250 g.
	Dissolve.	
b.	Lanolin, Anhydrous	100 g.
	Vaseline, White	600 g.
	Melt gently.	
c.	Rose Oil, Artificial	10 cc.
	or Eau de Cologne Oil	20 cc.

Cream with Diglycol Stearate

Diglycol Stearate	12 g.
Ammonium Stearate	1.2 g.
Cetyl Alcohol	2 g.
Mineral Oil	3 g.
Stearic Acid or Beeswax	1 g.
Starch	0.5 g.
Glycerin, or Glycol Bori-Borate	5 g.
Water, Distilled	75.3 g.

Four Purpose Creams

Four purpose creams are sold on the "platform" that they combine the properties of a cold-, cleansing-, nourishing- and vanishing cream in one preparation. This is patently contradictory.

Mineral Oil	3 pt.
Petrolatum (white) (heat to 140° F.)	½ lb.
Water	4½ pt.
Glycosterin	5 oz.
Preservative	½ oz.

Heat to 140° F. and add slowly with stirring to oil mixture. As the temperature falls, a gelatinous mass forms at 120° F. One oz. perfume oil is added while stirring and the gelatinous mass changes to a white cream. Slow stirring is continued until cold. This cream may be packed either in tubes or jars.

This cream can be modified by various coloring agents and perfumed as under cold cream to obtain specialty creams. Since it is neutral there may be incorporated in it viosterol, or gland or hormone extracts.

Another type of cream is that in which the emulsifying agent is either glyceryl monostearate or glycosterin.

These creams are emulsions of oil in water and for that reason evaporate quickly, and produce a cooling effect. They are much more water soluble than the beeswax type creams. These creams should be packed in air tight jars as there is a tendency for a small amount of water to separate from them.

Cold Cream (Non-Greasy)

1. Glycery Monostearate	22 g.
2. Petrolatum	16 g.
3. Paraffin Wax	12 g.
4. Mineral Oil	30 g.
5. Water	98 g.

Heat first four ingredients to 170° F. and stir together. Then slowly with stirring pour in the water which has been heated to the same temperature. Stir thoroughly and then allow to stand (hot) until air bubbles are gone. Add perfume and stir and pour at 110–130° F. Cover jars as soon as possible.

June Type Cream

The most recent advance in an all purpose cream, sold in tubes, is exemplified by the following formula which claims a waxless cleansing, nourishing, stimulating and softening cream which also acts as a powder base.

A.	Glycosterin	16	lb.
	Mineral Oil, White	3	gal.
	Petrolatum, White	6	lb.
	Parachol (Absorption Base)	2	lb.
B.	Water	7½	gal.
	Polyglycol or Triethylene Glycol	4	lb.

In separate vessels heat A and B to 160° F. Add B to A slowly while stirring vigorously. A jelly like mass results. Add 4 oz. perfume and continue stirring. As temperature drops to 110° F. a transformation takes place—a beautiful white cream results; stirring is continued until cold when it is packed into tubes or jars. It may be packed warm by heating, with stirring, to 105–110° F.

This cream wipes off the skin without leaving a greasy film. It, nevertheless, penetrates and is readily absorbed by the skin.

To give a cooling effect on the skin, 1–2 oz. of menthol may be added with the perfume.

Modified forms of this cream may be made by the addition of water soluble colors and appropriate perfumes, oils or other materials to produce

Lemon Cream
Strawberry Cream
Cucumber Cream
Turtle Cream
Viosterol Cream
Lecithin Cream
Hormone Cream
Olive Oil Cream
Almond Oil Cream

Yeast Four Purpose Cream

A	Mineral Oil	18	oz.
	Paraffin Wax	18	oz.
	Petrolatum, White	4½	oz.
	Glycosterin	18	oz.
B	Triethanolamine	2	oz.
	Yeast Solution (5%)	71	oz.
	Moldex (Preservative)	¼	oz.

Heat both parts to 65–70° C. and add A to B slowly with good mixing. Perfume to suit is added at 55° C.

Special Skin Creams

Formula No. 1

a.	Stearin	85 g.
	Lanolin	5 g.
	Cetyl Alcohol	10 g.
	Melt together.	
b.	Glycerin (28° Bé.)	36 g.
	Triethanolamine	5 cc.
	Borax	knifepointful
	Water	250 cc.
	Boil.	

Add *b* slowly to *a*, stir until cold. Perfume as desired is added at the end.

Formula No. 2

Glyceryl Mono Stearate	100 g.
Spermaceti	50 g.
White Petrolatum	30 g.
Mineral Oil	20 g.
Stearic Acid	20 g.
Titanium Dioxide	5 g.
Potassium Hydroxide	1 g.
Glycerin	30 g.
Distilled Water	701 g.

Witch Hazel Extract	40 g.
Perfume	3 g.

(a) Boil the glyceryl mono stearate in 400 pts. of the water with stirring until "dissolved."

(b) Heat the remainder of the water with the glycerin, dissolve the potassium hydroxide, and add to this the witch hazel.

(c) Melt spermaceti, petrolatum, stearic acid together.

(d) Run the waxes (c) into the solution (b) with heating and good stirring.

(e) Grind the titanium dioxide in the mineral oil, and pour this suspension into the saponified cream (d) with stirring.

(f) Add (a) to the cream.

Cool with stirring. At 25° C. add perfume. Homogenize.

SKIN "FOODS"

This type of cream is based on the erroneous impression that certain ingredients will actually "feed" and revitalize the skin.

Skin "Food" Creams

Formula No. 1

Lanolin	20 g.
Petrolatum, White	57 g.
Paraffin Wax	2 g.
Spermaceti	1 g.
Borax	0.2 g.
Water, Distilled	19.8 g.

Formula No. 2

Lanolin (Anhydrous)	36.4 g.
Spermaceti	6.4 g.
Snow White Petrolatum	48.2 g.
Distilled Water	7.875 g.
Perfume Oil	1.125 g.

Formula No. 3

Almond Oil	24 g.
Lanolin	22 g.
Soft Paraffin Wax	11 g.
White Beeswax	3 g.
Rose Water	40 g.
Perfume	to suit

Turtle Oil Creams

Formula No. 1

1. Diglycol Stearate	14 lb.
2. Mineral Oil	3¾ gal.
3. Lanolin	6 lb.
4. Petrolatum (White)	2 lb.
5. Water	6 gal.
6. Turtle Oil	5½ fl. oz.
7. Perfume Oil	5½ fl. oz.
8. Solution Yellow Color Made by Dissolving Yellow Dye 2 drams in Mineral Oil 14 fl. oz.	8¼ fl. oz.

Method of manufacture:

a. Melt 1, 2, 3, 4, 6 and 8 at 170° F.

b. Heat 5 to 180° F.

c. Add *b* to *a* while mixing. Allow mixer to run until batch is completely emulsified.

d. Allow batch to cool to 125° F. and add 7, and mix at low speed.

e. Batch should be allowed to cool without stirring to 100° F. at which temperature it is poured.

Formula No. 2

Diglycol Stearate	11.6 g.
Mineral Oil, White	31.5 g.
Lanolin	4.7 g.
Water, Distilled	49.75 g.
Petrolatum, White	1.65 g.
Turtle Oil	0.50 g.
Perfume	0.3 g.

Emulsify at 75–78° C., perfume at 50° C., stir until cooled to 38° C.

Formula No. 3

Turtle Oil	8.0 g.
Beeswax	20.0 g.
Paraffin Wax	15.0 g.
Mineral Oil	80.0 g.
Borax	2.0 g.
Distilled Water	50.0 g.
Perfume Oil	1.5 g.

Melt the first three ingredients at about 60° C. and strain the mixture into another container in which is the mineral oil, slightly warmed. Dissolve borax in the water and add to the cream slowly, stir well, and when cooled to 40° C., add perfume, and package. Excess heat must be avoided at all stages of the operation.

Liquid Turtle Oil Cream

Trihydroxyethylamine Stearate	20 g.
Turtle Oil	50 g.
Paraffin Oil (White)	40 g.
Diglycol Stearate	5 g.
"Carbitol"	20 g.
Water (distilled)	300 cc.

Preservative	5 g.
Perfume Oil	to suit

Melt together the first four of these ingredients, and slowly add the water, which has been heated to 50° C., with constant stirring. Continue stirring until cool, and then add "Carbitol," containing the perfume and preservative.

Hormone Creams

Day Cream

Semi-Fatty Stearate Cream	87.0 g.
Female Hormonal Material	6.0 g.
Male Hormonal Material	1.5 g.
Lanolin, Anhydrous	5.0 g.
Cholesterin	0.5 g.

Day Cream

Semi-Fatty or Dry Stearate Cream	91.5 g.
Female Hormonal Material	4.0 g.
Male Hormonal Material	1.0 g.
Lanolin, Anhydrous	3.0 g.
Cholesterin	0.5 g.

Night Cream

Cold Cream or Semi-Fatty Stearate Cream	87.0 g.
Female Hormonal Material	6.0 g.
Male Hormonal Material	1.5 g.
Lanolin, Anhydrous	5.0 g.
Cholesterin	0.5 g.

Night Cream

Cold Cream	83.3 g.
Female Hormonal Material	8.0 g.
Male Hormonal Material	2.0 g.
Lanolin, Anhydrous	5.0 g.
Cholesterin	1.0 g.
Lecithin	0.2 g.

Vitamin "F"

(Essential Linoleic Unsaturate)

Soluble in oils, alcohol, acetone, organic solvents generally and hydrocarbons such as petrolatum and mineral oil.

Should be biologically assayed and potency expressed in Shepherd-Linn units per gram.

Tabular summary of suggested levels at which to incorporate vitamin F in various cosmetic preparations.

Expressed in vitamin F units per gram or cubic centimeter of preparation.

Creams:	
Cleansing	240
Nourishing (Tissue or Lubricating)	120
Vanishing	120
Acne, Eczema, etc.	2,500
Hair Preparations:	
Hair Tonics	50
Special Tonics Designed for Dandruff Cures	2,500
For Baldness Remedies	2,500
Manicure Preparations:	
Special Pomade for Brittle Finger Nails	25,000
Nail Polish	5,000
Nail Polish Remover	5,000
Nail Pastes	5,000
Sun-Preparations:	
Remedial	500
Preventive	500

Vitamin D Cream

Parachol (Absorption Base)	25 kg.
Peanut Oil, Hydrogenated, or Pig Fat, Hydrogenated	5 kg.
Mineral Oil	5 kg.
Lanolin, Anhydrous	2 kg.
Cetyl Alcohol	1 kg.
Witch Hazel Extract	5 kg.
Glycerin	3 kg.
Water, Distilled	54 kg.
Perfume	0.1 kg.
Vitamin D-Preparation 2–5mg.	1 kg.

Vitamin F Cream

A	White Bee's Wax	12 oz.
	Anhydrous Lanolin	8 oz.
	Ceresin	14 oz.
	White Petrolatum	9 oz.
	Mineral Oil	24 oz.
	"Isovitafol L" (Vitamin F Concentrate)	4 oz.

Melt these all together.

B	Water	24 oz.
	Borax	1 oz.

Have both A and B at 180° F. Then mix and beat till cold.

Radioactive Cream for Dry Skin

Radium Solution (1 mg. of Radium Salts per 1 l. of Water)	1 g.
Thorium Chloride	0.25 g.
Rose Water	20 g.
Absorption Base	79 g.

Work the solution into the absorption base a little at a time in a mortar with a pestle.

Peroxide Creams

Most peroxide creams do not retain the peroxide as such for very long as it decomposes on contact with organic matter. A typical peroxide cream is made by adding 2% hydrogen peroxide (20–30 volume) to any cream containing water when the cream is no longer warm. It may be stabilized somewhat by the addition of 2/10ths of 1 percent of Moldex or similar preservative.

Wrinkle "Removers"

Wrinkling is caused by loss of elasticity of the skin through degeneration of its fibers. No treatment can cure it or restore to the skin its youthful elasticity and smoothness. Slight inflammation causes swelling and temporarily smoothes out the wrinkles, but with its subsidence they return. Such an inflammation, followed by exfoliation, can be caused by ultra-violet radiation, by freezing with carbon dioxide snow or by chemical irritants.

Formula No. 1

Betanaphthol	10 g.
Precipitated Sulphur	40 g.
Soft Soap, U.S.P.	25 g.
Petrolatum	25 g.

If this turns dark it does not indicate any loss of activity. It must not be used in cases in which the kidneys are impaired, and during its use the urine must be watched for signs of kidney irritation. It must be used on small areas only and not given to the patient to apply; but she must come daily to the doctor for the application.

The area should be washed with ether or benzine and the paste should be spread thickly and allowed to remain from twenty to thirty minutes, when it is removed thoroughly. Soon after application a slight burning sensation is felt, but this ceases in a few minutes. After the removal of the paste, the skin is red for a few hours. The treatment should be repeated each day until a tightening sensation or the onset of exfoliation shows that treatment has been sufficient. Five days is usually enough. During treatment no soap or water is to be used on the areas treated, but they may be cleansed by 0.5 per cent salicylic acid in alcohol.

Formula No. 2

Distilled Extract of Witch Hazel	500 cc.
Boric Acid	20 g.
Menthol	1 g.
Glycerin	50 cc.
Perfume (with a spirit basis)	100 cc.
Elderflower water	329 cc.

Dissolve the menthol in the perfume and add to the mixed liquids. Make up to volume as directed.

First requirements of skin creams for removing wrinkles is that they must be greaseless. These creams are naturally used as massage creams, for the process of removing wrinkles involves massaging.

Formula No. 3

1600 cc. of rose water and 350 cc. of glycerin. This mixture is brought up to boiling and 40 g. of potash soap added. The solution is boiled again and 18 g. of purified calcined potash added. In another vessel 180 g. of white stearin are melted. The first solution is filtered through cloth to remove impurities. Then it is brought to boiling and the molten stearin allowed to flow into the vessel in a thin stream while the solution is vigorously agitated. A large vessel must be used for carrying out this operation, for the mass must not be allowed to boil over due to evolution of large quantities of carbon dioxide. If contents of the kettle boil over, the result is an insufficient saponification of contents and a poor product. This is noticed by formation of small lumps in the cream. These lumps cannot be properly rubbed into the skin and spoil the entire action of cream. This cream is really a soft soap. The mass is cooled after being boiled long enough and is agitated thoroughly and perfumed with 15 g. of rose oil and 1 g. of vanillin. A small amount of alcohol may be added either after or during the addition of the stearin. This is effective in preventing formation of lumps.

Formula No. 4

Lanolin anhydrous 20 (parts by weight), cocoa butter 10, stearin 10, olive oil 12, cholesterol 2, lecithin 4, water 60, "Moldex" 0.4, sodium benzoate 1. According to another method, a melted base is first prepared with white wax 60 (grams), spermaceti 10, stearin 50, lanolin 60, cocoa butter 40, and sweet almond oil 180. In this melt are dissolved 1.2 grams cholesterol, with further addition, after complete solution, of 170 g. water, 1.5 g. sodium benzoate and "Moldex," the mass being stirred until it thickens.

Witch Hazel Snow or Foam

Stearic Acid	2	oz.
Potassium Carbonate	2⅓	oz.
Wool Fat	½	oz.
Liquid Paraffin	144	oz.
Glycerin	1	oz.
Witch Hazel Extract	10	oz.
Distilled Water	20	oz.

Dissolve the potassium carbonate in 6 oz. of hot water and gradually add the solution to a mixture of the stearic acid, wool fat and liquid paraffin, previously melted together with the aid of gentle heat. Stir vigorously for three or four minutes; add the glycerin, previously mixed with the solution of hamamelis and heated to 90° C.; stir until cold and beat to a foam.

Ruggles' Cream

Stearic Acid	75 g.
Potassium Carbonate	15 g.
Distilled Water	320 g.
Powdered Borax	5 g.
Quince Jelly	75 g.
Distilled Water	100 g.
Powdered Zinc Oxide	10 g.
Glycerite Starch	400 g.

Melt the stearic acid. At the same time dissolve the potassium carbonate in 320 cc. of distilled water and heat to about 170° F. on water bath. Bring stearic acid to the same temperature and mix them. Continue this temperature on the water bath, with occasional stirring, until the reaction is perfectly complete.

Dissolve the powdered borax in 100 cc. of distilled water, add the quince jelly and heat on water bath to about 170° F. Add this mixture to the first, which should be at the same temperature, and again leave on water bath until reaction is complete.

Heat the glycerite of starch to the same temperature, stir in the powdered zinc oxide with a glass stirring rod and add to the other mixture, stirring occasionally.

Let cool and add perfume (oil ylang ylang recommended).

The most important essential is to employ a perfect glycerite of starch. Use Kingsford's or other suitable grade of corn starch and U. S. P. Glycerin and make it up fresh for each batch.

It is also essential to have all three batches at exactly the same temperature when mixing them.

Modern Grease Paint

Stearic Acid	12.25 g.
Diglycol Stearate	6.12 g.
Caustic Potash	0.50 g.
Glycerin (30° Bé)	2.10 g.
Water, Distilled	15.34 g.
Erythrosin, or Tartrazine	0.12 g.
Zinc Oxide	6.12 g.
Lake Color, to suit	3.10 g.
Perfume, to suit	0.75 g.

Almond Pastes

Formula No. 1

Stearic Acid	8.5 g.
Beeswax	0.5 g.
Spermaceti	1.5 g.
Almonds, Peeled	10 g.
Glycerin	1 g.
Alcohol	1 g.
Ammonia (0.910)	0.5 g.
Borax	0.5 g.
Water, Distilled	76.5 g.

Make a paste of the almonds, the glycerin, and some of the water and add to the cream after it is stirred until cold.

Formula No. 2

Triethanolamine Stearate	20 g.
Beeswax, White	5 g.
Spermaceti	15 g.
Almonds, Peeled	30 g.
Mineral or Almond Oil	50 g.
Glycerin	2 g.
Water	105 g.

Honey-Almond Paste

Formula No. 1

Bitter Almonds, Peeled, Ground	250 g.
Honey, Purified	500 g.
Egg-yolks	8
Bergamot Essence	7 g.

Clove Essence	7 g.
Sweet Almond or Peanut Oil	500 g.

Grind the bitter almonds in the honey, work in the egg-yolks, the perfume oils, and ultimately the vegetable oil.

Formula No. 2

Almonds, Peeled	8.0 g.
Rose Water	30.0 g.
Soap, White	7.0 g.
Borax Solution (1:30)	15.0 g.
Honey, Purified	5.0 g.
Geranium Oil	a few drops

Formula No. 3

Bitter Almonds, Peeled	30.0	g.
Egg-yolk	1	
Honey	60.0	g.
Almond Oil	60.0	g.
Bergamot Oil	15	drops
Lemon Oil	12	drops
Neroli Oil	12	drops

Crack up the almonds in a little of water, grind the paste through a fine strainer, add the honey-eggyolk-oil mixture. Whip until the salve is formed.

"Honey and Almond" Type Cream

Cold Cream	½	oz.
Almond Oil	½	oz.
Glycerin	½	oz.
Boric Acid	1	oz.
Solution of Soda, B.P.	1½	oz.
Quince Mucilage	5	oz.
Water to make	5	pt.

Stir the cold cream, almond oil, and solution of soda together until a uniform soapy emulsion is obtained. Dissolve the boric acid in 60 ounces of warm water; to this add the glycerin and quince mucilage, and add the mixture slowly, and with constant stirring, to the mortar contents. Perfume with spirits of almonds and rose when cold, and make up.

Amandine

Honey	16	cc.
Soft Soap	8	g.
Balsam of Peru	1	cc.
Bergamot Oil	1.5	cc.
Bitter Almonds Oil	1.5	cc.
Clove Oil	1	cc.
Sweet Almond Oil	56	cc.
Preservative	1.5	g.

Toilet-Cream with Locust Bean Gum

Locust Bean Gum	10	g.
Glycerin	120	cc.
Water, Distilled	240	cc.
Alcohol, 90%	20	cc.
Perfume	2–3	g.
Preservative	0.8	g.

Skin Cream
(Type Crême Mouson)

(a)	Stearic Acid	800 g.
	Water	1000 g.
(b)	Potassium Carbonate	80 g.
	Water	2300 g.
(c)	Alcohol	100 g.
(d)	Woolfat, Purified	240 g.
	White Beeswax	60 g.
(e)	Glycerin	1250 g.
	Water	4000 g.
(f)	Perfume	170 g.

Heat the stearic acid and the water (a) on the waterbath, and add the hot (b) to it at a temperature higher than the melting point of the stearic acid. The kettle should be only partly filled, because the saponification is accompanied by strong foaming. Add (c) to help the gelling. Mix. Add the melted fats (d), mix thoroughly again, add (e).

Keep stirring until well emulsified and take off the waterbath. Add (f), stirring until cold.

Skin Cream with Sericin

Stearic Acid	15	g.
Sodium Hydroxide	0.7	g.
Borax	0.5	g.
Sericin, Purified	1	g.
Glycerin	10	g.
Perfume	0.5	g.
Water, Distilled	72.3	g.

Cream Containing Pancreatin

German Patent 283 923

Absorption Base	30 g.
Woolfat, Neutral	3 g.
Mineral Oil	5 g.
Pancreatin, Purified	1 g.
Glycerin	5 g.
Water, Distilled	56 g.

Formalin Cream (Patented)

Formalin (40%)	80 oz.
Diglycol Stearate	15 oz.
Diglycol Laurate	5 oz.

Creme Kaloderma

Gelatin	25 g.
Distilled Water	275 g.
Honey	100 g.
Glycerin	600 g.
Preservative	15 g.

Quinto Cream

Quince Seed	90 gr.
Boric Acid	30 gr.
Salicylic Acid	20 gr.
Glycerin	1.5 oz.
Cologne Water	4 oz.
Boiling Water	4 oz.
Spirit of Lemon	to suit

Triturate the quince seed with the boiling water, add the acids, and strain through muslin.

Creams with Cetyl Alcohol

Formula No. 1

(a)	Cetyl Alcohol	150 g.
	Petrolatum, White	240 g.
	Beeswax, White	250 g.
	Woolfat Anhydrous	350 g.
(b)	Perfume	10 g.
(c)	Water	up to 1500 g.

Melt (a) at lowest possible temperature, cool to just above the chilling point, add (b). Add luke-warm water (c) in small portions, with long intermissions. Mix thoroughly.

Formula No. 2

(a)	Cetyl Alcohol	120 g.
	Woolfat, Anhydrous	50 g.
	Paraffin Wax (52/54° C.)	200 g.
	Mineral Oil, White	620 g.
(b)	Perfume	10 g.
(c)	Water	up to 2500 g.

Formula No. 3

(a)	Cetyl Alcohol	60 g.
	Cholesterol	40 g.
	Beeswax, White	50 g.
	Woolfat, Anhydrous	100 g.
	Mineral Oil, White	290 g.
	Petrolatum	450 g.
(b)	Perfume	10 g.
(c)	Water	up to 2500 g.

Substance	Formula No. 4	Formula No. 5	Formula No. 6	Formula No. 7
Cetyl Alcohol	10	10	10	20
Liquid Paraffin	10	40	40	20
White Soft Paraffin	80	50	15	60
Water	—	—	35	60

No. 4. Translucent. Of consistency somewhat stiffer than soft paraffin.

100 g. + 60 g. water (37.75 per cent.) give a creamy-white cream.

No. 5. Translucent. Consistency that of soft paraffin.

100 g. + 60 g. water give a creamy-white cream somewhat softer than A.

No. 6. Creamy-white soft cream.

No. 7. Creamy-white cream, somewhat stiffer than 5.

These hydrous creams can be rubbed quickly and smoothly into the skin, in fact, they are vanishing creams. The liquid paraffin may be replaced in part by vegetable oil. Every 100 g. of the above preparations will take up to a maximum of 65 g. of water. By an addition of 10 per cent. of wool fat the ability to take up more water can be increased.

Emulsion with Cetyl Alcohol

Cetyl Alcohol, Pure	3–5 g.
Paraffin Oil and Fatty Oil	65–67 g.
Water, Distilled	30 g.

Absorption Base Cream

Absorption Base Creams are coming to the fore because of their beneficial effect on the skin because of their cholesterin and oxycholesterin content.

Parachol is a highly refined absorption base of the Eucerin type, which is used in producing high grade creams which are pure white—not yellow like most creams of this type and which are also free from the objectionable lanolin odor. Such creams do not dry out and will not corrode metal containers. The following formula may be used as a starting point. For special purposes, sulphur, bismuth subnitrate, mercury salts, titanium dioxide, salicylic and thymol or other products may be introduced.

Absorption Base Cream.

1.	Parachol	10 lb.
	Parasterin	20 lb.
	Mineral Oil	10 lb.
2.	Water	25 lb.

Heat (1) in water, both, till melted, allow to cool to 45–47° C. Warm (2) to 45–47° C. and add in 7 or 8 different portions to (1), stirring vigorously, taking care not to add more water until previous portions are absorbed.

Creams with Pearly Lustre

Stearin	85	g.
Lanolin	5 (or less)	g.
Myristic Alcohol	10	g.
Glycerin	36	cc.
Triethanolamine	5	cc.
Borax	a knife-tip full	
Water	250	cc.
Perfume [*no* Alcohol]	2	g.

Lily Toilet Cream

Carob, Bean Powdered	10.0 g.
Glycerin	120.0 cc.
Water	240.0 cc.
Lily Perfume	5.0 cc.
Alcohol (90%)	20.0 cc.
Benzoic acid	0.5 g.

Greaseless Cream

Agar-Agar Solution, (1:20 glycerin:79 water)	63 g.
Sodium Cetyl Sulphonate	10 g.
Glyceryl Monostearate	5 g.
Water, Distilled	22 g.

Greaseless Quinosol Cream

180 grams stearin are melted in a 6 to 7 liter vessel on a water bath with 400 grams of water. Melted mass is allowed to remain on water bath and is mixed with a boiling solution of 18 grams potassium carbonate in 400 grams water and stirred constantly with a wood stirring rod, while carbonate solution is added in small portions. This is continued until a uniform mass is obtained. Excess alkali in product must be neutralized with a little stearin. Then 300 grams glycerin, 40 grams lanolin and 10 grams beeswax are added and finally 1 to 2% (20 to 40 grams) perfume bouquet usually used in perfuming soap. When a homogeneous product is obtained, the vessel is removed from the water bath and cooled to 55° C. while being constantly stirred. Then a solution of 12 grams quinosol in 800 grams water, heated to the same temperature, is added in portions. Mixture is agitated while being cooled to room temperature. It is permitted to stand for 1 to 2 days, then worked up again and finally filled into tubes or jars.

Soothing Cream

Used to relieve skin irritation, especially after a depilatory has been used.

A zinc oxide paste, containing 28 parts almond oil, 60 parts zinc oxide, 15 parts talc and 60 parts cold cream is useful; also a mixture of 30 parts lanolin and 90 parts soap-camphor liniment perfumed with oil of lavender.

Soothing and Softening Cream

Glyceryl Mono-Stearate	12 g.
Cetyl Alcohol	4 g.
Cocoa Butter	13 g.
Lanolin	3 g.
Balsam of Peru	4 g.
Witch Hazel	15 cc.
Water	49 cc.

Put the first four ingredients into the water and heat with constant stirring until the solids have melted. Warm and stir in the witch hazel and finally stir in the balsam of Peru. About one tenth per cent of a good preservative should be added.

Baby Skin Cream

Cetyl Alcohol	20 g.
Mineral Oil	15 g.
Lanolin	5 g.
Petrolatum, White	50 g.
Glycerin, C.P.	10 g.
Rose Water	60 g.
Perfume	to suit

Menthol Cream

Menthol	0.2 g.
"Moldex" or Other Good Preservative	0.2 g.
Perfume Oil	0.3 g.
Alcohol	5 g.
Dissolve and add	
Glycerin	5 g.
Add	
Tragacanth-Glycerin Base (See)	100 g.

Petrolatum Cream

Glyceryl Monostearate	10 g.
White Petrolatum	20 g.
Mineral Oil	10 g.
Water	60 cc.

Translucent Jelly Cream

Stearic Acid	6 g.
Spermaceti	15 g.
White Petrolatum	30 g.
Mineral Oil	49 g.
Perfume Oil to Suit.	

Melt the stearic acid and the spermaceti, add the petrolatum and when melted stir in the mineral oil which has first been heated. When almost set stir in perfume.

Tragacanth-Glycerin Base

Tragacanth, White, Fine Powder	1 g.
Glycerin	5 g.
Grind thoroughly in mortar and add:	
Water, Warm	94 g.

Add while stirring and in small portions, warm up to 40° C. Stir until paste is homogeneous.

Glycerin Jelly for the Hands

a.	Wheat Starch } grind	10 g.
	Water } grind	15 g.
	Glycerin	100 g.
b.	Tragacanth, White	2 g.
	Alcohol (90%)	5 g.
	Methyl-*p*-Hydroxybenzoate	0.5 g.

Grind *a* and *b* separately, mix, warm then on the water bath until odor of alcohol disappears.

Glycerin-Honey Jelly

Honey	20 g.
Water	500 g.
Glycerin	450 g.
Agar-Agar, Cut	15 g.
Methyl-*p*-Hydroxybenzoate	1 g.

Warm to complete swelling and solution percolate, if necessary. Stir, and add:

Formaldehyde (40%)	1 g.
Perfume Composition	1 g.

Almond Hand-Cleansing Paste

The "*Almond Bran*" is made out of two equal parts of sweet and bitter almonds. One can make a "Glycerin Paste" or a "Camphor Paste."

Glycerin Type

Two hundred fifty pounds of the bran are pounded with 5 lb. of rose water and mixed with the following:

One-quarter pound bean or cornflour, 1–2 chicken eggs, 15 lb. borax, 5 lb. fine potassium carbonate, and about 50 lb. glycerin.

The Camphor Paste is made by adding to the pounded "Almond Bran" a mixture of 25 lb. each of 10% camphor oil and spermaceti, molten together.

After cooling, add a powderized mixture of 100 lb. potato flour and 50 lb. talc, and 100 lb. rose water. Mix well altogether. Color with alkannin or curcuma.

Astringent Cream

Formula No. 1

Diglycol Stearate	10 g.
Lanolin Anhydrous	5 g.
Mineral Oil	3 g.
Heat to 170° F.	
Tannic Acid	2 g.
Water	70 cc.

Heat to 170° F. and add to above at that temperature with agitation.

Perfume as desired.

Formula No. 2

Paraffin	15 g.
Lanolin	10 g.
Mineral Oil	60 g.
Cetyl Alcohol	15 g.

Heat to 150°. Then add a heated solution of:

Alum	15 g.
Tannic Acid	15 g.
Water	280 cc.

Agitate until the cream congeals.

Astringent Cream

1. Glycosterin 3 lb.
2. White Petrolatum 1 lb.
3. Astringent Powder No. 1 4 oz.
   (Aluminum Cetyl Acetate)
4. Water 15 lb.
5. Perfume 1 oz.

Heat (1) and (2) to 160° F. and add to it slowly (4) which has been heated to 200° C. Stir and work in (3) until uniform; add (5) just before pouring.

Alloxan—Make up
(Blush Cream)

(a white cream reddening on the skin)

(a)	Almond Oil	180 g.
	Spermaceti	30 g.
	White Beeswax	30 g.
	Water	50 g.
(b)	Alloxan (in Alcohol)	5 g.

This is prepared in a similar manner to cold cream; the alloxan is dissolved in alcohol and added last. The product should be stored in well-closed containers.

Make-up Base

a	Glyceryl Monostearate	10 g.
a	"Carbitol"	7 g.
a	Stearic Acid	1 g.
	Water	76 g.
	Alcohol	5 g.
	Perfume	to suit

Warm (a) and mix until uniform; dissolve perfume in alcohol and add to (a) which has been cooled.

Make-up Remover

Mineral Oil	2 gal.
Stearic Acid	1 lb.
Water	3 gal.
Triethanolamine Stearate	3 lb.
"Carbitol"	2 lb.
Perfume	2 oz.

"Bear Grease" Cosmetic

Formula No. 1

Beef Marrow	4 g.
Veal Suet	2 g.
Preservative	.1 g.

Color and perfume as desired.

Formula No. 2 (Stick Form)

Beef Marrow	4 g.
Veal Suet	2 g.
Ceresin	2 g.
Preservative	.1 g.

La Rouce Bath Cream

Tannic Acid	4 g.
Expressed Oil of Almonds	160 g.
Hydrous Lanolin	240 g.

Melt, mix and beat until smooth.

The preparation made from this French recipe is much used to close the pores, constrict the skin and make the flesh firm after the hot or Turkish bath. It is also used as a wrinkle cream.

Ink Removing Cream

U. S. Patent 1,968,304

A substantially non-aqueous cream for the removal of ink stains from the skin contains about 500 g. of zinc stearate, about 300 g. of citric acid, about 500 cc. of 95 per cent ethyl alcohol and about 2000 cc. of diethylene glycol.

Protective Hand Creams

Formula No. 1

Zinc Stearate, U.S.P.	10 g.
Aluminum Subacetate Solution N.F. (7½–8%)	15 g.
Gum Camphor	3 g.
Menthol Crystals	1 g.
Acid Carbolic, U.S.P.	½ g.
Glycerin, U.S.P.	½ g.
Lanolin, Anhydrous	½ g.
Gum Tragacanth	4½ g.
Soap (Low Alkali Content)	18 g.
White Mineral Oil Technical	½ g.
Triethanolamine	½ g.
Water	46 g.

Formula No. 2

Zinc Stearate, U.S.P.	10 g.
Aluminum Subacetate Solution N.F. (7½–8%)	15 g.
Gum Camphor	3 g.
Menthol Crystals	1 g.
Acid Carbolic, U.S.P.	½ g.
Glycerin, U.S.P.	½ g.
Lanolin (Anhydrous)	½ g.
Gum Tragacanth	4½ g.
Soap (Low Alkali Content)	18 g.
White Mineral Oil Technical	½ g.
Triethanolamine	½ g.
Water	44¼ g.
Sulpho Ammonium Ichthyolate	2 g.

Formula No. 3

White Mineral Technical Oil	35 g.
Paraffin Wax	55 g.
Ammonium Sulpho-Ichthyolate	2 g.
Stearic Acid	1 g.
Triethanolamine	½ g.
Water	7½ g.

Formula No. 4

Glyceryl Monostearate	8 lb.
Magnesium Stearate	14 lb.
Beeswax	3 lb.
Petrolatum	10 lb.
Mineral Oil, White	5 lb.
Water	60 lb.

Formula No. 5

(a)	Petrolatum, White	61 g.
	Lanolin, Anhydrous	10 g.
	Beeswax, White	4 g.
	Cetyl Alcohol	13 g.
(b)	Bismuth Subnitrate	4 g.
	Zinc Stearate	4 g.
	Zinc Oxide	4 g.
	Perfume, to suit	4 g.

Melt up (a), adding the waxes in the order of their melting points.

Add (b), which has been thoroughly mixed and sifted before.

If necessary, mill to make smooth.

Formula No. 6

(a)	Glyceryl Monostearate	12 g.
	Cetyl Alcohol or Spermaceti	10 g.
	Mineral Oil, White	7 g.
	Petrolatum	5 g.
	Glycerin	3 g.
	Titanium Dioxide	5 g.
	Water	58 g.
(b)	Perfume	to suit

Heat up altogether, and stir, when melted, to form emulsion. Stir while cooling. Add (b), mix thoroughly, and pour.

Formula No. 7

(a)	Petrolatum	35 g.
(a)	Cetyl Alcohol	5 g.
(b)	Butyl Stearate	5 g.
(a)	Lanolin, Anhydrous	4 g.
(c)	Zinc Stearate	5 g.
(c)	Talcum	17 g.
(a)	Mineral Oil, White	25 g.
(c)	Titanium Dioxide	4 g.
(d)	Perfume	to suit

Melt all materials (a) on waterbath, add (b). Mix in the sifted mixture of (c). Mix two hours, perfume, and pour near titer.

Skin Protective Film

Soap Flakes	7.48 g.
Glycerin	26.40 g.
Sodium Silicate	24.20 g.
Tragacanth, Gum	0.21 g.
Lemon Oil	0.16 g.
Water	41.60 g.

Mechanic's Protective Hand Cream

Glyceryl Monostearate	8 g.
Magnesium Stearate	14 g.
Beeswax	3 g.
Petrolatum	10 g.
Mineral Oil	5 g.
Water	60 cc.

Heat together to 70° C. and stir until cool.

Mechanics Hand Protective Coating

U. S. Patent 2,021,131

Water	1600 oz.
Sodium Stearate	288 oz.
Glycerin	1155 oz.
Sodium Silicate	906 oz.
"Lemenone" (A stabilized lemon odor)	1 oz.

Housewives Protective Hand Cream

Pulverized Neutral White Soap	10 oz.
Triethanolamine	2 oz.
Titanium Dioxide	2 oz.
Lanolin	2 oz.
Glycerin	4 oz.
Gum Arabic	4 oz.
Water	76 oz.

Massage Preparations

These substances are dispensed in ointment, mixture or solution form, and applied before or after treatment, usually with a vibrator.

Formula No. 1

Menthol	2.5 g.
Tragacanth	4 g.
Glycerin	12 cc.
Alcohol	15 cc.
Water	300 cc.

Formula No. 2

Gelatin	2 g.
Water	48 cc.
Glycerin	5 cc.
Glycerite of Boroglycerin	45 g.

Formula No. 3

Fluid Extract of Witch Hazel	10 cc.
Wool Fat	60 g.
Petrolatum	30 g.

Formula No. 4

Menthol	0.8 g.
Camphor	0.8 g.
Eucalyptol	3 g.
Petrolatum	96 g.

Massage Creams

Formula No. 1

65 g. mineral oil, 35 g. cetyl alcohol and 10 cc. water.

Formula No. 2

90 g. stearic acid, 9 g. potassium carbonate, 800 cc. water are used to make a soapy mixture by first melting the stearic acid and then adding the solution of carbonate in water and stirring until all carbon dioxide evolution has ceased. Then the mass is cooled. It is mixed with 5 g. white beeswax, 20 g. anhydrous lanolin, 150 g. glycerin and perfumed with 6 g. oil of eucalyptus, 5 g. oil of pinus sylvestris and 1 g. camphor.

Formula No. 3

65 g. mineral oil, 7.5 g. stearic acid, 7.5 g. white beeswax, 6 g. solid paraffin wax, 9 g. liquid paraffin, 0.5 g. sodium carbonate, 0.5 g. borax and 35 cc. water are mixed together.

Formula No. 4

500 g. lanolin, 500 g. rose water, 500 g. lard, 200 g. glycerin, 15 g. cheiranthus, and 5 g. dianthus (clove pink).

Formula No. 5

Spermaceti	10 g.
Solid Paraffin	15 g.
Mineral Oil	45 g.
Lecithin	1.5 g.
Cholesterin	0.5 g.
Borax	1 g.
Water	30 g.
Perfume	as required

The solution of lecithin and cholesterin is accomplished best in the liquid or melted fats and waxy constituents. The melted mass is permitted to be cooled at 40° C. and the hot solution of borax in water is poured first in small portions and then in larger portions into the fused mass while stirring thoroughly. Then it is stirred cold.

In the case of vanishing cream, it is somewhat more difficult to work in the lecithin. The simplest way is to dissolve the lecithin in the melted stearic acid (overheating should be prevented) and to mix the potash solution into it by stirring in the usual way. On the other hand saponification and emulsification might be affected by the lecithin. If any oil is permitted in the vanishing cream, lecithin is ground fine with warm mineral oil (1 part of lecithin to say ½–1 part of mineral oil), so that a mass is produced that can be distributed. As soon as the cream has been mixed and while it is still warm, the warm lecithin oil is stirred thoroughly into it. The whole of it is stirred cold.

Formula No. 6

Glycerin	1 oz.
Borax	2 dr.
Boracic Acid	1 dr.
Rose Geranium Oil	30 drops
Anise Oil	15 drops
Bitter Almond Oil	15 drops
Milk	1 gal.

Heat the milk until it curdles and allow it to stand 12 hours. Strain it through cheese-cloth and allow it to stand again for 12 hours. Mix in the salts and the glycerin, and triturate in a mortar, finally adding the odors and the coloring. The curdled milk must be as free from water as possible in order to avoid separation.

Formula No. 7

"Ceraflux"	13
Beeswax	12
Mineral Oil	50
Water	26
Borax	1
Perfume	½

Procedure as for Cold Cream, A

Formula No. 8

White Beeswax	12.5 g.
Paraffin Wax	10 g.
White Mineral Oil	50 g.
Distilled Water	26 g.
Borax	1 g.
Perfume	0.5 g.

Formula No. 9

"Parachol" (Absorption Base)	70 g.
Cocoa Butter	370 g.
Mineral Oil, White	370 g.
Water, Distilled	190 g.

Peanut Oil Massage Cream

White Beeswax	20 g.
Spermaceti	20 g.
Peanut Oil	45 g.
Lanolin	12 g.
Water	45 g.
Borax	3 g.
Camphor	1 g.

Melt the wax over a water bath, add the lanolin and oil, and heat to 80° C. The camphor is dissolved in the oil with gentle heat, the borax is dissolved in the water and heated to 80° C. At this temperature the water is added to the wax oil mixture at the same temperature with vigorous stirring; best done with a motor stirrer.

Massage Cream with Cetyl Alcohol

Beeswax	5 g.
Cetyl Alcohol	12 g.
Carnauba Wax, White	3 g.
Vaseline, White	6 g.
Olive Oil, Preserved	9 g.
Paraffin Oil	65 g.

Rolling Massage Creams

Formula No. 1

Stearic Acid	8 g.
Paraffin Oil	2.7 g.
Cocoa Butter	1 g.
Starch	14.3 g.
Boric Acid	2.8 g.
Glycerin	3.3 g.
Water, Distilled	66.7 g.
Ammonia (26%)	0.9 g.
Perfume	0.3 g.

Formula No. 2

1.	Stearic Acid	6.75 lb.
	Cocoa Butter	13.50 oz.
	Mineral Oil	2.25 lb.
2.	Corn Starch	12.00 lb.
	Boric Acid	2.40 lb.
	Water	5.60 gal.
	"Moldex"	1.50 g.
3.	Glycerin	45 fl. oz.
	Ammonia (26° Bé)	12 fl. oz.
	Perfume (Rose)	4 oz.
	Color (Rose)	1 oz.

Mix the corn starch with the cold water until smooth (no lumps). Add the boric acid. Heat until it forms a thick translucent paste, stirring continually, taking care to avoid overheating and burning the bottom of the pan. Take off the heat and add No. 3. Stir. Then add No. 1, which has previously been melted together at 200° F. Stir rapidly for about 1½ to 2 hours. Add color and perfume, and 2 oz. sodium benzoate dissolved in 4 oz. water. Pack cold.

Glycerite of Starch

The following method is recommended as being simpler than the U. S. P. X method and giving better results: Mix 10 g. starch with 20 cc. cold water to a homogeneous mixture, add to 70 cc. glycerol in a porcelain dish and stir till homogeneous, place on a sand bath heated with an electric hot plate or a Bunsen burner, regulating the temperature so that the heat increases rather slowly and stirring almost constantly. Do not heat above 144° F.

CHAPTER II

LOTIONS

LIQUID preparations, either clear or milky used to keep the skin soft, smooth and white, are called lotions. They are also used to alleviate and soothe skin which has been irritated, burned or chapped. Many of the formulae given under liquid creams are used as lotions.

Hand Lotions

Formula No. 1

Castile Soap, Neutral White Powdered	90 gr.
Lanolin	2 oz.
Borax	2 dr.
Water	1 pt.
Perfume Oil	¼ to ½ oz. to the above amount or to suit individual requirements

Directions: Dissolve soap and Borax in ½ pint water. Mix Lanolin with the remainder of the water (hot). Mix two solutions, shaking well. This produces a finished milk white product.

Formula No. 2

No. 1.	Quince Seed	10 oz.		425 gr.
	Water	2 gal.		
No. 2.	Spermaceti	1 lb.	13 oz.	113 gr.
	Beeswax, White		3 oz.	288 gr.
No. 3.	Soap, Powdered	2 lb.	11 oz.	389 gr.
	Borax, Powdered		7 oz.	138 gr.
	Salicylic Acid		1 oz.	160 gr.
	Water	5 gal.		
No. 4.	Glycerin	5½ lb.		
	Water to make	10 gal.		
	Alcohol	1 gal.		
	Perfume Oil to suit			

Directions: Take No. 1 and soak in water about 4 hours, then strain off the mucilage. Take No. 2 and melt together. Take No. 3 and dissolve in the water. Then take No. 2 and No. 3 and mix with constant stirring. Then add No. 4 and use small amount of Ultramarine Blue color to make the preparation white.

Formula No. 3

Quince Seed	31.2 g.
Soap Powdered	68.0 g.
Borax	20.7 g.
Sodium Benzoate	5.7 g.
Spermaceti	306.0 g.
White Wax	10.4 g.
Glycerin	454.4 g.
Alcohol	180 g.
Perfume Oil	22.0 g.
Sodium Tribenzoate	7.5 g.
Water to make	1 gal.

Make mucilage from the quince seed and add this to a solution which has been made by first dissolving the soap and the powders in water, together with the glycerin, which is then added, to the melted waxes. This is thoroughly stirred together and the perfume oil added when almost cold.

Formula No. 4

Stearic Acid	234.0	g.
Trihydroxyetheleneamine Stearate	58.4	g.
"Carbitol"	116.8	g.
Zinc Sulphocarbolate	7.36	g.
Quince Seed	29.20	g.
Glycerin	596.0	g.
Perfume Oil	15.0	g.
Alcohol	180	g.
Sodium Tribenzoate	7.5	g.
Water to make	1	gal.

Formula No. 5

Stearic Acid	65	g.
Trihydroxyetheleneamine Stearate	4	g.
"Carbitol"	4	g.
Menthol	1.5	g.
Water	1265	cc.
Quince Seed Mucilage (made from 8 g. of seed)		
Glycerin	2	oz.
Perfume to suit		

Formula No. 6

Hand Cleanser and Conditioner

1. Mineral Oil	70	lb.
2. Olive Oil	8	lb.
3. Trihydroxyethylamine Stearate	14	lb.
4. Water	70	lb.
5. Perfume	2	lb.

Heat Nos. 1, 2 and 3 together to 140° F. and stir until homogeneous. Add No. 4 slowly while stirring and then stir in the perfume. Continue stirring until cool. By varying the amount of water a thicker or thinner preparation will be formed. The thicker preparations are put up in tubes and are now carried by men and women, especially motorists, who, when water is not available, merely put a little of this cleaner on their hands, rub it in and then wipe off with it the grease, oil, paint or dirt present. Not only is this an excellent detergent but it leaves the skin smooth, and produces a cooling sensation and prevents chapping during cold weather.

Formula No. 7

Alcohol	600	cc.
Glycerin	100	cc.
Menthol	5	g.
Perfume, Rose Oil, Etc.	1	cc.
Salicylic Acid	2	g.
Water	300	cc.

Formula No. 8

Alcohol	550	cc.
Glycerin	175	cc.
Menthol	3	g.
Perfume, as desired, about	1	cc.
Salicylic Acid	2	g.
Water	275	cc.

Formula No. 9

Alcohol	500	cc.
Glycerin	250	cc.
Menthol	1	g.
Perfume, as desired, about	1	cc.
Salicylic Acid	2	g.
Water	250	cc.

A lavender coloration of varying intensity may be obtained by adding traces of ferric chloride solution. Formula No. 3 gives a rather oily lotion.

Formula No. 10

Boric Acid	1	dr.
Glycerin	6	dr.

Dissolve by heat and mix with

Lanolin	6	dr.
Petrolatum	1	oz.

The borated glycerin should be cooled before mixing. Add any perfume desired.

Formula No. 11

1. Trihydroxyethylamine Stearate	7	g.
2. Lecithin	1	g.
3. Lanolin	2	g.
4. Cetyl Alcohol	3	g.
5. Mineral Oil	15	g.
6. Water	71.5	cc.
7. Perfume	0.5	g.

Heat (1) in (6) till dissolved. Heat (5) and (3) and add (2) and (4). Stir well and add to (1), (6). Add perfume.

Formula No. 12

Gum Tragacanth, Powdered	1	g.
Alcohol	5	g.

Mix the above until uniform, then add

Water	93	cc.
Salicylic Acid	0.4	g.
Perfume	0.6	g.

Mix until uniform

Formula No. 13

Witch Hazel	58 cc.
Bay Rum	58 cc.
Spirits of Camphor	20 cc.
Tincture of Benzoin	4 cc.
"Carbitol"	180 cc.

Formula No. 14

Macerate 3 oz. of quince seed in 2 quarts of cold water for 24 hours. Strain through linen cloth with force and add 1 quart of water to the strained mucilage. Mix: Bay Rum, 16 oz; glycerin, 8 oz.; orange flower water, 12 oz.; alcohol, 26 oz. and add to the mucilage, followed by sufficient water to make 1 gal. of finished product.

Formula No. 15

Tragacanth, Powdered	28 g.
Alcohol	336 cc.
Tincture Benzoin Compound	4 cc.
Glycerin	140 cc.
Rose Water	308 cc.
Distilled Water Sufficient to Make	2240 cc.

1. Shake tragacanth with warm alcohol.
2. Dilute tincture benzoin compound with some alcohol.
3. Mix glycerin, water and rose water.
4. Mix all and mix until uniform.

Formula No. 16

Triethanolamine Stearate	7 g.
Lecithin	1 g.
Lanolin	2 g.
Cetyl Alcohol	3 g.
White Mineral Oil	15 g.
Water	71.5 cc.
Perfume	.5 g.

Put the triethanolamine stearate into the water and heat with constant stirring until it dissolves. Meanwhile heat the mineral oil and lanolin, add the lecithin and cetyl alcohol. Stir well and slowly add this mixture to the triethanolamine stearate solution. Finally add perfume.

Formula No. 17

Gum Tragacanth, Powdered	2.0 g.
Glycerin	10.0 g.
Olive Oil	8.0 g.
Tincture of Benzoin	3.0 g.
Alcohol	10.0 g.
Triethanolamine	1.0 g.
Rose Water	65.9 cc.
Formaldehyde	1. g.

Mix the tragacanth in half the alcohol and stir the mixture into half the rose water. Stir the glycerin and triethanolamine into the remainder of the rose water and heat the mixture to about 125° F. Stir in the olive oil, previously heated to the same temperature. Warm and add the mucilage of tragacanth. Stir well and add the benzoin and formaldehyde mixed with the remainder of the alcohol.

Formula No. 18

Tincture of Benzoin	21.5 g.
Spirits of Camphor	1.5 g.
Glycerin	5. g.
Witch Hazel	32. cc.
Rose Water	40. cc.

Procedure: Mix the last three and stir in the first two ingredients.

Formula No. 19

Karaya Gum	2 g.
Glycerin	10 g.
Alcohol	5 g.
Distilled Water	82 g.
Methyl-para-oxy-benzoic Acid	0.1 g.
Perfume	to suit

Formula No. 20

Gum Tragacanth (Ribbon No. 1)	25 g.
Glycerin	500 cc.
Water, Distilled	3500 cc.
Benzoic Acid	3 g.
Salicylic Acid	1 g.
Perfume	to suit
Coloring	to suit

Dissolve the benzoic and salicylic acids in the glycerin at low heat, stirring well.

The gum tragacanth used should be of finest grade, Aleppo type, No. 1. Stir gum into the water, allow to stand for a minimum of 24 hours, with occasional stirring. Add color in solution, if desired. Mix until uniform. Pass through double-thickness of fine-mesh cheesecloth. After straining stir the glycerine-acid mixture into the gum-water mass. Mix with mechanical mixer for 30 minutes. Strain through single-thickness cheesecloth. Add perfume, and mix until mass is well blended. Bottle.

This lotion is stable, and will not separate. It will keep indefinitely when corked.

Formula No. 21

1.	Mineral Oil	70 lb.
2.	Olive Oil	8 lb.
3.	Trihydroxyethylamine Stearate	14 lb.
4.	Water	70 lb.
5.	Perfume	2 lb.

Heat Nos. 1, 2 and 3 together to 140° F. and stir until homogeneous. Add No. 4 slowly while stirring and then stir in the perfume. Continue stirring until cool. By varying the am^unt of water a thicker or thinner preparation will be formed. The thicker preparations are put up in tubes and are now carried by men and women, especially motorists, who, when water is not available, merely put a little of this cleaner on their hands, rub it in and then wipe off with it the grease, oil, paint or dirt present. Not only is this an excellent detergent but it leaves the skin smooth, and produces a cooling sensation and prevents chapping during cold weather.

Formula No. 22

Lanolin, Anhydrous 1 lb.
Glycosterin 1¼ lb.
Heat to 170° F. and to it add slowly with stirring.
Water 4 gal.
Deramin ½ lb.
Heated to 170° F.
To the above add slowly with stirring.
Water 12 gal.
Heated to 130° F.
In a separate vessel mix:
Witch Hazel 32 gal.
Tragacanth, Gum 1 oz.
Moldex 1 oz.

Allow to stand overnight and heat to 110° F. and then mix into above.

Various modifications of the above can be made by adding color and perfume. This lotion is an effective sun-burn preventive and alleviator. For this purpose it is perfumed with a medicated perfume oil containing Benzocaine, Thymol, etc.

Formula No. 23

Stearic Acid	3.15 g.
Glycerin	6.00 g.
Potassium Hydroxide	.15 g.
Water	80.30 cc.
Alcohol	8.50 g.
Perfume	.50 g.
Quince Seed	1.25 g.
Preservative	.15 g.

Dissolve the potassium hydroxide in one-third of the water, bring the rest of the water to a temperature of 80° C.; add the quince seed and soak for six hours. Melt the stearic acid in the glycerin, dissolve the perfume in the alcohol. Add the potassium hydroxide solution to the melted fatty substance and boil for a minute. Allow the temperature to drop to about 70° C. and then stir it into the quince seed mucilage. Stir occasionally until cool; then slowly add the alcohol, perfume and preservative.

Formula No. 24

Stearic Acid	3.00 g.
Alcohol	5.00 g.
Mineral Oil	5.00 g.
Triethanolamine	2.00 g.
Glycerin	5.00 g.
Water	75.85 cc.
Quince Seed	3.50 g.
Perfume	.50 g.
Preservative	.15 g.

Melt the stearic acid in the mineral oil and glycerin. Bring the temperature to about 70° C.; boil the triethanolamine in the water and add the melted fats. Stir vigorously until the temperature drops to about 50° C., then slowly stir in the quince seed mucilage and then slowly add the perfume and preservative dissolved in alcohol.

Formula No. 25

Stearic Acid	1.50 g.
Soap, Powdered Neutral	1.00 g.
Alcohol	2.00 g.
Glycerin	4.90 g.
Boric Acid	2.50 g.
Borax	2.50 g.
Quince Seed	2.50 g.
Water	82.45 cc.
Perfume	.50 g.
Preservative	.15 g.

Put the quince seed into half the water to which the preservative has been added. Allow to soak 24 hours and strain through muslin. Heat the rest of the water and dissolve in it the borax. Add the melted stearic acid and stir vigorously. Add the soap, boric acid and glycerin. Agitate until cool. Add the quince seed mucilage and the perfume dissolved in alcohol.

Formula No. 26

Beeswax, White	1.00 g.
Quince Seed	2.75 g.
Stearic Acid	1.65 g.
Borax	2.50 g.
Glycerin	3.00 g.
Water	85.45 cc.
Perfume	.50 g.
Alcohol	3.00 g.
Preservative	.15 g.

Melt stearic and beeswax in glycerin. Add borax dissolved in hot water. Add mucilage and other ingredients as before.

Formula No. 27

Powdered Tragacanth	1.75 g.
Pulverized Neutral White Soap	3.00 g.
Glycerin	7.00 g.
Alcohol	8.00 g.
Borax	.50 g.
Preservative	.15 g.
Boric Acid	1.00 g.
Water	78.10 cc.
Perfume	.50 g.

Dissolve the preservative in half the water and add the tragacanth and allow it to stand until dissolved, stirring it occasionally. Heat the remainder of the water; add the glycerin, borax and boric acid, and when dissolved, add the soap and stir until cool, then add the mucilage. Stir gently and add the perfume dissolved in the alcohol, a little at a time.

Formula No. 28

Spermaceti	2.00 g.
White Beeswax	.25 g.
Glycerin	6.00 g.
Soap	3.00 g.
Borax	.50 g.
Sodium Benzoate	.20 g.
Quince Seed	3.40 g.
Alcohol	4.00 g.
Water	80.00 cc.
Perfume	.50 g.
Preservative	.15 g.

Add the quince seed to two-thirds of the water in which the preservative has first been dissolved. Allow to soak for 24 hours and strain. Add the glycerin, borax and sodium benzoate to the remainder of the water and stir until dissolved. Melt and add the spermaceti and white wax, stir rapidly for one or two hours then add the soap. Add the mucilage next and finally add the perfume dissolved in the alcohol, in a very thin stream.

Formula No. 29

Spermaceti	3.75 g.
White Beeswax	.75 g.
Glycerin	2.00 g.
Pulverized Neutral White Soap	1.50 g.
Borax	.35 g.
Almond Oil	3.00 g.
Quince Seed	1.50 g.
Alcohol	1.50 g.
Water	84.00 cc.
Preservative	.15 g.
Perfume	.50 g.

Proceed as in Formula No. 28.

Formula No. 30

White Beeswax	4.125 g.
Glycerin	2.000 g.
Pulverized Neutral White Soap	3.375 g.
Borax	.375 g.
Almond Oil	3.000 g.
Honey	1.250 g.
Quince Seed	1.50 g.
Alcohol	1.500 g.
Water	80.550 cc.
Witch Hazel	1.500 g.
Boric Acid	.175 g.
Perfume	.500 g.
Preservative	.150 g.

Add the quince seed to two-thirds of the water in which the preservative has been dissolved; allow to stand 24 hours and strain through muslin. Boil the remainder of the water, add the soap, boric acid, witch hazel, glycerin, borax. Melt and add the beeswax, spermaceti, oil of almond, and the honey. Add the quince seed solution quickly. Agitate slowly until cool, then add the perfume and alcohol.

Formula No. 31

Citric Acid	1.00 g.
Glycerin	5.00 g.
Alcohol	6.00 g.
Boric Acid	.50 g.
Lemon Oil	1.00 g.
Benzoate of Soda	.50 g.
Quince Seed	2.50 g.
Water	83.50 cc.

Dissolve the benzoate of soda in two-thirds of water, add the quince seed and allow to soak 24 hours, then strain through muslin. Heat the remainder of the water and dissolve the boric and citric acids in it. Add the glycerin; then add the quince seed mucilage. Mix the oil of lemon in the alcohol and add it slowly with continuous stirring.

Formula No. 32

Bay Rum	2 oz.
Alcohol	2 oz.
Witch Hazel	2 oz.
Glycerin	3 oz.
Gum Tragacanth	1/6 oz.
Water	1 qt.

Soak the gum in the water for 24 hours, then stir until thoroughly dispersed, add remaining ingredients, scent as desired.

Formula No. 33

Water	100 lb.
Diglycol Stearate	5.6 lb.
Preservative	1/4 lb.

Heat to 160° F.; turn off heat and begin stirring; when temperature drops to 140° F. add

Water	50 lb.
Alcohol	7 lb.
Perfume	to suit

Formula No. 34

A.	Lanolin	12 lb.
	Mineral Oil	20 lb.
	Trihydroxyethylamine Stearate	4 1/4 lb.
	Glycosterin	2 lb.
B.	Glycerin	8 lb.
	Water	200 lb.
	Benzoate of Soda	1/4 lb.
C.	Perfume to suit.	

Heat A and B separately to 180° F. and run B into A slowly while stirring. When temperature has dropped to 100° F. add perfume. Continue stirring until COLD.

The low cost and high quality of these lotions make them of great interest. This eliminates the use of spermaceti, almond oil and gums which are prone to spoilage and the technique is very simple.

These formulae can be made thinner by increasing the amount of Glycerin or thicker by decreasing the amount of Glycerin. They have excellent smoothing and nourishing properties for the skin because of their Lanolin and Glycerin content.

1. Lanolin	1 lb.
2. Tincture of Benzoin	20 oz.
3. Glycosterin	10 lb.
4. Witch Hazel	250 lb.

Melt 1, 2 and 3 together and run into this slowly with stirring 4 heated to 140° F.

Formula No. 35

Mace Oil	10 oz.
Olive Oil	10 oz.
Ammonia	15 oz.
Essence of Rosemary	5 oz.
Rose Water	50 oz.
Lecithin	1/2 oz.
Chloroform	3 oz.
Perfume to suit.	

Add the olive oil to the mace and mix thoroughly, add the ammonia water and keep stirring until a saponaceous mass is evolved. Dissolve the lecithin in the chloroform. Mix the rosemary with the rose water and add the lecithin solution. Then add this to the first mixture very slowly; keep up a very slow mixing for about an hour afterward.

Formula No. 36

Castor Oil	6 oz.
Tar Oil Rectified	10 oz.
Phenol	1 oz.
Formalin	1 oz.
Sesame Oil	160 oz.
Soft Soap	10 oz.
Alcohol	30 oz.
Perfume	to suit

Dissolve the soap in part of the alcohol using slight heat. Dissolve the formalin and the phenol in the rest of the alcohol. Mix the sesame, castor and tar oils, add the soap and then the formalin-phenol.

Other materials utilized in the preparation of ointments and lotions of this kind are: storax, creosote, ammoniated mercury, sulphonated bitumen, procaine hydrochloride, copper oleate, sublimed sulphur, balsam of Peru, titanium oxide, silver lactate, alcohol, olive oil, sesame oil, benzoated lard and a number of absorption bases.

Formula No. 37

Oxyquinoline Sulphate	1 oz.
Tincture of Fish Berries	10 oz.
Glycerin	30 oz.
Tincture Benzoin	8 oz.
Witch Hazel	150 oz.
Water	10 oz.
Perfume to suit.	

Dissolve the sulphate in water. Mix the fish berries with the glycerin, add the benzoin and the witch hazel. Then add the sulphate solution. Other chemicals used in the manufacture of eczema preparations are: calomel, iodoform, oil of wormwood, silver protein, sodium iodide, potassium iodide, pine tar, bismuth resorcinate, mercuric salicylate, bismuth subnitrate, red mercuric iodide, basic aluminum acetate, benzocaine, bismuth oxyquinolate, and various absorption bases.

Formula No. 38

Gum Tragacanth, Powdered	4	lb.
Sweet Almond Oil	12½	pt.
Water	37	gal.
Benzoate of Soda	2	lb.
Alcohol	6	gal.
Perfume Oil		to suit
Tincture Benzoin	26	oz.
Glycerin	6	gal.

In a large mixing kettle mix tragacanth with sweet almond oil to a thin paste.

Dissolve preservative in water, in a separate kettle.

Add alcohol, perfume oil, benzoin and glycerin to the gum and mix well.

Finally add the water with very rapid stirring, being careful to keep the two batches at substantially the same temperature, for best results.

Best results will be obtained if a propeller type mixer is used. The secret of a good lotion of this type is to use extremely high speed stirring during the addition of the first portion of the water.

The consistency can be varied to suit by varying the quantity of gum.

Face Lotions

Formula No. 1

Triethanolamine	0.5	cc.
Glycerin	4	cc.
Alcohol	33	cc.
Distilled Water	62	cc.
Perfume	0.5–1	cc.

Formula No. 2

Triethanolamine	0.5 cc.
Glycerin	4 cc.
Alcohol (30%)	95.5 cc.
Perfume	to suit

Formula No. 3

Orange Flower Water	800 cc.
Eau de Cologne	200 cc.
Triethanolamine	6 cc.
Spirits of Camphor	20 cc.
Glycerin	100 cc.

Formula No. 4

Camphor	20 cc.
Alcohol (96%)	850 cc.
Glycerin (28° Bé.)	50 cc.
Perfume	30 cc.
Distilled Water	1500 cc.
Triethanolamine	15 cc.

Formula No. 5

Triethanolamine	5 cc.
Alcohol (96%)	500 cc.
Spirits of Camphor	100 cc.
Perfume	10 cc.
Glycerin	20 cc.
Witch Hazel, Distilled	1000 cc.

Formula No. 6

For Dry Skin

Mineral Oil, White	35 cc.
Beeswax	20 g.
Aminostearin	8 g.
Water	50 cc.

Warm together and mix vigorously until emulsified.

Formula No. 7

Mineral Oil	72 cc.
Aminostearin	14 g.
Water	200 cc.

Formula No. 8

Triethanolamine	5	cc.
Aromatic Spirit	30	cc.
Bergamot Oil	12.5	cc.
Orange Flower Oil	0.5	cc.
Lemon Oil	2	cc.
Rosemary Oil	15	cc.
Alcohol (70%)	940	cc.

Formula No. 9

Camphor	25 g.
Alcohol	850 cc.

Glycerin	25 cc.
Perfume Mixture	30 cc.
Distilled Water	1570 cc.

Formula No. 10

Boric Acid	10 g.
Glycerin	29 cc.
Menthol	1 g.
Perfume	5 cc.
Alcohol	255 cc.
Hamamelis Distillate	300 cc.
Rose Water	400 cc.

Formula No. 11

Alcohol	450 cc.
Camphor, Spirits of	100 cc.
Perfume	10 cc.
Hamamelis Distillate	440 cc.

Formula No. 12

Potassium Carbonate	400 g.
Distilled Water	2000 cc.
Orange Flower Water	1000 cc.
Alcohol	100 cc.
Perfume	to suit

Formula No. 13

Borax	50 g.
Sodium Thiosulphate	500 g.
Distilled Water	8500 cc.
Glycerin	500 cc.
Eau de Cologne	500 cc.

Formula No. 14

Alcohol, 96%	450 g.
Camphor, Spirits of	100 g.
Perfume Composition	10 g.
Witch Hazel, Distilled	430 g.
Glycerin	10 g.

Dusty Odor Face Lotions

Formula No. 1

Glycerin	1 cc.
Lactic Acid	0.2 cc.
Menthol	0.5 g.
Opoponax—Perfume with Violet Root Oil, etc.	0.5 cc.
Alum	0.3 g.
Alcohol (35%)	97.5 cc.

Formula No. 2

Glycerin	1 cc.
Citric Acid	0.2 g.
Aluminum Acetate	0.3 g.
Menthol	0.5 g.
Hamamelis Water	5 cc.
Perfumes (as above)	0.5 cc.
Alcohol (40%)	92.5 cc.

Formula No. 3

Glycerin	1 cc.
Alum	1 g.
Zinc Sulphophenylate	0.5 g.
Perfumes (as above)	0.5 cc.
Menthol	0.5 g.
Isopropyl Alcohol	10 cc.
Rose Water	10 cc.
Alcohol (30%)	76.5 cc.

Face Lotion
(For Oily Skin)

Sulphur, Precipitated	2 g.
Glycerin	5 g.
Camphor Spirits (10%)	3 g.
Lavender Water	10 g.
Borax	1 g.
Distilled Water	81 g.

Face Lotion
(For Dry Skin)

Lanolin or Cholesterol	0.05 g.
Lecithin	0.05 g.
Alcohol	6 g.
Glycerin	3 g.
Almond Oil	10 g.
Distilled Water	about 85 g.

Face Water for Mottled Skin or Freckles

Zinc Sulphate	1 g.
Citric Acid	0.5 g.
Hydrogen Peroxide (3–10%)	89.5 cc.

Astringent Lotions

Astringent lotions are usually based on alcohol as the active ingredient or on an alcohol containing product, such as: witch hazel.

Formula No. 1

Mild

Menthol	4 oz.
Zinc Phenolsulphonate	5 lb.
Camphor	4 oz.
Perfume	8 oz.
Alcohol	10 gal.

All of the above are dissolved together and 90 gallons of witch hazel is added to it. The product may be colored slightly by the use of a water soluble color.

Formula No. 2

Water	24	oz.
Glycerin	½	oz.
Alum	1	oz.
Isohol (or Alcohol)	4	oz.
Lavender Oil	1	dr.
Zinc Phenolsulfonate	¼	oz.

Dissolve the lavender oil in the Isohol and stir into the water containing the other ingredients.

Formula No. 3

Glycerin	2.00 g.
Potassium Alum	3.50 g.
Zinc Sulphocarbolate	0.10 g.
Water	94.40 g.
Perfume } Color }	to suit

Formula No. 4

Alum	1	oz.
Potassium Carbonate	0.25	oz.
Glycerin	0.50	oz.
Rose Water	10.00	oz.

Water to make 1½ pints. Some of this water can be replaced by witch hazel.

Formula No. 5

Witch Hazel Extract	5 gal.
Zinc Phenolsulfonate	8 oz.
Color and Perfume	to suit

Formula No. 6

Mild

Witch Hazel	1 gal.
Aquaresin G.M.C.	2 oz.
To above add	
Menthol	⅛ oz.
Dissolved in	
Alcohol	1 pt.
Color	to suit

This may be perfumed by absorbing the perfume oil in powdered charcoal and filtering the above through it.

Formula No. 7

Mild

Alcohol	3½	gal.
Glycerin	4	pt.
Orange Flower Water	20	gal.
Zinc Phenolsulfonate	1	lb.
Color		to suit
Perfume		to suit

Formula No. 8

Medium Strength

Alcohol	35	gal.
Borax	2	oz.
Zinc Phenolsulphonate	4	lb.
Perfume	2	lb.
Camphor	8	oz.
Glycerin	3	gal.

All of the above are dissolved together and water sufficient to bring the volume to 100 gallons is added.

Formula No. 9

Strong

Lavender Oil	1	lb.
Vanillin	1	oz.
Isohol (or Alcohol)	5	gal.
Menthol	1	oz.

Mix the above until dissolved and to it add slowly with stirring

Polycol	2	pt.
Aquaresin G.M.C.	1	pt.
Water	5	gal.

Allow to stand over-night; filter through magnesium carbonate and color to suit.

Formula No. 10

Strong

Alcohol	50	gal.
Ethyl Aminobenzoic-acid	8	oz.
Parachlormetaxylenol	8	oz.
Menthol	8	oz.
Thymol	4	oz.
Lavender Oil	3	lb.
Glycerin	5	gal.
Vanillin	8	oz.

All of the above are dissolved together. Water is added to make 100 gallons.

Other materials, such as: resin, benzoin, peru or styrax may be used in small quantities.

Propylene glycol, or diethylene glycol may be used in place of the glycerin.

Formula No. 11

Strong

Salicylic Acid	3¼	lb.
Benzyl Cinnamate	2½	oz.
Acetone	1	gal.
Alcohol	1	gal.

The quantity of salicylic acid may be reduced ½ if a milder agent is desired.

Pearly Finishing Astringent Lotion

Gum Tragacol	½ oz.
Moldex	1 g.
Water (warm)	5 pt.
Allow to stand for a day and stir into it Isohol	3 pt.

To 20 pounds of soft vanishing cream (see Vanishing Cream formulae) which has stood long enough to develop a pearly sheen, there is added slowly a gallon or more, if desired, of the above gum solution. Stirring must be slow but thorough. Filter through cheesecloth and bottle. This lotion may be colored if desired.

This lotion is shimmering and pearly. It is quick drying and leaves the skin in a fresh soft condition ready for the application of powder.

Astringent Lotion (Non-Alcoholic)

Water	1 gal.
Aquaresin G.M.C.	2 oz.

Allow to stand over-night

Perfume by filtering through powdered charcoal in which perfume oil has been absorbed.

If a non-resinous astringent is desired the Aquaresin G.M.C. may be replaced by zinc phenolsulfonate.

Astringent Lotion Cleanser

Alcohol	5 gal.
Glycopon S	4 lb.
Water	5 gal.
Phenol	2 oz.
Perfume	5 oz.
Color	to suit

Skin Lotion

(For Chapping, Sunburn, Dry Skin, etc.)

Formula No. 1

Diglycol Stearate	2.66 g.
Glycopon S	5.00 g.
Glycerin	12.00 g.
Water	80.33 cc.
Perfume, Color, Medicaments	to suit

Formula No. 2

Gum Tragacanth	4 oz.
Glycerin	3 oz.
Phenol	1 oz.
Teel Oil	120 oz.
Water	360 oz.
Perfume	2 oz.

Formula No. 3

Zinc Phenolsulfonate	30 gr.
Alcohol	4 dr.
Glycerin	2 dr.
Tincture of Cochineal	1 dr.
Orange Flower Water	1½ oz.
Rose Water to make	6 oz.

Lotion for Oily Skins

Formula No. 1

Boric Acid	1 dr.
Alcohol	0.5 oz.
Rose Water	5.5 oz.

Formula No. 2

Alcohol	40 g.
"Carbitol"	10 g.
Betanaphthol Disulphonate	0.5 g.
Water	48 g.
Perfume	to suit

Skin Toning Lotion

Boric Acid	1 g.
Witch Hazel	15 cc.
Rose Water	15 cc.
Alcohol	10 cc.
Orange Flower Water	59 cc.

Warm the witch hazel and dissolve the boric acid in it. Mix the rest of the ingredients with the orange flower water and add the boric acid solution. Mix, age and filter.

Skin Cleansing Lotion

British Patent 423,426

Borax	1.33 g.
Potassium Alum	2.30 g.
Soda Ash	1.75 g.
Water	100 cc.

Evaporate down to half of volume.

Foundation Lotion

Mineral Oil	1 lb.
Glycosterin	1 lb.
Parachol (Absorption Base)	½ lb.

Heat to 150° F.

Deramin	½ lb.
Water	10 pt.
"Moldex" (Preservative)	1 oz.

Heat to 150° F. and add slowly with stirring to oil mixture. Stir while cooling and add 2 oz. perfume oil at 110° F. Then add 5 gallons water heated to 110° F. and stir until cold.

This makes a fine skin softener and conditioner.

Non-Perspiring Lotion

Alcohol	20 g.
Betnaphthol Disulphonate	2 g.
Water	78 g.
Perfume	to suit

Antiseptic Drying Lotion

Chlorbutanol	1 oz.
Salicylic Acid	1 oz.
Peppermint Oil	½ oz.
Alcohol	30 oz.
Water	66 oz.

Almond Lotion

1. Mineral Oil	35 lb.
2. White Wax	2 lb.
3. Trihydroxyethylamine Stearate	8 lb.
4. Perfume (Almond)	1 lb.
5. Water	50 lb.

Heat Nos. 1, 2 and 3 together to 140° F. and stir until homogeneous. Heat No. 5 to 140° F. and run in slowly to the above mixture, stirring thoroughly. When the temperature has dropped to 105° F. add the perfume drop by drop, stirring until completely absorbed. Continue stirring until cool and package.

Low Cost Almond Lotion

1. Diglycol Stearate	7	lb.
2. Water	30	gal.
3. Gum Tragacanth Solution	6	gal.
4. Benzaldehyde	3	fl. oz.
5. Bergamot Oil	1½	fl. oz.

Method of manufacture:

a. Melt No. 1 at 160° F.

b. Heat No. 2 to 205° F. and run into stone jar (note final temperature of water after dumping into jar must not be below 170° F.).

c. With high speed agitator running, add *a* (molten at 160° F.) to *b*, at at least 170° F. and allow mixer to run until temperature has dropped to 140° F.

d. Add 3 to batch while mixture is still running.

e. Add 4 and 5 immediately after 3 and allow mixer to continue running until temperature has dropped to 90° or 95° F.

The gum solution is made as follows:

Gum Tragacanth	2½ lb.
Water	50 gal.

Allow the gum to soak for several hours and beat into solution.

Rose Lotion

1. Diglycol Stearate	7	lb.
2. Water	30	gal.
3. Gum Solution	6	gal.
4. Rose Oil	3	fl. oz.
5. Red Color Solution Made by Dissolving Red Dye, 1 oz., in Water, 1 qt.	¾	fl. oz.

Method of manufacture:

a. Melt No. 1 at 160° F.

b. Heat No. 2 to 200° F. and run into stone jar (note: final temperature of water after dumping into jar must not be below 170° F.).

c. With high speed agitator running add *a* (molten at 160° F.) to *b* at at least 170° F. and allow mixer to run until temperature has dropped to 140° F.

d. Add 3 to batch while mixer is still running.

e. Add 4 and 5 immediately after 3 and allow mixer to continue running until temperature has dropped to 90° or 95° F.

The gum solution is made as explained under low cost almond lotion.

Glycerin and Cucumber Lotion

	Cucumber Perfume	5 g.
b.	Alcohol	50 g.
	Benzoic Acid	0.3 g.
	Cucumber Perfume	5 g.
c.	Tragacanth, Fine, White	5 g.
	Glycerin	100 g.

Grind *c* together, then add *a* and *b* in small portions, grinding to get homogeneous paste.

Cucumber and Egg Lotion

Cucumber Juice	400 g.
Alcohol	50 g.
Benzoic Acid	0.25 g.
Egg Yellow Color	1–2 g.
Lavender Oil	3 g.

Rose Oil, Artificial	1	g.
Glycerin	100	g.

Lemon Juice Lotion

Glycerin	2	g.
Lemon Juice	5	g.
Water	88½	g.
Lemon Oil	½	g.
Acimul	4½	g.

Melt the above together at lowest possible temperature and stir till cold.

Lemon Lotion

1. Diglycol Stearate	7	lb.
2. Water	30	gal.
3. Gum Solution	6	gal.
4. Lemon Oil	1½	fl. oz.
5. Yellow Dye	¾	oz.

Method of manufacture:

a. Melt No. 1 at 160° F.

b. Heat No. 2 to 200° F. and run into stone jar (note: final temperature of water after dumping into jar must not be below 170° F.).

c. With high speed agitator running add *a* (molten at 160° F.) to *b* at at least 180° F. and allow mixer to run until temperature has dropped to 145° F.

d. Add 3 to batch while mixer is still running.

e. Add 4 and 5 immediately after 3 and allow mixer to continue running until temperature has dropped to 95° or 100° F.

The gum solution is made as explained under almond lotion.

Lemon Juice Lotion

Pectin	2.5	g.
Lemon Juice	9.5	g.
Water	88	cc.
Preservative	0.15	g.

Carob Lotion

Carob Bean Mucilage	45.0	cc.
Tincture of Benzoin	2.0	cc.
Glycerin	5.0	cc.
Lily Perfume	2.5	cc.
Water to make	100.0	cc.

Larkspur Lotion

Larkspur, Coarse Powder	100	g.
Potassium Carbonate	10	g.
Alcohol	500	cc.
Water	500	cc.

Boil the larkspur for 15 minutes in an aqueous solution of the potassium carbonate. Filter and while cooling pass the alcohol through the drug while in the filter. Add enough water through the filter to bring up to 1000 cc.

Lanolin Lotions

Formula No. 1

Lanolin, Anhydrous	0.9	g.
Borax	0.1	g.
Sodium Soap Powder, or Potassium Soap	0.2	g.
Distilled Water	98.8	g.

Formula No. 2

Lanolin	8	g.
Ammonium Linoleate	3	g.
Borax	1	g.
Distilled Water	87	g.
Paraffin Oil	1	g.

Formula No. 3

Lanolin, Anhydrous	7	g.
Soap Powder	2	g.
Cocoa Butter	3	g.
Borax	1	g.
Distilled Water	7	cc.
Rose Water	80	cc.

The lanolin (together with the other fats or oils) is melted up to about 60° C., and into it, the soap water, at the same temperature, is poured with stirring.

Formula No. 4

Lanolin, Anhydrous	12	g.
Paraffin Oil	20	g.
Diethylene Glycol Stearate	2	g.
Triethanolamine Stearate	4.25	g.
Distilled Water	200	g.
Glycerin	8	g.

Melt up the first four ingredients and heat them to 82° C. The glycerin-water is heated to an equal temperature and stirred into the oil. Stir until cold. Perfume at 36° C.

Lecithin Lotion

Milky lotions (emulsions) are produced by dissolving lecithin in oil and agitating or churning the oil solution with neutral soap solution containing water or glycerin. In this way they form emulsions that are not too stable. Far more stable is the following emulsion:

Two parts of glyceryl monostearate ester, 1 part stearin alcohol, 5 parts stearin, 2 parts lanolin, 5 parts mineral oil (according to the particular fattiness desired 10–15 parts) and 2 parts lecithin are melted and 1 part potash in 5 parts glycerin and 40 parts hot water is stirred during heating into the fused mass. It is further heated until the mass no longer rises thick. Then it is stirred cold. It is then thinned after cooling with more water until the particular thin liquid state desired is attained. Instead of or in conjunction with the first two constituent parts a glycol stearate may be used.

Modern Glycerin-Sulphur Lotion

Colloidal Sulphur in Glycerin (24%)	100 g.
Tincture of Green Soap	100 g.
Eau de Cologne—Oil	1 g.
Water, Distilled	799 g.

Methyl Cellulose Lotions

Formula No. 1

(Viscous)

Methyl Cellulose	0.75 g.
Paraffin Oil	36.5 g.
Distilled Water	62.25 g.
Perfume	to suit

Formula No. 2

(Thin)

Methyl Cellulose	0.75 g.
Paraffin Oil	36.5 g.
Distilled Water	60.0 cc.
Alcohol	2.25 cc.
Perfume	0.5 g.

Preparation: Prepare a 4% solution of methyl cellulose as follows:

Methyl Cellulose, Dry, shredded	1
Water, Distilled, Boiling	24

Stir well. The methyl cellulose dissolves while the solution is cooling. Let stand 24 hours; stir up again.

The required amount of this solution is put into a container, and the paraffin oil is added in a thin jet, very slowly, stirring thoroughly. It is best to add only a part of the oil, forming an "emulsion nucleus," and to add the rest then.

The remaining water is stirred in under equal conditions. Perfume homogenize.

Sulphur, Castor Oil and Tragacanth Lotion

Tincture Quillaja	3 g.
Salicylic Acid	1 g.
Precipitated Sulphur	2 g.
Alcohol	20 g.
Castor Oil	10 g.
Tragacanth	0.5 g.
Water to make	100 cc.

Triturate the salicylic acid, precipitated sulphur and tragacanth with the castor oil, and the tincture of quillaja, and gradually add most of the water, triturating constantly. Add the spirit, shake vigorously, and make up to volume with water.

Wrinkle Lotion

Alum	20 gr.
Zinc Sulphate	5 gr.
Glycerin	2 fl. dr.
Tincture of Benzoin	2 fl. dr.
Perfume	to suit

Distilled water sufficient to make 1 quart.

Lotion for Hives or Prickly Heat

Menthol	2 g.
Alcohol	3 oz.
Sodium Bicarbonate	10 g.
Witch Hazel	3 oz.
Water to make	1 pt.

Dissolve menthol in alcohol, add sodium bicarbonate and witch hazel. When dissolved add the water, stirring vigorously. Should not be used near the eyes, delicate skin, cuts, etc.

Face Water

Triethanolamine	0.5 g.
Glycerin	4 g.
Alcohol	33 g.
Perfume	0.5 g.
Distilled Water	62 g.

Modern Neutral Face Water

Alcohol (40%)	920 cc.
Diethylene Glycol	30 g.
Glycerin	50 g.

Face Water, Acid

Alcohol (45%)	900 cc.
Tri- (or Di-) Ethylene Glycol	30 g.
Citric Acid	5 g.
Glycerin	30 g.
Witch Hazel	35 cc.

Face Water, Astringent

Alcohol (35%)	950 cc.
Diethylene Glycol	30 g.
Glycerin	15 g.
Tannic Acid, Pure	3 g.
Phosphoric Acid	2 g.

Face Water with Witch Hazel

Alcohol (40%)	920 g.
Witch Hazel	50 cc.
Glycerin	30 g.

Sulphur Face Water

Sulphur, Colloidal	3 g.
Potassium Carbonate	1.5 g.
Glycerin	5 cc.
Spirits of Camphor	4 cc.
Alcohol	10 cc.
Distilled Water	76.5 cc.

Kummerfeld's (Face) Water

Sulphur, Colloidal, or Finely Precipitated	2 g.
Glycerin	12 cc.
Spirits of Camphor	4 cc.
Eau de Cologne	20 cc.
Distilled Water	100 cc.

Optionally: Addition of Borax, or Potash, or Triethanolamine (intensifies effect).

Prophylactic Face Waters

Formula No. 1

Ammonium Chloride	0.5 g.
Witch Hazel	20 cc.
Rose Water	10 cc.
Distilled Water	69.5 cc.

Formula No. 2

Ammonium Chloride	2.5 g.
Cherry Laurel Water	10 cc.
Witch Hazel	10 cc.
Rose Water	20 cc.
Distilled Water	57 cc.
Diethylene Glycol	0.5 cc.

Facial and Body Reducer

Camphor	5 oz.
Epsom Salt, Powdered	10 oz.
Isohol	85 oz.
Tincture Iodine	1 cc.
Water	5 oz.
Perfume	2 oz.

Stir quickly while bottling as this preparation separates quickly. Bottles should be labeled "Shake before using."

Coloring Toilet Lotions

Spirit soluble burnt sugar can be used in all dilutions of alcohol containing over 40 per cent of alcohol. However, for tinting lotions, dry extract of quassia is in many cases useful, particularly since it serves at the same time as a denaturant. The following is an example:—

Dry Extract of Quassia	1 dr.
Borax	15 gr.
Alcohol	12 oz.
Water	8 oz.

Heat 1 oz. of water to boiling, add the borax and the dry extract of quassia and triturate. Add the remainder of the water, then the spirit; set aside for one day and filter.

If a dye is preferred use Caramel B.

EMOLLIENT LOTIONS

Glycerin Milk

Mucilage of Quince Seed	70 g.
Powdered Soap	1 g.
Boric Acid	2½ g.
Alcohol	2 g.
Glycerin	25 g.

Perfume and Color, as desired.

Tragacanth Lotion

Tragacanth, Ribbon	0.8 g.
Boric Acid	1.6 g.
Glycerin	12.0 g.
Alcohol	12.0 g.
Water	75.0 cc.

Perfume and Color, as desired.

Quince Lotion

Quince Seed	1.6 g.
Boric Acid	0.6 g.
Sodium Borate	0.6 g.
Glycerin	12.0 g.
Alcohol	12.0 g.
Water, to make	100.0 cc.

Perfume and Color, as desired.

Almond Lotion

Blanched Almonds	4 oz.
Curd Soap	½ oz.
Bitter Almond Oil	10 min.
Bergamot Oil	1 dr.
Alcohol	4 oz.
Rose Water	12 oz.

Lanolin Skin Milk

Wool Fat	50 g.
Medicinal Soap	3 g.
Glycerin	20 g.
Rose Water	300 g.
Benzoin, Tincture	5 g.
Perfume Composition	10 g.
Water, Distilled	612 g.

Face Milk

Beeswax	1 g.
Spermaceti	1 g.
Olive, Almond, or Maize Oil	8 g.
Olive Oil Soap, Powdered	2 g.
Corn or Maize Starch	3–3½ g.
Distilled Water	25 g.
Glycerin	5 g.
Witch Hazel Extract	10 g.
Iris Tincture	1 g.
Lactic Acid	1 g.
Distilled Water	48 g.

Cucumber Face Milk

(a)	Wool fat, Anhydrous	30 g.
(b)	Rose Water	200 g.
	Potash Soap	10 g.
	Glycerin	20 g.
(c)	Perfume (Oil Eau de Cologne, Chypre, Fougère, etc.)	10 g.
	Benzoin, Tincture	30 g.
(d)	Cucumber Juice, Fresh, Percolated	700 g.

Melt (a) on the water-bath, and add to it the luke-warm (b) in small portions. (c) is added to the emulsion, and all are mixed through thoroughly. Take off the water-bath and stir in slowly the luke-warm (d). Stir until cold.

Almond Milk

Formula No. 1

(a)	Almonds, Peeled,	70 g.
	Rose Water	to paste
(b)	Benzoin, Tincture	20 g.
	Benzaldehyde	2 g.
	Rose Oil	1 g.
(c)	Borax	7 g.
	Glycerin	50 g.
	Rose Water, to make	10000 g.

Grind (a) to a fine paste, mix with (b), and ultimately add the solution (c). Strain after a few days standing.

Formula No. 2

(Lait Naturel d'Amande)

Sweet Almonds, Peeled	23 g.
Water, Distilled or Rose	70 g.
Alcohol	7 g.
Preservative	0.2–0.3 g.
Perfume	

The peeled almonds are crushed, and ground finely in the roller mill. The alcohol-water mixture is added very slowly to this almond paste, stirring thoroughly. The whole is driven through a pigment grinding mill with discs of hard porcelain. The emulsion is poured through finest linen cloth, to remove the coarse particles.

To thicken this emulsion, and to stabilize it, 0.1% tragacanth, can be worked in (also flea seed—emulsone, pectin, etc.).

Milk of Almonds, Artificial

Paraffin Oil (Viscosity 30–32)	35 g.
Beeswax	2 g.
Triethanolamine Stearate	8 g.
Perfume	1 g.
Water, Distilled	50 g.

Melt the first three ingredients together to 60° C., and stir in the water which has been previously warmed to the same temperature.

Perfume at about 40° C., stirring and adding drop by drop. Stir until cold.

Benzoin Milk

Formula No. 1

Mix in a mortar or dish:

a.	Tincture of Benzoin	50 cc.
	Alcohol	200 cc.
b.	Glycerin	100 cc.
c.	Water, Distilled	700 cc.

First grind *a*, add *b*, and pour slowly under stirring *c* into *a* and *b*. Let stand a week. Filter. Shake before use.

(Lait de Benzoin, Lait Virginal)

Formula No. 2

Tincture of Benzoin, Siam, 5%	50 g.
Infusion of Panama-Bark, 1:5	50 g.
Witch Hazel Extract	100 g.
Rose Water, or Other Flower Waters	800 g.

Formula No. 3

Tincture of Benzoin, 5%	50 g.
Saponin, White	5 g.
Diethylene Glycol	25 g.
Distilled (or Flower) Water	920 g.

Formula No. 4

Tincture of Benzoin, 10%	80 g.
Tincture of Quillaja-Bark (1:5)	20 g.
Glycerin	100 g.
Distilled (or Flower) Water	800 g.

Preparation: Mix tincture of benzoin with the saponin-extracts, or dissolve the saponin in some of the distilled water, and mix this with the tincture of benzoin. This mixture is to be poured slowly into the water with good agitation.

In case further additions of alcohol is planned, the water can be added to the tincture of benzoin.

Formula No. 5

Tincture of Benzoin, 10%	50 g.
Tincture of Quillaja-Bark (1:5)	20 g.
Alcohol, 90%	100 g.
Distilled Water	830 g.

Benzoin Milk with Eau de Cologne

Tincture of Benzoin (5%)	50 g.
Eau de Cologne, Containing about 1% Essential Oils	300 g.
Tincture of Quillaja Bark, 1:5	20 g.
Diethylene Glycol	150 g.
(or Glycerin)	300 g.
Distilled or Flower Water	350–500 g.

Mix the benzoin with the eau de Cologne, add the quillaja, and thereafter the diethylene glycol. The whole is added slowly to the water.

Milky Lotion with Pectin

Base Emulsion (See Below)	550 g.
Distilled Water	445 g.
Perfume	5 g.

Base Emulsion

Distilled Water	710 g.
Mineral Oil	180 g.
Dried Pectin	50 g.
Citric Acid	10 g.
Extract Chamomile Flowers	50 g.

Moisten the pectin with a little alcohol and then rub with a little water in which the citric acid is dissolved until a fine mucilage is obtained. The pectin swells to a large extent. In the rest of the water dissolve the liquid chamomile extract and the warm solution a little at a time to the pectin mucilage. When all the water has been added, heat until a uniform solution results, avoiding overheating. The oil is then emulsified with this solution, preferably in a colloid mill or a homogenizer.

Lait de Jour

Formula No. 1

Stearic Acid	5 g.
Spermaceti	1 g.
Beeswax, White	1 g.
Di (or Tri) Ethylene Glycol	5 g.
Triethanolamine, Purified	1 g.
Water, Distilled	87 g.
Perfume	0.3 to 0.5 gr.

Formula No. 2

Glyceryl Mono Stearate	4–5
Diethylene Glycol	2
or Glycerin	4
Water, Distilled	94–93

Heat the wax to 70–80° C., and do the same with the water-diethylene glycol mixture.

Pour glycerol monostearate into water with good stirring until cooled. Homogenising is very helpful to stabilize the emulsion.

Advisable is the addition of very little Ammonia (0.05%). Small amounts of Cetyl alcohol, myristyl alcohol, Stearin, paraffin beeswax can be added.

Lait de Jour with Glycosterin

Glycosterin	4–5 g.
Ammonium Stearate or Triethanolamine Stearate, Oleate, or Potassium Soap	0.4–0.5 g.
Water, Distilled	95.6–94.5 g.

Lait de Jour with Witch Hazel

Stearin	6 g.
Cetyl Alcohol	1 g.
Beeswax, White	1 g.
Triethanolamine, Purified	1 g.
Glycerin or Diethylene Glycol	2 g.
Witch Hazel Extract	40 g.
Water, Distilled or Rose	49 g.
Perfume	to suit

Method: Melt the waxes together, and heat to 60–70° C. Dissolve the triethanolamine and the other ingredients in the water and heat this solution to 60–70° C.

Stir in the waxes slowly. Cool stirring, and add the perfume very slowly. Homogenizing is advisable.

Skin Hardener

Alum	30 g.
Water and Alcohol (Equal Parts)	250 cc.

Skin Smoothener

Formula No. 1

Boric Acid	3 dr.
Tragacanth	8 g.
Glycerin	3 dr.
Distilled Water	16 oz.

Boil—stir until a clear jelly is obtained.

Skin Smoothener

Boric Acid	2 g.
Gum Tragacanth	8 g.
"Carbitol"	3 g.
"Moldex"	1 g.
Distilled Water	250 cc.
Perfume and Color to suit	

Soak the gum in cold water for one hour, then heat to boiling, add the boric acid and the moldex, and cool. Add the perfume and color to the "Carbitol," and pour this into the mixture. Then add the balance of the distilled water.

Liquid Deep Pore Cleanser

Witch Hazel Extract	50 oz.
Alcohol	28 oz.
Polyglycol	15 oz.

Almond Cream Liquid

Sweet Almond Oil	1 lb.
Spermaceti	2 lb.
Beeswax	2 lb.
Castile Soap, Powdered	3 lb.
Borax	2 lb.
Quince Seed Jelly	1 lb.
Alcohol	1 pt.
Water	4 pt.

Melt the spermaceti and wax together. Dissolve the soap and borax in hot water. Mix these together and add balance of ingredients. Stir and filter through cloth.

Cholesterol Emulsions

Type "Nivea Oil"

Formula No. 1

Paraffin Oil	55 g.
Cholesterol	4–5 g.
Water, Distilled	40 g.

Formula No. 2

Paraffin Oil	65 g.
Oxycholesterol	5 g.
Water, Distilled	30 g.

Locust Bean Mucilage, 4%

Locust Bean (Carob) Gum	4 g.
Alcohol	to wet
Benzoic Acid	0.15 g.
Water, to make	100 g.

Locust Bean Gum Paste

Locust Bean Mucilage, 4%	100 g.
Glycerin	5 g.
Boric Acid	5 g.

Glycerin Jellies

Formula No. 1

Gelatin, White	2.5 g.
Honey	10. g.
Glycerin	57. g.
Alcohol	1. g.
Water, Distilled	29.5 g.

Formula No. 2

Gelatin, White	1.8 g.
Glycerin	30 g.
Alcohol	1 g.
Water, Distilled	67.2 g.

Use preservatives (boric acid—hydroxy benzoic acid but no formaldehyde or salicylic acid). Perfume 0.5% (Rose, Violet).

Agar-Agar Jelly

Agar-Agar	1 lb.
Glycerin	30 lb.
Water, Distilled	69 lb.

Soak the agar-agar in water over night. Take up to a boil cautiously. When the solution is clear, add the glycerin, and the evaporated water.

Quince Seed-Glycerin Jelly

Quince Seed Slime *	41 lb.
Glycerin	19 lb.

Water, Distilled	18	lb.
Alcohol	22	lb.
Preservative	0.5	lb.

* The *slime* is made from

Quince Seed	25	lb.
Water, Distilled	925	lb.

Gelatin-Agar Jellies

Formula No. 1

Gelatin, White	1.0 g.
Agar-Agar, Best	0.5 g.
Glycerin	30.0 g.
Water, Distilled	68.4 g.
Perfume	0.1 g.
Preservative	to suit

Formula No. 2

Gelatin, White	1.0 g.
Agar-Agar	0.5 g.
Glycol Bori-Borate	15.0 g.
Witch Hazel	60.0 g.
Distilled or Flower Water	23.5 g.
Preservative	to suit

Glycerin-Starch Jelly

(Starch-Glycerite)

Formula No. 1

Wheat or Rice Starch	6.7 g.
Glycerin	86.7 g.
Water, Distilled	6.6 g.

Wet the starch with a part of the glycerin, then add the remainder of the glycerin together with the water. Heat on waterbath to clarity and high viscosity.

Formula No. 2

Rice Starch	300–750 g.
Glycerin	1300 g.
Water, Distilled	100 g.

Arrow Root-Glycerin Jelly

Arrow Root Powder	50 g.
Water, Distilled	100 g.
Glycerin	1300 g.
Preservative (Sodium Benzoate, Borax, etc.)	

Glycerin-Starch Cream

(Type "Crême Simon")

Rice Starch	6 g.
Water, Distilled	12 g.
Glycerin	71 g.
Zinc Oxide	5 g.
Talc, Very Fine	0.5 g.
Tincture, Quillaja Bark 1:50	2 g.
Tincture of Benzoin 1:50	1.75 g.
Tincture of Tonka Beans	1.75 g.

Procedure: The zinc oxide and the talc are mixed thoroughly with the tinctures. To this paste, the glycerin-starch jelly is added in small portions, while still hot.

Run between stone rollers and homogenize in a pigment mill. The quillaja bark tincture can be substituted by a saponin-solution. Color is given by addition of small quantities of dyes or pigments, such as eosin or ultramarine.

Perfume: 0.1–0.3%

CHAPTER III

SKIN TREATMENTS

SKIN BLEACHES

Formula No. 1

A mild skin bleaching lotion that is absolutely harmless may be prepared from lemon juice with addition of 15 per cent alcohol to preserve it and 1 per cent glycerin.

Formula No. 2

A very good bleach for removing summer tan may be made by mixing 5 per cent of zinc peroxide or sodium perborate with 95 per cent magnesium carbonate or calcium carbonate. This should be mixed to a paste with water and then applied.

Formula No. 3

Local treatment may be tried by combining "Perhydrol" 1 part, (a 30 per cent solution of hydrogen dioxide,) anhydrous wool fat 6 parts and petrolatum sufficient to make 10 parts. This should be applied to a small area once a day. If irritation results, cease the application and wait for the reaction to subside. If no result is obtained, the strength of the perhydrol can be cautiously increased. After a small area is bleached somewhat, the next area may be treated until a satisfactory result is obtained.

Bleaching Creams

Formula No. 1

1. Borax	50 g.
2. Hydrogen Peroxide, 30%	150 g.
3. Wool Fat, Anhydrous	300 g.
4. Water, Distilled	170 g.
5. Vaseline, Yellow	100 g.
6. Ceresin	30 g.
7. Mineral Oil	200 g.

Melt 3., 5., 6., 7 on the water bath, add the solution of 1. in 4. with stirring and finally 2., and perfume (1%).

Formula No. 2

Borax	50 g.
Hydrogen Peroxide	150 g.
Wool Fat, Anhydrous	50 g.
Distilled Water	44 g.
Petrolatum, White	230 g.
Parachol (Absorption Base)	50 g.
Wool fat, Synthetic	25 g.
Perfume	to suit

Melt fats and oils, stir in borax-solution, add peroxide and perfume.

Formula No. 3

Petrolatum, White	850 g.
Sodium Perborate	150 g.
Perfume	to suit

Formula No. 4

Lanolin	250 g.
Almond Oil	125 g.
Rose Water	125 g.
Borax	10 g.
Sodium Perborate	10 g.
Geranium Oil	2 g.
Bergamot Oil	2 g.
Neroli Oil	0.3 g.
Wintergreen Oil	0.2 g.

It is important to choose oxidation-resistant perfumes, such as: Lavender, Chypre, Fongère, Opoponax, Patchouli, Peau d'Espagne, Bornyl Acetate, Eucalyptol, Thymol, Menthol.

Formula No. 5

1.	White Beeswax	25 g.
	Ceresin	25 g.
	Arachis Oil	80–100 g.
2.	Sodium Perborate	1 g.
	Hydrogen Peroxide (3%)	5 cc.

Melt waxes (1.) together on the water bath, cool, and stir in the solution (2.) of oxidants. Perfume.

Formula No. 6

Sodium Perborate	100 g.
Citric Acid	5 g.
Vaseline Oil	100 g.
Paraffin Wax	50 g.
White Vaseline	250 g.
Lanolin, Anhydrous	50 g.
Perfume	to suit.

Formula No. 7

Zinc Peroxide	20 g.
Citric Acid Powder	12 g.
Lanolin Anhydrous	77 g.
Perfume	to suit.

Formula No. 8

Hydrogen Peroxide, Concentrated	50 g.
Borax	20 g.
Mineral Oil	50 g.
Lanolin, Anhydrous	150 g.
Petrolatum, White	50 g.
Ceresin	50 g.

Formula No. 9

Petrolatum, White	150 g.
Sodium Perborate	50 g.
Citric Acid	50 g.
Mineral Oil	50 g.
Wool fat	50 g.

Formula No. 10

White Mercury Ointment	480 g.
Bismuth Subnitrate	30 g.
Lavender Oil	2.5 g.
White Petrolatum	110 g.

Formula No. 11

("Marylan" Type Crême)

Stearin, Best	125 g.
Water	300 g.
Caustic Potash	enough to saponify the stearin to 30 per cent.
Rice Starch	120 g.
Glycerin	60 g.
Water	390 g.
Aluminum Hydroxide	½–1%
Perfume	½–1%

Melt the stearin at 85° C. and stir into the potash solution of the same temperature. Make up starch solution by wetting the starch with glycerin, and adding the boiling water. Stir the starch solution into the stearin cream, add freshly precipitated aluminum hydroxide (allowing for its water content).

Cool, and perfume at about 40/35° C. Homogenize thoroughly.

Formula No. 12

Hydrogen Peroxide	10 oz.
Lanolin (Anhydrous)	30 oz.

Formula No. 13

Citric Acid	2 oz.
Bismuth Oxychloride	2 oz.
Rose Ointment	30 oz.

Formula No. 14

White Petrolatum	57.50 g.
Beeswax	29.00 g.
Mineral Oil	3.50 g.
Zinc Oxide	5.00 g.
Ammoniated Mercury	5.00 g.
Perfume, Color	to suit

Formula No. 15

White Wax	1½ oz.
White Petrolatum	12½ oz.
Ammoniated Mercury	1¼ oz.
Bismuth Subnitrate	¾ oz.
Red Rose Oil	40 drops

Melt the white wax in a double boiler. Add the petrolatum and stir until melted. Cool. Mix the ammoniated mercury and bismuth subnitrate. Add ¼ pound cold petrolatum mixture and mix in a paint mill. When smooth, add the balance of the petrolatum mixture and perfume.

Skin Whitener (Liquid White)

(Night White or Powder Base)

Formula No. 1

1. Glycosterin	10 lb.
2. Water	60 lb.
3. Titanium Dioxide	3 lb.

Heat 1 and 2 to 150° F. and stir until cold. Allow to stand overnight (very important). Stir the next morning and make sure that it is COLD. Then stir in Titanium Dioxide until uniform. In place of titanium, talc or zinc stearate may be used.

Formula No. 2

A lotion for hands and arms contains 2,500 parts witch hazel extract, 5,000 parts rose water, 1,000 parts alcohol, 1,800 parts glycerin, 100 parts tallow, 100 parts magnesium carbonate, 50 parts magnesium stearate and 1,000 parts antipyrine. First the antipyrine is dissolved in witch hazel extract and rose water. Then glycerin is added. The perfume used is absorbed by the magnesium carbonate, magnesium stearate and tallow. Then alcohol is added. This suspension is strongly shaken for two days. The milk is filtered through coarse filter paper. The two preparations are united with vigorous stirring and decanted. This preparation is applied with cotton. Skin is rubbed and preparation is allowed to dry. The skin remains white the entire evening. Advantage of this preparation over ordinary liquid powder is that a dull white effect is obtained, lasting 4 to 6 hours.

Leg and Arm Blemish Covering

Stearic Acid	4 lb.
Diethylene Glycol	16 lb.

Heat to 180° F. and to this add while stirring the following solution heated to 140° F.

Caustic Potash	4 oz.
Water	16 pt.

When uniform work in following:

Zinc Oxide	15 lb.
Yellow Lake	12 oz.
Persian Lake	4 oz.
Perfumed Oil	4 oz.

The colors may be varied to give more suitable shades.

Mole and Blotch Covering

Collodion	1 gal.
Zinc Oxide	1 lb.
Geranium Lake	½ oz.
Yellow Ochre Lake	1½ oz.

Black Eye Paint

For bleaching out the discoloration popularly known as a "black eye" the black-eye "artists" use solutions of oxalic acid or a compress of scraped bryony or Solomon's seal root. The covering-up treatment of the barber shop "expert" usually consists in bathing the part with a lotion composed of glycerin and hamamelis water in the proportion of 1 of glycerin to 5 of the "witch-hazel"; and then frescoing the discolored area with an adhesive powder or a grease paint.

The typical formulas for the powder follow:

Formula No. 1

Bismuth Subcarbonate	2 dr.
French Chalk	1 dr.
Carmine } Yellow Ochre }	to suit

Formula No. 2

Zinc Oxide	215 g.
Talc	345 g.
Magnesium Carbonate (Heavy)	35 g.
Color	to suit

This is colored with carmine and ochre or tincture of saffron to a flesh tint.

The paints are made by massing one of these powders with petrolatum.

Facial Masks (Mud Packs)

Formula No. 1

Mix to a paste about 15% bentonite with witch hazel or other aromatic water. A balsamic perfume may be added, or bay rum may be used instead. The preparation should be tinted as the mass is of a dull gray-green color. Powdered calamine may be added to both color the preparation and increase its value as a mask.

Formula No. 2

A	Acacia, Gum U.S.P.	37.00 g.
	* Dextrin	2.00 g.
	Boric Acid	0.5 g.
	Distilled Water	50.00 g.

* optional.

B	Alcohol	9.00 g.
	Glycerin	1.00 g.
	Cetyl Alcohol	2.00 g.
	Preservative	0.15 g.
	Camphor	0.2 g.
	Lavender Oil	0.3 g.
	Menthol	0.1–0.2 g.
	Distilled Water to make	100.00 cc.

A small amount of tincture of benzoin may be added if a more opaque product is wished. In manufacturing this product the ingredients comprising A and B are mixed separately, and then B is poured slowly, and with constant stirring, into the aqueous mixture. The use of a colloid mill, if possible, will ensure a very fine product.

Using this formula, and varying the different ingredients, a commercial product of any desired consistency may be evolved. The above preparation is removed by water.

Formula No. 3

Clay	100 lb.
Water (Cold)	20 gal.
Tincture of Benzoin	3 pt.
Perfume	3 oz.

Add the water to the clay and grind till smooth. Evaporate until 150 lb. remain. Run through mill to smooth clumped particles; cool and mix in the benzoin and perfume. Fill in collapsible pure tin tubes.

Formula No. 4

Sodium Benzoate	0.5 g.
White Bolus	150.0 g.
Zinc Oxide	30.0 g.

This powder is mixed with water before use to give a paste.

Formula No. 5

White Bolus	995 g.
Sodium Benzoate	5 g.
Cold Cream	125 g.
Water	to desired consistency
Perfume	to suit

Formula No. 6

Put on face for 20 minutes a mixture of

Oat Flour	20 g.
Arnica Flowers	2 g.
Chamomile Flowers	2 g.
Hamamelis Leaves	2 g.
Rosemary Leaves	2 g.
Camphor Water	30 cc.

Treat afterwards with astringent lotion of

Tannic Acid	0.25 g.
Rose Water	25 g.
Hamamelis Water	50 g.
Orange Flower Water	25 g.

Formula No. 7

Tragacanth	25 g.
Alcohol	40 g.
Calamine	80 g.
Zinc Oxide	30 g.
Zinc Stearate	50 g.
Glycerin	60 g.
Lime Water	1000 cc.

Mix the tragacanth in the alcohol. Then add to the lime water. Rub up zinc stearate, zinc oxide and calamine with glycerin. Add tragacanth, alcohol, lime water mixture to calamine, zinc oxide, zinc stearate and glycerin mixture.

Formula No. 8

Colloidal Clay	50 oz.
Citric Acid	5 oz.
Hydrogen Peroxide	5 oz.
Magnesium Sulphate	5 oz.
Glycerin	10 oz.
Water	25 oz.

Formula No. 9

Fuller's Earth	50.0 g.
Calamine	15.0 g.
Tragacanth (Powder)	0.2 g.
Magnesium Sulphate	5.0 g.
Extract of Witchhazel	15.0 g.
Water	5.0 g.
Glycerin	15.0 g.
Perfume	to suit

The earth tragacanth and calamine should be mixed, sieved and rubbed down with the glycerin and witchhazel. Add to these the magnesium sulphate dissolved in the water.

Formula No. 10

Gelatin, White	40 g.
Zinc Oxide	30 g.
Glycerin	50 g.
Water, Distilled	40 g.
Rose Oil	to suit
Boric Acid	15 g.

---

or:

Bean Meal	20 g.
Rice Meal	20 g.
Chicken Egg White	10 g.
Tincture of Benzoin	5 g.
Honey	10 g.
Rose Water	20 g.

Formula No. 11

Tragacanth	25 g.
Alcohol	40 g.
"Carbitol"	40 g.
Calamine	80 g.
Zinc Oxide	30 g.

Zinc Stearate	50 g.
Glycerin	20 g.
Lime Water	1000 cc.

Dissolve the tragacanth in the alcohol and carbitol. Then add to the lime water. Rub up zinc stearate, zinc oxide and calamine with glycerin. Add tragacanth, alcohol, lime water mixture to calamine, zinc oxide, zinc stearate and glycerin mixture.

Oxygen Liberating Face Masks

Formula No. 1

Talcum	300 g.
Infusorial Earth	250 g.
White Bolus	150 g.
Sea Sand	200 g.
Sodium Perborate	100 g.

Formula No. 2

Talcum	500 g.
Infusorial Earth	250 g.
White Bolus	150 g.
Sodium Perborate	100 g.

All components should be dry; the earth-ingredients can be rendered dry and sterile by heating.

To make a paste and to wash the mask off, use a toilet vinegar.

Freckle Preventive Treatment

Sulphur lotions should not be used as these tend to increase the pigmentation, neither should tar preparations, ichthyol, or resorcin be ingredients of the lotions. Before the hot weather comes the following ointment should be used:

Formula No. 1

Quinine Bisulphate	1.5 g.
Aesculin	1.0 g.
Simple Ointment	27.5 g.

The following ointment, to be applied twice a day, left on for thirty minutes, and then wiped off with a cleansing tissue, is recommended by Continental dermatologists:

Formula No. 2

Zinc Peroxide	20 g.
White Soft Paraffin Wax	70 g.
Anhydrous Lanolin	10 g.

The affected parts are then powdered with a powder composed of magnesium peroxide 30 parts, talc 50 parts, zinc oxide 20 parts.

Formula No. 3

Alcohol	4 oz.
Stronger Rose Water	2 oz.
Tincture of Benzoin	15 dr.

Apply every night after scrubbing.

Freckle "Removers"

Formula No. 1

Two grams of zinc phenol sulphate, 30 grams of distilled water, 2 grams of ichthyol, 30 grams each of anhydrous lanolin and petroleum jelly and 2 grams of lemon oil or other suitable perfume, will give good results.

Formula No. 2

Preparations with a bleaching action are made containing 1500 grams of wool grease, 530 grams of almond oil, 110 grams of beeswax, 150 grams of borax, 150 grams of hydrogen peroxide (100% by volume) and 10 grams of yellow petrolatum.

Formula No. 3

Chloral Hydrate	7.8 g.
Phenol	3.9 g.
Tincture of Iodine	60 drops
Glycerin	1 fl. oz.

Apply nightly with a brush. This solution is corrosive and must be used with discretion.

Skin-Peeling Lotion

Mercuric Chloride	1 oz.
Salicylic Acid	5 oz.
Chloral Hydrate	5 oz.
Glycerin	25 oz.
Acetone	10 oz.
Alcohol	200 oz.
Water	825 oz.

Perfume to suit.

Procedure: Take part of the petrolatum, add the salicylic, the phenol and the camphor and mill thoroughly. Melt the lanolin, the rest of the petrolatum and the beeswax, stir in the milled base and add the oil of eucalyptus.

Honey Freckle Cream

Honey	8 oz.
Glycerin	2 oz.
Alcohol	2 oz.
Citric Acid	6 dr.
Ambergris Tincture	15 drops

To be applied morning and night.

Freckle Lotion

Dissolve:

Potassium Carbonate	60 g.
Potassium Chlorate	20 g.
Borax	15 g.
Sugar	60 g.

In:

Rose Water	330 g.
Orange Flower Water	355 cc.
Glycerin	150 cc.

Chamomile Skin Paste

Chamomile Powder	150 g.
Zinc Oxide	100 g.
Talc	247 g.
White Petrolatum	450 g.
Mineral Oil	50 g.
Perfume	3 g.

Mix the powders and sift them into the melted petrolatum and oil. Mix until cold. Only small quantities of this material can be made homogeneous without the help of an ointment mill.

Almond Meal

Borax	2 lb.
Bicarbonate of Soda	2 lb.
Powdered Castile Soap	2 lb.
Fine Yellow Corn Meal	33 lb.
Wheat Flour	61 lb.
Perfume	5 oz.

Mix all the dry ingredients together and spray the perfume oils into the mixture with an atomizer.

Make-up Gum

(For attaching hair to skin)

½ oz. each of resin, tolu balsam, benzoin, sandarac mixed with 3 ozs. of alcohol.

SKIN OILS

Lecithin Skin Oil

Formula No. 1

Lecithin from Eggs	10–30 g.
Paraffin Oil	170–190 cc.
Olive Oil, Preserved	800 cc.
Perfume, to suit	5 g.

Formula No. 2

Lecithin from Brain Substance	20 g.
Paraffin Oil	180 cc.
Olive or Peanut Oil, Preserved	800 cc.

Cholesterin Oil

Fatty Oil, Pure, or in Mixture with Paraffin Oil	1000 cc.
Cholesterin, C.P.	5–10 g.

Cholesterin-Lecithin Oil

Same as Cholesterin Oil, but besides add Lecithin (Eggs, Brain-Substance) 20–30 g.

Skin Oil with Isocholesterin

Paraffin Oil plus Preserved Fatty Oil	97 cc.
Isocholesterin, Technically Pure	3 g.
or Same, Chemically Pure	2 g.

Skin Oil with Lanolin

Lanolin, Bleached	5 g.
Paraffin Oil or Fatty Oils	95 cc.

Skin Oil with Wool Wax

Wool Wax, Bleached, Purified	5 g.
Fatty Oil	35 cc.
Paraffin Oil	60 cc.

Skin Oil with Cetyl Alcohol

Cetyl Alcohol, Pure	3–5 g.
Paraffin Oil plus Fatty Oil, Preserved (1:1)	97–95 cc.

Skin Oil with Triethanolamine Oleate

Triethanolamine Oleate, Pure	2 g.
Fatty Oil	98 cc.

Non-Irritating Skin Oil

Diglycol Laurate Neutral	4 g.
Olive Oil	96 cc.
Perfume	to suit

External Antiseptic Oil

Phenol	5 g.
Olive Oil	to make 100 cc.

Antiseptic Baby Oil

White Mineral Oil (65–75)	45. oz.
Refined Peanut Oil	54.7 oz.
Oxyquinoline Benzoate	.2 oz.
Maleic Anhydride	.1 oz.

The maleic anhydride and the oxyquinoline benzoate are dissolved in the peanut oil and the mineral oil is added.

The preparation is then filtered. While there is still some discussion as to the effectiveness of the test for oil soluble antiseptics, those who have worked with oxyquinoline benzoate have testified to its effectiveness. The maleic anhydride is an antioxidant designed to prevent rancidity.

Astringent Skin Oil

Aluminum Stearate	3 g.
Fatty Oil	97 cc.

Warm together with good mixing until dissolved.

Skin Oil "Huile Ambrosiaque"

Ambergris, Best Quality	10 g.
Olive Oil	990 cc.
Perfume	to suit

Grind the amber with glass-powder and introduce into the warmed oil. Shake well. Filter after 3–4 weeks.

Skin Oil with Wool Fat Alcohols

Parachol (Absorption Base)	5–10 g.
Paraffin Oil	95–90 cc.

Skin Cleansing Oil

Parachol (Absorption Base)	2 g.
Triethanolamine Oleate	0.5 g.
Fatty Oil, Preserved	97.5 cc.

Add a little Triethanolamine.

Skin Nourishing Oil

Egg Oil	5 g.
Parachol (Absorption Base)	5 g.
Lecithin	1 g.
Sperm (Whale) Oil, Genuine, Deodorized	20 cc.
Fatty Oil, Preserved	69 cc.

Skin "Stimulating" Oils

Formula No. 1

Parachol (Absorption Base)	5 g.
Oxycholesterin, Artificial	3 g.
Fatty Oil (Olive, Sesame, Peanut), Preserved	92 cc.

Formula No. 2

Parachol (Absorption Base)	5 g.
Cetyl Alcohol, Pure	3 g.
Fatty Oil, Preserved	91 cc.

Witch Hazel Skin Oil

Witch Hazel Leaves, Powder	100 g.
Fatty Oil, Preserved	900 cc.

Pour hot oil over leaves, let stand for 8 days. Filter.

Massage Oil

Paraffin Oil	75 cc.
Parachol (Absorption Base)	5 g.
Olive Oil, Preserved	20 cc.

Muscle Oil

Formula No. 1

Castor Oil, Deodorized	66.6 cc.
Alcohol (92–95%)	33.3 cc.
Cholesterin, Pure	0.1 g.

Formula No. 2

Castor Oil Odorless	10 gal.
Alcohol	5 gal.
Perfume Oil	5 oz.

Sport Oil (for Swimmers)

Formula No. 1

Octadecyl Alcohol (Pure)	5 g.
Fatty Oil, Preserved	55 cc.
Paraffin Oil	40 cc.

Formula No. 2

Glycosterin	4 g.
Peanut Oil	50 cc.
Mineral Oil	35 cc.
Deramin	2 cc.
Perfume	to suit

Insect Repellent Creams

Formula No. 1

Beeswax	3–4 g.
Citronella Oil	15 g.
Spirits of Camphor	8 g.
Cedar Wood Oil	8 g.
White Petrolatum	60 g.

Melt petrolatum and beeswax, then add other constituents and stir until smooth.

Formula No. 2

A

Castor Oil	15.00 g.
Pennyroyal Oil	3.75 g.
Pine Tar Oil	3.75 g.
Camphor Oil	7.50 g.
Citronella Oil	3.75 g.

B

Beeswax	6.625 g.
Lanolin (Anhydrous) / Petrolatum	59.625 g.

Melt (B) and then add above oils (A).

Insecticide Cream

U. S. Patent 2,041,264

Diethyl Phthalate	50 g.
Sodium Oleate	0.5 g.
Sodium Stearate	4 g.
Water	45.5 g.

Insect Repellents for Campers

Oils of citronella, pennyroyal, cloves, lavender, eucalyptus, sassafras, and cedar are successful in keeping insects away. However, they (along with spirits of camphor) must be combined with a base to keep them from evaporating too quickly.

Citronella and lavender are mild, bland oils. Most of the others are somewhat irritating and should be kept away from the eyes.

Light Oil Combination

Formula No. 1

Castor oil, 2 ounces; pennyroyal, 1 dram; citronella, 1 dram; pure pine tar, 2 drams; sassafras oil, 1 dram; camphor, 2 drams. This preparation has many ingredients that repel insects.

Formula No. 2

Another having a thick dope with a vaseline base includes pure pine tar, ½ ounce; pennyroyal oil, ½ ounce; carbolated vaseline, 1½ ounces. Mix cold in a mortar.

Either castor oil, olive oil, or mineral oil can be used in preparing a heavy liquid mosquito dope. Castor oil is the best of the three to use for a heavy base, because insects do not like it, even without other ingredients.

Genuine oil of lavender will keep insects away. It is, of course, a de luxe oil to use in a mosquito dope. For women who want something fragrant, soothing, and healing to the skin, the combination of borated lanolin and oil of lavender is effective. When put up in tubes to keep out moisture an excellent preparation instantly is available.

Cedar oil is used in mosquito dopes.

Formula No. 3

Castor oil, 2 ounces, oil of cedar, 1 dram; pennyroyal, 2 drams; pine tar, 2 drams, and oil of sassafras, 1 dram is another good formula.

Insect Bite Lotion

Epsom Salt	20 g.
Camphor	3 g.
Menthol	1 g.
Glycerin	1 g.
Alcohol	25 g.
Water	50 cc.

Dissolve the camphor and menthol in the alcohol. Add the glycerin. Dissolve the salt in the water. Then add the alcohol solution gradually to the water solution. Mix well.

Pyrethrum Ointment

Pyrethrum Extract	27 g.
Absorption Base (Parachol)	73 g.

Mix until smooth. Useful in treating scabies and other insect infestations.

Mosquito Preparations

The following application is suggested as a means of preventing insect bites:

Cedar Oil	2 dr.
Citronella Oil	4 dr.
Spirits of Camphor	add 1 oz.

This should be smeared on the skin of the exposed parts as often as is necessary. Cod-liver oil used in the same way has been highly recommended, and in combination with quinine it makes an effective "sunburn and midge cream," a formula being as follows:

Quinine Acid Hydrochloride	5 g.
Cod-Liver Oil	20 g.
Anhydrous Wool Fat	75 g.
Lavender Oil (or Geranium)	to suit

The irritation of a mosquito or fly bite may be allayed by gently rubbing the puncture with a moist cake of soap, or by applying a 1 per cent alcoholic solution of methol, or 1–20 aqueous carbolic lotion. Hydrogen peroxide or weak ammonia solution dabbed on is also useful. If the bite shows signs of sepsis, constantly renewed hot boric fomentations should be applied, or if a limb is implicated, hot saline arm or leg baths.

Mosquito Protection Cream

(Non-Greasy)

Formula No. 1

Soak

a.	Agar-Agar	2 g.
	Water, Cold	400 g.

Then warm slowly over gentle heat:

b.	Melt Stearin	60 g.
c.	Alcohol	10 g.
d.	Potassium Carbonate	6 g.
	Water	440 g.
	Glycerin	68 g.

Make up emulsion by warming and stirring.

Add *a* to the emulsion of *b-c* in *d*, both should be 80° C.; stir continously. When cold, add 12 g. of the following mixture:

Cedar Oil	7.5 g.
Citronella Oil	15 g.
Camphor	2 g.
Eucalyptus Oil	4.5 g.
Alcohol	7 g.

Formula No. 2

Treatment as above:

Agar-Agar	2.2 g.
Stearin	60 g.
Potassium Carbonate	4 g.
Sal Soda	2 g.
Alcohol	12 g.
Beeswax, White	8 g.
Lanolin (Anhydrous)	8 g.
Glycerin	60 g.
Water	830 g.
Betanaphthol	1 g.

Essential Oils as in Formula No. 1

Treatment as in No. 1, saponify the fats (wax, lanolin, stearin) together.

Formula No. 3

a.	Agar-Agar	2.5 g.
	Glycerin	100 g.
	Water	750 g.
b.	Glyceryl Monostearate	120 g.
	Spermaceti	100 g.

Melt.

Pour *a* hot into *b*, make emulsion, stir. Add boiling water up to 980 g. Add, when cold:

Moldex or Other Good Preservative	2 g.
Essential Oils	12 g.

(See Formula No. 1)

Formula No. 4

Glyceryl Monostearate	11.0 g.
Cedar Leaf Oil	4.0 g.
Pennyroyal Oil	4.0 g.
Linalyl Acetate	3.0 g.
Gasoline	5.0 g.
Menthol	0.5 g.
Phenol	2.0 g.
Glycerin	5.0 g.
Water	65.5 g.

Put the glyceryl monostearate into the water, add the glycerin and bring the mixture to the boiling point with constant stirring. Keep stirring and when the temperature drops to about 45° C. add the rest of the ingredients which have been mixed together.

Formula No. 5

a.	Wheat Starch	5 g.
	Water	10 g.
b.	Glycerin	45 g.
c.	Lanolin	30 g.
d.	Clove Oil	5–10 g.

Grind *a* until homogeneous, add *b*, and warm gently until a homogeneous jelly is formed. Cool, and grind now with *c* and *d* in a mortar very thoroughly until distribution is satisfactory. Fill at once into collapsible tubes.

Formula No. 6

a.	White Wax	50 g.
	Spermaceti	50 g.
b.	Borax	4 g.
	Ammonia (0.96)	40 g.
c.	Water	510 cc.
	Wheat Starch	1 g.
	Gelatin	4 g.
	Sodium Benzoate	0.5 g.

Make up cream as usual pouring *b* into *a*, then add the solution *c* which is to be made up before (soak cold, then warm to clear solution, if necessary, pour through a fine sieve), stir thoroughly, stop heating, stir until cooled, and add

Eucalyptus Oil 50 cc.

Formula No. 7

Eucalyptus Oil	0.5 cc.
Caryophyllum Oil	0.5 cc.
Lavender Oil	0.5 cc.
Quinine Sulphate	1 g.
Glycerin Salve to make	100 g.

Formula No. 8

Tragacanth	3 g.
Alcohol	5 g.
Soap Solution	2.5–25 g.
Glycerin	45 g.

To this cream add:

Menthol	1 g.
Sodium Benzoate	1 g.
Citronella Oil	1 cc.
Caryophyllum Oil	0.5 cc.
Alcohol	10 cc.
Tincture of Green Soap	10 cc.

Mosquito Bite Ointment

Boric Acid Ointment U.S.P.	95 g.
Phenol	5 g.

Triturate phenol into ointment cold.

Mosquito & Insect Repelling Ointment

Pyrethrum Extract in Deodorized Kerosene	25 oz.
Parachol (Absorption Base)	75 oz.
Perfume	to suit

Mix until smooth. If a lower priced and lighter color product is wanted work in a little water at a time, not adding additional water until previous portion has been absorbed. This preparation will actually keep insects off the skin.

Mosquito Powder

Formula No. 1

Eucalyptus Oil	1 oz.
Powdered Talcum	2 oz.
Powdered Starch	14 oz.

This powder is to be rubbed into the exposed parts of the body to prevent the attack of the insect.

Formula No. 2

Pennyroyal Oil	4 oz.
Powdered Naphthaline	4 dr.
Starch	16 oz.

Mix well and sift. This is to be used like the preceding.

Mosquito Repellents

Formula No. 1

Pennyroyal Oil	5 cc.
Sandalwood Oil	5 cc.
Elore Oil	3 cc.
Peppermint Oil	5 cc.
Eucalyptus Oil	2 cc.
Linoloc	2 cc.
Citranel Oil	3 cc.
Camphor Oil	1 cc.

The above blend is stirred in the following emulsion

Parachol or other Absorption Base	15 g.
Petrolatum (White)	5 g.
Triethanolamine	5 cc.
Water	100 cc.

Each application is effective for about 20 minutes.

Formula No. 2

Pyrethrum Flowers	10 g.
Isopropyl Alcohol, or Alcohol with Thymol	100 g.
Cloves Oil	2 g.

Formula No. 3

Eucalyptus Oil	45 g.
Thuia Oil	20 g.
Laurel Oil	5 g.
Phenol	3 g.
Camphor	20 g.
Alcohol	100 g.
Turpentine Oil	50 g.
Quassia, Tincture	40 g.
Pyrethrum Extract	50 g.
Xylol	to make 1000 cc.

Formula No. 4

Pyrethrum Extract	0.5 g.
Amyl Salicylate	3.5 g.
Petroleum (b.-p. 182–292°; sp. gr. 0.801)	96 g.

Formula No. 5

Pyrethrum Powder	1 g.
Derris-Root Powder	1 g.
Tobacco Powder	0.5 g.
Alcohol, Diluted	25 g.

Percolate thoroughly and filter; add: oil of eucalyptus or menthol to suit.

Formula No. 6

White Mineral Oil	95 oz.
Hexyl Salicylate	5 oz.

The above product is not malodorous or very volatile.

CHAPTER IV

DEPILATORIES AND DEODORANTS

Depilatories

DEPILATORIES are used for the removal of hair from the face and limbs. Any preparation which will dissolve hair will also dissolve or irritate the skin. For this reason depilatories must be used with caution and completely removed as soon as possible after use.

Most depilatories contain sulphides of barium, strontium, calcium or sodium. All of these are caustic and evil smelling. The latter property may be tempered with glycerine. The odor is covered with certain odorous materials mentioned later. The wax type of depilatory doesn't act on the hair but after melting and cooling it grips the hair, which is pulled out by tearing off the wax mass.

Depilatory

Formula No. 1

Strontium Sulfide	50 g.
Zinc Oxide	50 g.
Rice Flour	60 g.
Perfume	to suit

Formula No. 2

Calcium Sulphide	4 lb.
Wheat Starch	12 lb.
Powdered Acacia	1 lb.

Formula No. 3

German Patent 601,078

Barium Sulphide	100 oz.
Starch	60 oz.
Magnesium Silicate	30 oz.
Pyrogallol	10 oz.

Make into a paste with water before using.

Odorless Depilatory

Hydrogen Peroxide (40 vol.)	3.5–5 g.
Polychol (or Polyglycol)	5 g.
Lanolin Anhydrous	20 g.

Rub together till uniform.

Depilatory Powder

30 parts strontium sulphide, 20 parts calcium sulphide, 30 parts starch, 16 parts talc, 3 parts aluminum acetate and one part menthol, all by weight.

Adhesive Depilatory

U. S. Patent 2,013,928

Rosin	90 g.
Cottonseed Oil	10 g.

Warm together and stir until uniform. This is applied warm and allowed to "set." When cold it is pulled off taking the hairs with it.

Depilatory Cream

Formula No. 1

One part gum tragacanth, 10 parts water, 10 parts glycerin and six parts starch, together hot, and intimately mixed with 35 parts strontium sulphide, 3 parts sodium sulphide, 30 parts zinc oxide, 10 parts lanolin, 15 parts water and 0.2 part menthol.

Formula No. 2

Titanium Dioxide	15 g.
Barium Sulphide	37 g.

Starch	50 g.
Phenol	1 g.
Lanolin	26 g.
Stearic Acid	5 g.
Triethanolamine	1.6 g.
Water	137.4 g.

Add the triethanolamine and the stearic acid to half the water. Heat the mixture until the stearic acid melts and then stir until a creamy soap forms. Allow the mixture to become lukewarm and then stir in starch and continue to stir until all lumps have disappeared. Dissolve the barium sulphide in the rest of the water and bring to a boil. Then stir in the soap-starch solution and continue stirring until the mixture thickens. Add the melted lanolin and stir. Then slowly sift in the titanium dioxide and mix until smooth. Finally add the phenol and perfume.

Liquid Depilatory

Sodium Sulphide	10 g.
Witch Hazel	100 g.

This solution is put on the desired spot with cotton, wiped off 2–3 minutes later with dry cotton.

The spot is to be washed with water thoroughly, or rather with a weak citric acid solution to destroy the irritating alkali.

Depilatory Paste

Strontium Sulphide	3 oz.
Zinc Stearate	¾ oz.
Starch	1¾ oz.
Glycerin	1¾ oz.
Water	to make a paste
Perfume	0.2 oz.

Depilatory Perfumes

The essential oils, which have been found suitable for perfuming depilatories include oil of wintergreen, vetivert oil, patchouly oil, oil of thyme, lavender oil; also the aromatics, amyl salicylate, terpineol, benzyl acetate, menthol. About 2% is usually added. Lavender oil, particularly terpeneless, is much liked for this purpose, as it alleviates skin irritation.

Deodorants

Deodorants are used to prevent or minimize objectionable body odors produced by perspiration. These odors differ with the individual and the state of health.

Commercial deodorants are of two kinds. One kind tends to deodorize the perspiration, while the other stops its flow as well as deodorizing it. Most of them contain antiseptics and astringents.

Deodorant Powders

Formula No. 1

Aluminum Stearate	12 oz.
Aluminum Sulfate (powdered)	12 oz.
Talc	25 oz.

Formula No. 2

Talc	90 oz.
Zinc Peroxide	10 oz.

Formula No. 3

Zinc Oleate	8 lb.
Sodium Perborate	3 lb.
Boric Acid, Powdered	5 lb.
Sodium Bicarbonate	2 lb.
Magnesium Carbonate	4 lb.
Italian Talc	18 lb.

Mix powders thoroughly and perfume to suit.

Formula No. 4

Methyl Salicylate	1.5 g.
Eucalyptus Oil	2.0 g.
Thymol	12.0 g.
Menthol	0.5 g.
Boric Acid	39.0 g.
Acetanilid	43.0 g.
Starch	2.0 g.

Formula No. 5

Zinc Peroxide	0.5 g.
Betanaphthol Benzoate	0.1 g.
Talcum	99.4 g.

Formula No. 6

Aluminum chloride 7 g., aluminum sulfate 8 g., boric acid 10 g., water 75 g.

Liquid Body Deodorant

A.

Aluminum Aceto-Tartrate	1 lb.
Rose Perfume (water soluble)	1 oz.
Water	5 gal.

B.

Aluminum Chloride (Crystalline)	8 lb.
Hydrochloric Acid	4 oz.
Phenyl Ethyl Alcohol	4 oz.
Water	5 gal.
Color	to suit

Perspiration Deodorants

A. Liquid Type

Salicylic Acid	2 g.
Aluminum Chloride	4 g.
Cologne Spirit	30 mil.
Rose Water	54 mil.
Glycerin	10 mil.
Rose Colour	a trace

Dissolve the salicylic acid in the Cologne spirit, and the aluminum chloride in the rose water. Mix and add the glycerin. A more delicate perfume may be used.

B. Paste Type

Salicylic Acid	10 g.
Levigated Zinc Oxide	60 g.
Greaseless Cold Cream	480 g.
Perfume	to suit

Deodorant Cream

Formula No. 1

Benzoic Acid	4 g.
Zinc Oxide	12 g.
Parachol (Absorption Base)	4 g.
Petrolatum, White	80 g.
Perfume	to suit

Warm together and stir until cold. This gives a soothing non-irritating cream of a most excellent appearance.

Formula No. 2

Benzoic Acid	4 g.
Zinc Oxide	12 g.
Lanolin	4 g.
Petrolatum (Snow White)	80 g.
Perfume	to suit

Formula No. 3

British Patent 425,059

Coconut Oil	63 g.
Lemon Oil	5.2 g.
Boric Acid, Powdered	21 g.
Starch, Powdered	10.5 g.
Lanolin	0.2 g.
Perfume	0.1 g.

Formula No. 4

Formaldehyde	1 oz.
Vanishing Cream	99 oz.

Formula No. 5

Cold Cream	84 g.
Zinc Oxide	15 g.
Formaldehyde	1 g.
Perfume	to suit

Anti-Perspiration Cream

1. Lanolin Hydrous	1.0 g.
2. Benzoinated Lard	90.0 g.
3. Zinc Oxide	6.5 g.
4. Salicylic Acid	1.2 g.
5. Benzoic Acid	0.9 g.
6. Perfume Oil	0.4 g.

Dissolve (4) and (5) in small amount of alcohol; mix into (1) and then work into (2). Grind in (3) until smooth and then work in (6).

Anti-Perspiration Liquid

Oxyquinoline Sulfate	1 g.
Rose Water	500 g.

Anti-Perspiration Powder

Oxyquinoline Sulfate	1 g.
Talc	10 g.

Perspiraton Deodorizing Cream

Beeswax	8 oz.
Liquid Petrolatum	24 oz.
Borax	100 gr.
Benzoic Acid	20 gr.
Salicylic Acid	400 gr.
Hot Water	16 oz.

Melt the wax and oil and heat to about 160 degrees F. Dissolve the other materials in the water, heat to the same temperatures as the wax solution, and pour it into the latter, beating briskly until the cream is formed. Here a comparatively high temperature of the solutions, plus a small amount of stirring, results in a glossy cream.

Perspiration Deodorant

Sodium Perborate	10 g.
Sodium Bicarbonate	2 g.
Glycerin	1 g.
Rose Water	98 cc.

Tint pink with eosin.

Vanishing Type Deodorant Cream

1. Stearic Acid	21	lb.
2. Trihydroxyethylamine Stearate	11	lb.
3. "Carbitol"	10.5	lb.
4. Zinc Sulphocarbolate	.75	lb.
5. Zinc Stearate	10.00	lb.
6. Benzoic Acid	2.00	lb.
Water (Distilled)	8.00	gal.
Perfume Oil	.75	lb.

This formula will make 100 lb. of finished cream. Melt 1 and 2 together, heat to 95° C. add 3, heat water to boiling, add to other ingredients above, mix in heated jacketed kettle, then sift in 4, 5 and 6. Mix thoroughly while hot until uniform consistency is obtained. Transfer to Day Mixer and continue mixing for 4 or 5 hours, add perfume when lukewarm.

Deodorant Pencil

(White product)

Formula No. 1

Zinc Phenolsulfonate	5 g.
Zinc Oleate	10 g.
Aluminum Palmitate	7.50 g.
Parachol	20.00 g.
Glyco Wax A	40.00 g.
Titanium Dioxide	

Formula No. 2

Zinc Phenolsulfonate	10 g.
Zinc Oleate	10 g.
Aluminum Palmitate	7.5 g.
Parachol	30 g.
Glyco Wax A	30 g.
Titanium Dioxide	15 g.

Rub the first three ingredients to a fine powder and add to liquified wax the Parachol mixture. Stir until just before solidification and pour into molds.

Magoffin's Perspirine

Powdered Talc	5 lb.
Corn Starch	5 lb.
Boric Acid	10 oz.
Rose Oil	1 dr.

Mix the first three ingredients. Triturate the oil with two ounces of the mixture and then mix all together. Run through a No. 60 sieve at least five times.

CHAPTER V

SUNBURN PREPARATIONS

Sunburn Products

THE most commonly used preparation depends on its ability to protect the skin from burning. The next type is an alleviator of pain after the skin has been burned. Finally there is the preparation which gives the skin a tanned appearance.

The first type incorporates materials which prevent the ultra-violet rays from the sun from reaching the skin. The second type has a cooling and soothing as well as an antiseptic action. It lessens pain and promotes healing. The last type depends on the use of pigments or dyes which color the skin.

Sun-Burn Preventive Preparations

Formula No. 1 (Cream)

Quinine Sulphate	3 g.
White Ceresin Wax	5.5 g.
White Petrolatum	20.5 g.
Mineral Oil	19.5 g.
Lanolin, Anhydrous	15.0 g.
Water	35.5 g.
Cassia Oil	1.0 g.

Heat the water to 70° C. and dissolve the quinine sulphate in it. Melt the ceresin, petrolatum, and lanolin together, stir in the mineral oil, bring the mixture to 65° C. and stir in the quinine solution. Continue stirring until the temperature drops to 45° C. and then add the oil of cassia.

Formula No. 2 (Cream)

Quinine Bisulphate	2.5 g.
Cholesterin Absorption Base	25.5 g.
Mineral Oil	12.5 g.
Alcohol	10.0 g.
Water	49.5 g.
Perfume	.5 g.

Dissolve the quinine bisulphate in the alcohol. Melt the absorption base and the mineral oil together. Heat the water to the same temperature and stir it into the melted fat. Continue stirring until the temperature drops to about 45° C. and add the quinine solution and the perfume.

Formula No. 3 (Cream)

Sodium Naphthol 6:8 disulphonate	3.0 g.
Borax	3.0 g.
Beeswax, White	20.0 g.
Mineral Oil	20.0 g.
Water	37.5 g.
Petrolatum	16.0 g.
Perfume	.5 g.

Heat the water and dissolve the borax in it. Add the sodium naphthol 6:8 disulphonate and stir until dissolved. Melt the beeswax, petrolatum, and mineral oil together. Add the liquids to the fats with constant stirring and when the temperature drops to about 45° C. add the perfume.

Formula No. 4 (Lotion)

Quinine Bisulphate	3.00 g.
Glycerin	5.50 g.
Gum Tragacanth Powder	2.50 g.
Alcohol	15.50 g.
Citric Acid	.75 g.
Water	72.25 g.
Perfume	.50 g.

Mix the gum tragacanth powder with one-half of the alcohol and add it to one-half of the water. Dissolve the quinine bisulphate in the remainder of the alcohol and add the perfume. Dissolve the citric acid in the remainder of the water. Add the glycerin to the citric acid solution then add the quinine solution and finally the mucilage. Mix well.

Formula No. 5 (Lotion)

Aesculin	3.5 g.
Glycerin	3.5 g.
Borax	4.0 g.
Alcohol	15.0 g.
Water	73.5 g.
Perfume	.5 g.

Heat the water, dissolve the borax in it and add the aesculin. Stir until dissolved. Mix the perfume with the alcohol, add the glycerin and stir this into the aesculin solution. Filter. If it is desired to color the solution add a sufficient quantity of spirits soluble brown.

Formula No. 6 (Oil)

Quinine Oleate	4.5 g.
Olive Oil	30.0 g.
Peanut Oil	64.5 g.
Cassia Oil	.5 g.
Perfume Oil	.5 g.

Dissolve the quinine oleate in the peanut oil; add the other oils and perfume. If it is desired a sufficient quantity of pigment brown may be added to this preparation.

Formula No. 7 (Powder)

Quinine Sulphate	3 g.
Zinc Stearate	10 g.
Titanium Dioxide	7 g.
Talc	58 g.
Colloidal Clay	13 g.
Precipitated Chalk	5 g.
Suntan Color Base	4 g.

Dissolve the quinine sulphate in a small quantity of alcohol and rub up this solution with the colloidal clay. Allow the alcohol to evaporate; add the other ingredients and proceed as in the manufacture of ordinary face powder. This powder differs from the suntan formulas given in the chapter on face powders in that it is much more opaque and possesses a substance which will prevent sunburn.

Formula No. 8

Zinc Oxide	26 g.
Lanolin	46 g.
Water	28 cc.

Rub together the zinc oxide and lanolin and then work in the water gradually.

Formula No. 9

Lanolin	2 lb.
White Petrolatum	8 lb.
Zinc Oxide	4 lb.
Glycerin	4 lb.

Mix the above thoroughly.

Formula No. 10

Beeswax	60 g.
Cocoa Butter	30 g.
Parachol (Absorption Base)	40 g.
Peanut Oil, Refined	300 g.
Glyceryl Tristearate	20 g.
Moldex	1 g.
Perfume and Color	to suit

Melt together everything but perfume and color. Stir until dissolved. Cool to 100° F. and stir in perfume and color. This preparation can be made firmer by reducing the amount of peanut oil. It penetrates the skin better than most similar preparations.

Formula No. 11

Petrolatum	87.5 g.
Lanolin	6.0 g.
Pigment Brown	6.0 g.
Perfume	.5 g.

Grind the color with a small quantity of petrolatum. Melt the petrolatum together with the lanolin, strain in the color base, mix, strain and perfume.

Formula No. 12

Ceresin Wax	15.0 g.
Beeswax	8.0 g.
Lanolin	10.0 g.
Petrolatum	10.0 g.
Mineral Oil	56.5 g.
Perfume	.5 g.
Color	Sufficient

Melt the waxes; add the lanolin and petrolatum. Mix, strain and perfume. Then add a sufficient quantity of brown.

Formula No. 13

Glyceryl Monostearate	14 g.
Lanolin	6 g.
Olive Oil	10 g.
Linseed Oil, Fatty Acids	4 g.

Cetyl Alcohol	6 g.
Water	136 g.

Heat the above to boiling while mixing mechanically. When homogenous shut off heat and continue mixing until thickening begins. Then run in, slowly

Picric Acid (20% solution)	20 g.

and then

Benzocaine	4 g.

Continue mixing until the cream "sets."

Sunburn Liniment

Water White Steam-distilled Pine Oil	75 cc.
Medicinal Olive Oil	25 cc.

The finished product will be almost water white and is an effective treatment for sunburn. The product is applied by rubbing directly on the sunburned surface of the skin.

Sun Burn or After-Shave Lotion

1. Emulsone B	50 g.
2. Boric Acid	50 g.
3. Alcohol	100 g.
4. Phenol	1 dr.
5. Menthol	1 dr.
6. Oil of Rose	1 dr.
7. Glycol	400 g.
8. Water	7 pt.
9. Titanium Dioxide	2 oz.

Rub No. 1 and No. 2 together with No. 3, add and mix in thoroughly Nos. 4, 5, 6 and 7. Mix Nos. 8 and 9 and stir into previous mixture rapidly for 4 minutes only. Strain through cheesecloth and bottle. This gives a thick soothing cream which is very popular.

Sun Burn—Protectors

Formula No. 1

Liquid

a. Triethanolamine	40 g.
Trihydroxyethylamine Stearate	40 g.

Melt on water bath, make emulsion in

Water (60° C.)	620–630 g.
b. Paraffin Oil	100 g.
Peanut Oil	150 g.
Oleic Acid	30 g.

Warm up on water bath to 40° C.

Preservative	1 g.

Pour *b* into *a,* perfume with

c. Perfume Oil	to suit

Stir until cold.

Formula No. 2

Cream

White Wax	60 g.
Cocoa Butter	30 g.
Lanolin, Anhydrous	40 g.
Peanut Oil	300 g.
Spermaceti	20 g.
"Moldex" or Other Preservative	1 g.
Perfume	5–10 g.

Formula No. 3

a. Gum Tragacanth (Powder)	15 g.
Glycerin	50 g.

Grind in mortar.

b. Quinine Acid Sulphate	100 g.
Citric Acid	100 g.
Water	1200 g.
Alcohol with Perfume	400 g.
c. Glycerin	150 g.

Grind *a,* then add the *b* solution, and finally add *c.*

Formula No. 4

a. Quinine Hydrochloride	4 g.
Alcohol	12 g.
b. Citric Acid	0.8 g.
Water	10 g.
c. Tragacanth Powder	3.5 g.
Glycerin	10 g.
Water	42.5 g.

Mix solutions *a* and *b* and then work into solution *c.*

Perfume Composition, with Fresh Perfume Odor	9 drops

Sunburn Healing Preparations

Formula No. 1 (Healing Oil)

Tincture of Benzoin	4 g.
Borax	4 g.
Olive Oil	40 g.
Lime Water	52 g.

Dissolve the borax in the lime water; add the olive oil with rapid agitation. When an emulsion is formed add the tincture of benzoin.

Formula No. 2 (Sunburn Lotion)

Zinc Sulphocarbolate	1 g.
Alcohol	8 g.
Glycerin	5 g.
Spirits of Camphor	1 g.
Rose Water	85 g.

Dissolve the zinc sulphocarbolate in the alcohol. Add the glycerin and the spirits of camphor, mix with the rose water.

Formula No. 3

Boric Acid	4 g.
Acetic Acid	2 g.
Citric Acid	1 g.
Alcohol	10 g.
Glycerin	5 g.
Water	78 g.

Heat part of the water and dissolve the boric acid in it. Dissolve the citric acid in the alcohol and the acetic acid in the remainder of the water. Add the glycerin, boric acid solution, the citric acid solution, mix and filter.

Formula No. 4 (Sunburn Salve)

Benzocaine	4 g.
Boric Acid	5 g.
Lanolin	15 g.
Petrolatum	76 g.

Mix the benzocaine and part of the petrolatum. Add the boric acid and run through an ointment mill until a smooth and impalable mass is formed. Melt the remainder of the petrolatum and lanolin, strain and add the milled medicament base.

Formula No. 5 (Sunburn Powder)

Boric Acid	10 g.
Bismuth Subnitrate	5 g.
Magnesium Stearate	10 g.
Preservative	5 g.
Talc	70 g.

Make the same as talcum powder.

Formula No. 6 (Sunburn Lotion)

Picric Acid Solution (20%)	1.5 g.
Alcohol (90%)	10 g.
Water	88 g.
Perfume	.5 g.

Dissolve the perfume in alcohol, add to the water and then dissolve the picric acid in the solution. This is excellent for sunburn but as it is will stain the skin yellow; it may be found objectionable for facial sunburn. As dry picric acid is explosive when heated quickly or subjected to percussion, it is safer to purchase the 20%.

Anti-Sunburn Cream (Greaseless)

Formula No. 1

Glyceryl Monostearate 10 g.
Stearic Acid 15 g.
Melt together and mix with
Diethylene Glycol 5 g.
Menthyl Salicylate 10 g.
Add while stirring
Water (boiling) 60 g.

Stir till thick.

Formula No. 2

Stearic Acid	96 g.
Trikalin	20 g.
Glycerin	32 g.
Water	400 g.
Aesculin	10–25 g.
Perfume	to suit

Formula No. 3

Subnitrate of Bismuth	1½ dr.
Powdered French Chalk	30 dr.
Glycerin	2 dr.
Rose Water	1½ oz.

Mix the powders, and rub down carefully with the glycerin; then add the rose water. Shake the bottle before use.

Formula No. 4

Glycerin Cream	2 dr.
Jordan Almonds	4 dr.
Rose	5 oz.
Essential Oil of Almonds	3 drops

Blanch the almonds, and then dry and beat them up into a perfectly smooth paste; then mix in the glycerin cream and essential oil. Gradually add the rose water, stirring well after each addition; then strain through muslin.

Lotion, Anti-Sunburn

Quinine acid sulphate is used in proportion of 4 parts, dissolved in 64 parts of water which also contains 1 part of citric acid and 12 parts of 95% alcohol. This solution is added to mixture of 4 parts of finest, pulverized gum tragacanth and 5 parts of glycerin. Solution is added to gum mixture in small portions with constant agitation. Preparation is easily made and is highly effective. It can be perfumed to taste.

Sunburn-Protecting Oil

Formula No. 1

Quinine Oleate	3–5 g.
Paraffin Oil	27 cc.
Peanut Oil	70–68 cc.
Dye (Oil-Soluble Red)	

Formula No. 2

Quinine Ricinoleate	3–5 g.
Olive Oil	97–95 cc.

Formula No. 3

Mineral Oil	75 g.
Sesame or Peanut Oil, Pale	23 g.
Thymol	0.5 g.
Lanolin, Anhydrous	1.5 g.
Perfume	1–2 g.
Made up of:	
Pine Oil	3 cc.
Lavender Oil	1 cc.
Rosemary Oil	1 cc.
Laurel Oil	3–5 cc.

Sun Tan Oil

The basis of all such bronzing preparations is generally a vegetable oil, preferably arachis oil (peanut oil), olive oil, or sesame oil. Arachis oil in particular is said to have a bronzing effect, but in nearly all cases it is accompanied by a special dye, such as the one indicated below.

The following formula may be used as a basis for experiments, and is said to have a bronzing effect as a result of direct application:

Formula No. 1

Arachis Oil	60 g.
Bergamot Oil	1 g.
Olive Oil	38 g.
Brown Oil Soluble Dye	1 g.

Formula No. 2

Mineral or Olive Oil	95–98 g.
Quinine Ricinoleate	5– 2 g.
Oil Soluble Red or Orange Dye	to suit

Formula No. 3

Olive Oil	50 g.
Peanut Oil, Refined	49 g.
Bergamot Oil	1 g.
Color	Sufficient

Mix the oils and add a sufficient quantity of pigment brown for a suitable shade.

Formula No. 4

Olive Oil	50 g.
Peanut Oil, Refined	43 g.
Sesame Oil	5 g.
Thuja Oil	1 g.
Bergamot Oil	1 g.

Mix the oils, filter and add a very small quantity of oil soluble brown.

Formula No. 4

Suntan oil containing turtle oil:

Coconut Oil, Edible Grade	42 lb.
Sesame Oil	50 lb.
Turtle Oil, Refined	2½ lb.
Salol	5 lb.
Perfume Oil	½ lb.

Mix the sesame and turtle oils, warm this mixture and dissolve it in the salol. Add the molten coconut oil and then perfume.

If coloring is desired, 1¼ ounces of a 1 per cent solution of oil soluble aniline dye is usually sufficient.

In the above formula, the salol, which is rated as possessing excellent protective qualities against sunburn, is used for this particular effect.

Formula No. 5

Paraffin Oil	20 cc.
Fatty Oils, Free from Acid, Preserved	80 cc.
Etheric Oils (Bergamot, Eau de Cologne [free from Methylanthranilic Ester] or Pine Needle Oil)	1 cc.

Dye with Chlorophyll, Oil-soluble.

Formula No. 6

Quinine Hydrochloride	3.0 g.
Peanut Oil	96.5 g.
Color Oil (Soluble)	As desired
Perfume	.5 g.

Formula No. 7

Cherry Kernel Oil	100 g.
Green Color (Oil Soluble)	to suit
Preservative	0.1 g.

Formula No. 8

Peanut Oil	98 g.
Quinine Oleate	2 g.
Perfume and color	to suit

Sun Tan Lotions

Fatty, for use during strenuous exercise such as golf or tennis, in which case the emulsion must be such that it will not be dissolved by perspiration:

Formula No. 1

Olive Oil 50; Sesame Oil 50; Perfume Compound 1.

Formula No. 2

Lanolin anhydrous 300; Petrolatum 700; Perfume Compound 5.

Formula No. 3

Petrolatum 20; Lanolin 20; Ceresin 15; Wax 30; Olive Oil 60.

Formula No. 4

Lanolin anhydrous 200; Water 220; Olive or Peanut Oil 200; Perfume to suit.

Formula No. 5

Glycerin 20; Peach kernel Oil 20; Liquid Petrolatum 10; Water 45; Emulsifying agent (Ethanolamine stearate or Glycol stearate) 5; Perfume to suit.

The above have a beneficial effect on the skin but will give protection for a short time only.

A lotion of the following composition will protect the skin over a longer period:

Formula No. 6

White Petrolatum 20; Liquid Petrolatum 10; Quinine Bisulphate 4; Water 50; Emulsifying agent 20.

The lotions given below are greaseless, glycerin being the base. The action of these lotions is due to quinine or aesculin which they contain in soluble form.

Formula No. 1

Glycerin 60; Water 30; Quinine Bisulphate 6.

Formula No. 2

Gelose (a product made from agar-agar) 2; Glycerin 40; Rose water 60; Quinine Bisulphate 5.

Formula No. 3

Glycerin 500; Water 500; Aesculin 50; Tragacanth 20; Gelose 15.

Formula No. 4

Water 10; Starch 10; Glycerin 120; Aesculin 4.

A preservative must be added to Formulas No. 2, 3, and 4. The action of the aesculin may be increased by the addition of potash. (Approximately 10 drops of a 10% solution). A lotion containing aesculin is generally more satisfactory than one containing quinine bisulphate since aesculin is non-irritating. Extended use of quinine bisulphate may cause a slight irritation.

The perfume used in all these preparations must be stable in water, acids, and alkalies; and, moreover, must not irritate. Special care must therefore be taken in compounding. Very light types are usually preferred. Eau de cologne types are particularly recommended.

Formula No. 5

Alcohol	15.0 g.
Glycerin	5.0 g.
Water	79.5 g.
Perfume	0.5 g.
Color	Sufficient

Add a sufficient quantity of spirit soluble brown to this lotion to produce the required shade. Then mix and filter the preparation. Owing to the difficulty of applying such lotions uniformly they are not particularly satisfactory.

Some manufacturers prefer to use a lotion with a sulfonated oil or sulfonated fatty alcohol base together with a small quantity of alcohol and water. This is colored with a spirit soluble color. Such a preparation is easy to apply and it does not give the skin an oily appearance because the sulfonated materials being water soluble are dissolved as soon as the user goes into the water leaving a brown precipitate on the skin.

Formula No. 6

Agar-agar	4 g.
Glycerin	40 g.
Rose-water	60 g.
Æsculin	5 g.
Extract of Tormentilla	40 g.

Vanishing Cream, for Sun and Wind Burn

Stearic Acid	14 oz.
Apricot Kernel Oil	5 oz.
Ethylamino Benzoate	½ oz.
Potassium Carbonate	1 oz. 175 gr.
Borax	1 oz.
Distilled Water	70 oz.
Glycerin	9 oz.

Melt stearic acid and apricot kernel oil together and add ethylamino benzoate. Stir until dissolved and strain through cloth. Dissolve potassium carbonate and borax in distilled water and filter then add glycerin. Adjust temperature of both the oil-stearic acid mixture and of the borax, potassium carbonate solution to 75° C. then add slowly while stirring the melted stearic acid and apricot kernel oil mixture to the aqueous solution. Stir until completely emulsified and until temperature has dropped to about 40–45° C. Fill into jars or tubes.

Cold Cream, for Sun and Wind Burn

Apricot Kernel Oil	54 oz.
White Beeswax	13 oz.
White Ceresin Wax	8½ oz.
Ethylamino Benzoate	½ oz.
Borax, Powdered	½ oz.
Distilled Water	25 oz.

Melt apricot kernel oil, beeswax and ceresin wax together and add ethylamino benzoate. Stir until dissolved. Adjust temperature to 65° C. Dissolve borax in hot distilled water and filter. Adjust temperature to 65° C. Then add borax solution slowly while stirring to the oil and wax mixture kept at the same temperature and stir until cold.

Artificial Sunburn Liquids

Formula No. 1

Powdered Cudbear	20 lb.
Powdered Henna	4 lb.
Peanut or Almond Oil	32 lb.

Macerate at 120° F. for 3 hours and filter.

Formula No. 2

Quinine Sulfate	2 lb.
Witch Hazel	5 lb.
Lanolin	10 lb.
Peanut Oil	92 lb.

Formula No. 3

Peanut Oil	60 lb.
Olive Oil	35 lb.
Bergamot Oil	1 lb.
Laurel Berry Oil	3 lb.
Chlorophyl	1 lb.

Formulae 2 and 3 above require exposure of skin to sun.

CHAPTER VI

LIPSTICKS AND ROUGES

Lipsticks

AN ideal lip-stick is uniform and has the highest melting temperature compatible with easy spreading qualities. It should not be too greasy or crumbly. It should not bleed or sweat. The most popular melting range is between 130 and 145° F. Odor and taste are very important factors. What may be a good lip-stick when made, may age poorly and develop bad characteristics.

The most popular dyestuff used in lipsticks is "bromo-acid," a fluorescein derivative. It is usually dissolved in castor oil, butyl stearate, or diglycol laurate (neutral). Many different waxes are used to give body. Every manufacturer has his own "pet" combination. Beeswax is the most frequently used wax.

"Bromo-Acid" lipsticks are orange in color but turn pink when applied to the lips. They produce indelible sticks. For getting other shades, pigments are incorporated.

Procedure: The dye is dissolved in the dye solvent heated to about 160° F.; then add the oils; fats and waxes are added and stirred in until dissolved. The pigments are next added and mixing is continued until the temperature drops to 130–140° F. The mix is passed through an ointment or color mill to properly distribute the colors. The sticks are cast in molds. For each formula it is necessary to determine the best casting temperature. The molds should be allowed to stand for an hour and then chilled.

Lipsticks

The composition of a really first class lipstick base requires study and experiments and it is not until many changes of the original formula have been effected that a product of the right consistency is found. Another factor to be considered is the climate. Lipsticks for use in tropical regions have to be of a different composition. The type and quantity of color will also influence the consistency somewhat. Modifications may be necessary which can only be determined by actual experiments.

Formula No. 1

White beeswax 300; Spermaceti 300; Peach kernel oil 600.

Formula No. 2

Lanolin anhydrous 150; White beeswax 500; Liquid petrolatum 600; Spermaceti 50.

Formula No. 3

Stearic acid 200; Liquid petrolatum 500; White beeswax 500; Ceresin white 200; Paraffin 400.

Formula No. 4

Stearic acid 150; Lanolin anhydrous 150; Liquid petrolatum 700; Beeswax 700; Ceresin white 400.

The addition of talcum or zinc oxide is often recommended to produce a dull effect and to increase the covering property of the stick. They are undoubtedly quite useful but make production somewhat difficult. Being of a higher specific gravity they may cause an uneven distribution of the color. Light kaolin is much more practical.

When perfuming a lipstick care must be taken to choose a compound which will cover the smell and taste of the fatty lipstick base. The perfume must also be fairly palatable.

Formula No. 5

Mineral Oil	1 lb.
Ceraflux	2 lb.
Beeswax	2 lb.
Stearacol	8 lb.

Heat to 160° F and to it add the following:

Lake color (any shade desired)	1 lb.
Bromo Acid G	½ lb.
Perfume Oil	4 oz.

It is then ground through a warmed ointment mill and is ready for moulding.

This formula can be modified by replacing the mineral oil with lanolin, parachol, petrolatum or similar material. The waxes can be varied to include spermaceti, ozokerite, etc.

Formula No. 6

White Beeswax	20 g.
Paraffin	5 g.
Spermaceti	8 g.
Cocoa Butter	10 g.
Benzoinated Lard	25 g.
Parachol	20 g.
Bromo Acid G	3 g.
Color Mixture for Shade	10 g.
Preservative	.05 g.
Perfume (with flavor character)	1 g.

Mix the colors first with the bromo acid. Melt the parachol and the lard, add the color mixture and grind through a paint mill three or four times. Meanwhile melt and mix the rest of the waxes, and, when the colors are ready, add the melted waxes and mix thoroughly. Heat should not be raised above the melting point of the waxes. As soon as the batch is finished it should be molded, keeping it so far as possible at a constant temperature.

Formula No. 7

1. Stearoricinol	4 to 6 oz.
2. Paraffin Wax	1 oz.
3. Beeswax	1 oz.
4. Bromo Acid G	½ oz.
5. Geranium Lake	½ oz.
6. Perfume to suit.	

Melt and grind above in heated ointment mill 160° F. and mold.

No alcohol or other solvent is necessary as 1 is a powerful solvent.

The above formula gives an indelible stick which goes on evenly to form a coating free from objectionable gloss. After it penetrates it does not come off easily.

In hot weather the above formula should be modified by increasing the amount of beeswax.

Formula No. 8

Vaseline	15 oz.
Beeswax	10 oz.
Spermaceti	400 gr.
Carmine	6 dr.
Perfume to suit.	

Melt and stir. Allow to cool some before adding perfume. Pour into molds.

Formula No. 9

Beeswax, White	33 g.
Benzoinated Lard	12 g.
Sesame Oil	20 g.
Castor Oil	29 g.
Perfume Oil	2 g.
"Bromo-Acid" G	4 g.

Formula No. 10

Paraffin	2 oz.
Vaseline Oil, White	3 oz.
Beeswax, White	1 oz.
Ozokerite	3 oz.
Titanium Dioxide	1 oz.
Colors: For 100 parts use:	
Fixation Red I No. 46	3.5 oz.
Medium Red No. 28	22 oz.

Other red dyes used: Carmine, Nakarat, Fixierrot, Cherry Red, Orient Red.

Formula No. 11

(Non-Indelible) For Theatrical Use

Petrolatum	4 lb.
Paraffin Wax	2 lb.
Mineral Oil	1 lb.
Carnauba Wax	6 oz.

Lanolin	8 oz.
Lake Color	1 lb.
Perfume	as desired

The same lake color mixtures as are used in the greasy cream rouges are suggested to secure the various shades. The procedure is the same.

Formula No. 12

Indelible

Stearoricinol	28 lb.
Mineral Oil	4 lb.
Lanolin (Anhydrous)	2 lb.
Petrolatum	2 lb.
Paraffin Wax	8 lb.
Beeswax	8 lb.
Bromo "Acid" G	1 lb.
Lake Colors	5 lb.
Perfume Oil	1 lb.

By varying the colors correspondingly different shades may be gotten.

Indelible

Formula No. 13

Castor Oil	4	lb.
Cocoa Butter	2	lb.
Stearic Acid	1½	lb.
Paraffin	2	lb.
Beeswax	1¾	lb.
Carnauba Wax	2	oz.
Lanolin	8	oz.
Bromo Acid G (tetrabrom fluorescein)	12	oz.
Lake Color (see cream rouge)	12	oz.
Preservative	1	oz.
Perfume	2	oz.

Formula No. 14

Castor Oil	6	lb.
Glyceryl-Monostearate	2	lb.
Stearic Acid	½	lb.
Cetyl Alcohol	½	lb.
Bromo Acid G (tetrabrom fluorescein)	10	oz.
Erythrosine	¼	oz.
Oil Soluble Red	16	gr.
Perfume	1½	oz.

The oils and waxes are heated together and the oil soluble color is dissolved therein. The bromo acid and erythrosine are then added and the entire mass is ground through an ointment mill. For this particular type lipstick, various shades may be secured by the use of various of the oil soluble colors, such as: yellow and orange in combination with the red, and the use of other water soluble dyestuffs in place of the erythrosine, such as: tartrazin, ponceau, etc.

Changeable Orange Lipstick

Formula No. 1

Cocoa Butter	1 lb.
Beeswax	2 lb.
"Ceraflux"	2 lb.
Stearacol	8 lb.
"Moldex"	1 oz.
Bromo "Acid G"	2 oz.
Perfume Oil	4 oz.

Heat gently and stir until dissolved and filter through a heated funnel.

Formula No. 2

Cocoa Butter	20 lb.
Castor Oil	12 lb.
Ceresin	15 lb.
Beeswax	5 lb.
Bromo "Acid G"	4 oz.
Perfume Oil	1 lb.

Formula No. 3

Changeable Orange

Castor Oil	5 lb.
Cocoa Butter	3 lb.
Ceresin	3 lb.
Beeswax	2 lb.
Bromo Acid G (tetrabrom fluorescein)	2 oz.
Preservative	2 oz.
Perfume	2 oz.

The oils and waxes are melted. The bromo acid and the benzoate are then added and the entire mixture is filtered hot.

Lip Pomade

Formula No. 1

Mineral Oil	6	lb.
Petrolatum	2	lb.
Paraffin	2	lb.
Ozokerite	¼	lb.
Beeswax	¾	lb.
Perfume	½	oz.

The materials are melted together and poured into a suitable mold. These sticks are intended for use in softening of lips and preventing chapping of the lips.

Materials such as: lanolin, absorption base, olive oil, cocoa butter, may also be introduced into the formula. From 2–4 oz. of zinc oxide ground into the product will give a whiter stick and will aid as a healing agent.

Materials such as: menthol, camphor, thymol and similar medicants, may be used in small quantities and most conveniently introduced into the product by molding them into the perfume and then adding the mixture to the melted oils and waxes.

Formula No. 2

Mineral Oil	1 gal.
Petrolatum White	2 lb.
Ozokerite White	5 lb.
Beeswax White	2 lb.
Perfume	1 oz.
Color	to suit

Lip Rouge—Indelible

Formula No. 1

Castor Oil	7 lb.
Lanolin	1 lb.
Beeswax	1 lb.
Bromo "Acid G" (tetrabrom fluorescein)	12 oz.
Lake Color	12 oz.
Perfume	as desired

Formula No. 2

Castor Oil	6 lb.
Cetyl Alcohol	1 lb.
Stearic Acid	4 oz.
Lanolin	1 lb.
Glyceryl Mono Stearate	1 lb.
Bromo "Acid G" (tetrabrom fluorescein)	8 oz.
Lake Color	4 oz.
Perfume	as desired

The lake color mixtures used in the previous formulae may be used to secure the various shades. The procedure is the same as in the above formulae.

Lipstick Perfume

Rhodinol	300 g.
Linalol	30 g.
Neroli Petals	20 g.
Heliotropin	200 g.
Phenylethyl alcohol	130 g.
Geraniol	320 g.
Vanillin	5 g.

Rouges

Dry Rouges

Dry rouges were originally made by mixing talc and carmine with a mucilage of tragacanth, placing the plastic mass in metal trays or cups and allowing them to harden. These products were then sold in these trays or cups.

The manufacturing technique was then developed to the point wherein with a slight modification of the formula, the plastic mass was placed on discs, allowed to dry and then turned into shape by a cutting tool.

The present day manufacture of rouges is done in several different ways. The most simple is a mixture of the following:

Talc	40 lb.
Kaolin	35 lb.
Zinc Oxide	15 lb.
Precipitated Chalk	10 lb.

Mix the above with sufficient dry color to give the desired shade (see following), grind in a ball mill for a period of time sufficient to distribute all color particles throughout the entire mass. The material is then bolted through at least a 140 mesh silk, and is then moistened with a tragacanth solution of a strength of ¼ oz. gum tragacanth and ¼ oz. boric acid to 1 gallon water. This solution is added to the powder mass at the rate of 1 oz. to every pound of dry material. The perfume oil is also incorporated at this stage.

The slightly wetted powder is brushed through at least a 30 mesh wire screen and bolted through at least a 60 mesh silk screen. The rouge material is then ready for pressing.

The type press used for this particular formula is a foot press which has a fast downward and upward stroke. The metal disc or cup onto or into which the rouge is to be pressed is moistened with a tragacanth solution of a strength of 1 oz. of gum tragacanth to 1 gallon of water.

Rouge Compacts

Carmine	1 oz.
Talc	21 oz.

Gum Acacia	1¾ oz.
Ammonia	a few drops

Mix first three items in a mortar, add a few drops of ammonia and some water. Pound into a fine mass adding more water in small portions to form a stiff paste. Fill into molds immediately. The amount of carmine can be increased to obtain different shades.

Rouge Compact Powders

Rouge Brunette

Rouge Brunette	12 g.
Alizarin Lake	2 g.
Rhodamin B	2 g.
Ultramarine	2 g.
Titanium Dioxide	22 g.
Powder Base	100 g.

Suntan

Light Ochre	30 g.
Burned Ochre	50 g.
Umber	15 g.
Powder Base	250 g.

Mandarin Red

Eosin	0.5 g.
Cadmium Yellow	5 g.
Alizarin Lake	2 g.
Mandarin Red	12 g.
Powder Base	200 g.

Solid "Make-Up"

(Rouge)

French Pat. 780,084

Dye (e.g. Cochineal)	1000 g.
Gum Arabic	250 g.
Honey	85 g.
Water	750 g.
Ammonia	55 g.

Evaporate to dryness, mold; moisten before use.

Non-Greasy Cream Rouges

The new non-greasy cream rouges are packed in air-tight jars in accordance with the following formula:

Stearic Acid	4 lb.
Glycosterin	2 lb.

Heat to 170° F.

Trikalin	13½ oz.
Polycol	17½ lb.
Water	½ gal.
Erythrosine or Tartrazine (certified)	1 oz.

Heat to 170° F and add slowly with stirring to melted stearic acid and glycosterin. When cool grind in the following mixture:

Zinc Oxide	2 lb.
Lake Color	1 lb.
Perfume Oil	4 oz.

Cream Rouge

The following is an excellent base:

Formula No. 1

Paraffin Wax	48 g.
White Beeswax	6 g.
White Mineral Oil	160 cc.
Perfume	5 cc.
Color	107–214 g.

The method of making is as follows:

Make a quantity of base and allow it to set. While the base is setting, sift the dry colour through the fine sieve, remembering that the colour cannot be too fine. Next weigh out the amount of base required and remelt. When liquid, add to it the previously sifted colour. Mix thoroughly, heating again, if necessary, to keep the whole mass in a pourable condition. Now strain through the silk which has been stretched over the receptacle. Any dry colour that has not passed through the silk is transferred to the mortar and ground as fine as possible, after which it is added to a small quantity of the molten mass, which is then strained. The perfume is added as usual when nearly cold.

Formula No. 2

(a)	Eosin	0.5 g.
	Alcohol	10 cc.
(b)	Stearate Cream	200 g.
	Spermaceti	5 g.

Mix (a) into (b) which has been made up on a waterbath. Keep warm and stir to drive off the alcohol.

Formula No. 3

Stearic Acid	25.0 oz.
Water	61.5 oz.
Glycerin	10.0 oz.
Potassium Hydroxide	1.0 oz.
Oil-Soluble Dyestuff	2.5 oz.
Perfume	to suit

Paste Rouge

Formula No. 1

Beeswax	8 lb.
"Stearoricinol"	28 lb.

Mineral Oil	4 lb.
Lanolin Anhydrous	2 lb.
Petrolatum	2 lb.
Bromo "Acid G"	1 lb.
Lake Colors	5 lb.
Perfume Oil	1 lb.

Formula No. 2

By decreasing the amount of waxes in a lipstick formula, a paste rouge is made.

Liquid Rouge

Erythrosine	0.25 g.
Eosin (Bluish)	0.40 g.
Glycerin	80.00 cc.
Alcohol	560.00 cc.
Simple Syrup	100.00 cc.
Heliotrope Bouquet	to suit
Distilled Water to make	1000.00 cc.

Dissolve dyes in glycerin-alcohol mixture. Add simple syrup and heliotrope; then add water.

Colors for Rouges

To Be Added to a 100 Pound Batch

Orange

Scarlet Lake	7 lb.
Yellow Ocher	8 oz.
Indian Red	4 oz.

Light No. 1

Indian Red	3 lb.
Burnt Sienna	1 lb.
Brilliant Lake	2 lb.
Maroon Lake	8 oz.

Light No. 2

Scarlet Lake	4 lb.
Brilliant Lake	2 lb.
Yellow Ocher	8 oz.
Indian Red	8 oz.
Geranium Lake	4 oz.

Geranium No. 1

Geranium Lake	5 lb.
Scarlet Lake	7 lb.
Brilliant Lake	3 lb.

Geranium No. 2

Geranium Lake	12 lb.
Orange Toner	4 oz.
Crimson Lake	8 oz.

Medium No. 1

Brilliant Lake	18 lb.
Scarlet Lake	2 lb.
Maroon Lake	1 lb.

Medium No. 2

Brilliant Lake	12 lb.
Geranium Lake	4 lb.
Maroon Lake	3 lb.
Indian Red	3 lb.

CHAPTER VII

EYE PREPARATIONS

Eyebrow Pencils

Apart from those methods which serve to preserve the eye region in good physical condition, actual beauty treatment is now practiced on a very considerable scale. Coloring of the eyebrows, painting of the eyelashes and shading of the eyelids are now important components of face cosmetics, the greatest attention being devoted to the first operation. Coloring of the eyebrows or their simulation after complete shaving is effected with colored wax pencils. Ordinary pure charcoal pencils tend to cause falling-out and drying of the hair.

Ingredients used in preparing the wax pencils are white wax, benzoinated tallow, cocoa butter, petroleum oil and olive oil. The pigments are lamp black, umber, and ochre. Large manufacturers find it economical to use pigment grinding machines and other equipment of the most modern design, but small concerns can nevertheless cope with the production of these cosmetics.

Formula No. 1

The base comprises a composition made up from 110 g. fine petroleum oil, 60 g. white ceresin, 15 g. white wax, 240 g. benzoinated tallow, and 1 g. coumarin. The fatty base is thoroughly ground with the pigments, the molten base being gradually stirred into the very finely powdered pigment contained in a mortar. After thorough trituration the mixture is again warmed, digested for about half an hour on a water bath, and again allowed to cool. As soon as the mass begins to thicken, it is again vigorously stirred and forced through a fine-mesh sieve by applying powerful pressure with the pestle. Lumps and impurities are retained upon the sieve. The preparation which passes through the mesh is then again thoroughly mixed, with gentle heating before casting. The mass should be neither too hot nor too fluid when being cast, since settlement of the insoluble pigment will result in lack of uniform coloration. Oil-soluble dyestuffs will certainly only enter into consideration in exceptional cases.

Formula No. 2

2 parts cocoa butter, 2 parts ceresin, and 1 part olive oil. Into this is stirred 0.6 part dyestuffs (i.e., about 10% of the total gross weight), which has previously been ground up with a little olive oil.

As soon as the mass has reached the state when it can just be cast, it is emptied into metal moulds. As a rule these impart the required taper to the pencils, but if this is not the case they are tapered after removing from the moulds and wrapped in thick metal foil while leaving the points exposed.

Wax Bases for Eyebrow Pencils

Formula No. 1

Mineral Oil, Yellow	210 g.
Ceresin, White	320 g.
Beeswax, White	30 g.
Benzoinated Tallow	440 g.

Formula No. 2

Beeswax, White	420 g.
Ceresin, White	105 g.
Paraffin Wax, Soft	135 g.
Wool Fat, Anhydrous	135 g.
Peanut Oil	205 g.

Formula No. 3

Ceresin, (50/52° C.)	30 g.
Japan Wax	20 g.
Beeswax	30 g.
Mineral Oil	20 g.

Colors:

Black

Lampblack, Oil-soluble black, animal charcoal; nigrosin.

Brown

Umber brown, etc., or a brown aniline dye.

Blonde

Mixture of brown with burnt ochre.

Eyebrow Pencils

Formula No. 1

Blonde

Wax Base	400 g.
Ceresin	100 g.
Ochre, Light	150 g.
Ochre, Dark	150 g.

Formula No. 2

Dark Brunette

Wax Base	400 g.
Ceresin	100 g.
Umber, Dark	300 g.
Lamp black	5 g.

Formula No. 3

Châtain (*chestnut*)

Wax Base	400 g.
Ceresin	100 g.
Umber, Light	200 g.
Umber, Dark	130 g.
Ochre, Burnt	40 g.

Formula No. 4

Black

Wax Base	400 g.
Ceresin	100 g.
Lampblack	30 g.

Formula No. 5

Brown

Burnt Sienna	80 g.
Burnt Umber	100 g.
Hard Paraffin Wax	420 g.
Soft Paraffin, Yellow	400 g.

Formula No. 6

Paraffin Wax	300 g.
Cocoa Butter	300 g.
Beeswax	100 g.
Petrolatum	100 g.
Carbon Black	sufficient

Mix thoroughly and run into molds to form sticks.

Eyelid Pencils

The production of shading tones on eyelids can be effected with pencils, the composition of which is very similar to that of the eyebrow pencils. The mass consists of the wax base detailed above with the addition of about 20% ceresin. The color scale is somewhat more varied in the case of these pencils, since a wider range of tones can be induced in the usual brown and bluish black shades. Chestnut is obtained by mixing 225 g. pale umber and 150 g. mahogany brown with 1000 g. of the molten wax mass. For dark brown tones mix with the same quantity of wax 300 g. of a brun foncé; black shades require for the same wax quantity 100 g. zinc white, 120 g. ultramarine, and 4 g. lamp black.

Regarding the perfuming of these preparations, these should generally be of a very refined character. About 5 to 10 g. of perfume are required for each kilogram of mass. In cases where a fancy perfume is desired, preference should be given to one with a fresh natural odor.

Eye Shadow

Formula No. 1

Gris d'Ombre (*gray*)

Fat Powder Base	150 g.
Ultramarine	125 g.
Lamp black	3 g.

Formula No. 2

Blen d'Ombre (*Blue*)

Fat Powder Base	150 g.
Ultramarine	120 g.
Lamp black	1 g.

Formula No. 3

Brun

Fat Powder Base	150 g.
Umber	180 g.
Burned Ochre	20 g.
Lamp black	0.5 g.
Ultramarine	50 g.

Formula No. 4

Dark Brown Shades

Fat Powder Base	150 g.
Umber	150 g.
Burned Ochre	50 g.
Lamp black	0.5 g.
Ultramarine	50 g.

Formula No. 5

Mineral Oil	5 lb.
Lanolin	2 lb.
Petrolatum	1 lb.
Beeswax	1 lb.
Paraffin	2 lb.
Perfume Oil	4 oz.

Color with any of following combinations:

Blue

Ultramarine Blue	2 lb.
Zinc Oxide	2 lb.

Green, Light

Zinc Oxide	3 lb.
Green Lake	1 lb.

Gray

Ultramarine Blue	1 lb.
Carbon Black	1 lb.
Zinc Oxide	2 lb.

Brown

Burnt Umber	3 lb.
Zinc Oxide	1 lb.

Green, Dark

Green Lake	3 lb.
Zinc Oxide	1 lb.

Violet

Violet Lake	1 lb.
Zinc Oxide	3 lb.

Heat colors and wax mixture and grind in ointment mill; pack by pouring hot.

Mascara is the name given to colorings for eye lashes. Some of these products are also useful for giving an upward turn to the lashes.

Formula No. 1

The following formula produces a non-irritating, waterproof mascara:

"Savolin"	4 lb. 5 oz.
Ceresin (high melting)	2 lb.
Carnauba Wax	1 lb.
Lanolin	5 oz.
Ivory Black	½ lb.
Perfume Oil	2 oz.

Formula No. 2

Trihydroxyethylamine Stearate	40 lb.
Carnauba Wax	10 lb.
Carbon Black	30–40 lb.

Melt with stirring and cast or extrude in sticks.

Mascara—Soapless Type—Poured

Triethanolamine	14 lb.
Stearic Acid	20 lb.
Oleic Acid	5 lb.
Ricinoleic Acid	5 lb.
Carnauba Wax	30 lb.
Ozokerite	15 lb.
Petrolatum	6 lb.
Perfume	1 lb.

These materials are all melted together.

The following colors are ground into the molten mass to secure the various shades:

Black

Charcoal Black	5 lb.

Brown

Burnt Umber	10 lb.
Burnt Sienna	1 lb.
Indian Red	3 lb.

Blue

Ultramarine Blue	12 lb.
Titanium Oxide	2 lb.

Liquid Mascara

Tincture of Benzoin (25%)
Black Dye (Oil Soluble) to suit

Black Eye Paint

Bismuth Subcarbonate	2 dr.
Talc	1 dr.

Mix and color with carmine or calamine to skin tint. Apply after washing the parts with a mixture of:

Glycerin	1 dr.
Water	5 dr.

Eye Lash Grower (Darkener)

Yellow petroleum jelly is supposed to have the property of stimulating the growth of lashes and brows, as well as darkening them at the same time. Two formulas will indicate the type:

Formula No. 1

Yellow Petrolatum Jelly	50 g.
Turtle Oil	50 g.

Melt and Perfume.

Formula No. 2

Yellow Petrolatum Jelly	50 g.
Castor Oil	49 g.
Paraffin Wax	1 g.

Either No. 1 or No. 2 can be modified to give a darker-looking preparation by the addition of burnt sienna and/or umber. In this instance the usual precaution will have to be observed regarding packaging products containing suspended materials. Use a preservative where there is a chance for the oils to decompose. Para-oxy-benzoic acid esters are suitable for this. Perfume with lavender or bergamot, or both.

Eyebrow and Eyelash Softener

Formula No. 1

Castor Oil	20	oz.
Almond Oil	60	oz.
Perfume	¾	oz.

Formula No. 2

Diglycol Laurate	100	oz.
Acetic Acid, Glacial	¼	oz.
Mineral Oil, Medicinal	200	oz.

Formula No. 3

Beeswax	200 g.
Cocoa Butter	300 g.

Melt together and add:

Peanut Oil	750 g.
"Moldex" or Other Good Preservative	2 g.

Formula No. 4

Oleic Acid, White	1 g.
Mineral Oil	200 g.

Mix cold and stir until complete solution is obtained.

Eye Oil (Balsamic)

Some women prefer to use an oil preparation on the lashes and brows. For this purpose the following is a type:

Castor Oil	24.5 cc.
Sweet Almond Oil	75.0 cc.
Perfume	.5 cc.

The perfume should consist of some mild stimulant, such as camphor oil, along with balsams. Oil storax, 10; oil camphor, 45; rose oil synthetic, 10. The preparation should be allowed to stand for some time before bottling. It should be crystal clear and just slightly aromatic. The addition of .5 per cent caritol is a wise one, especially so because vitamin A is very much concerned with the health of the eyes. Caritol is a .3 per cent solution of carotene in oil.

Plucking Cream

This is useful to apply as an anæsthetic cream on those parts of the eyebrow to be plucked. The instructions are to rub the preparation in well and leave on for half an hour previous to plucking. For manufacturing such a preparation use a cold cream base and 1 per cent ethyl aminobenzoate. The resulting cream will also facilitate plucking of undesirable hairs.

Eye Cream

The purpose of such a cream is to soften wrinkles, commonly called crowsfeet, around the eyes. The preparation must be rich in the so-called nutritives. The following are type formulas:

Formula No. 1

Lanolin	50 g.
Olive Oil	20 g.
Castor Oil	10 g.
Turtle Oil	20 g.
Preservative	Sufficient

Perfume as desired

Formula No. 2

Lecithin	5 g.
Cholesterol	1 g.
Lanolin	10 g.
Expressed Almond Oil	59 g.
Beeswax	25 g.
Preservative	Sufficient

Perfume as desired

One preparation of this type now on the market is perfumed with violet, the net result being that it is much different from the usual cream.

CHAPTER VIII

SOAPS AND CLEANERS

Soaps

CHEMICALLY, soaps are compounds of alkalies and fatty acids. Hard soaps are made with soda, and soft soaps with potash. The oils and fats that are saponified to make soap may be of vegetable or animal origin. What raw materials are used, is determined by the type of finished product desired. It is not economical to make soaps on a small scale. If the quantity required is not large it is better to buy from a large manufacturer, rather than to make them.

Toilet Soap Base

The following represent five standard and workable compositions of the stock used in making the soap base. The first mixture contains eighty per cent of fresh beef tallow, and twenty per cent of good grade coconut oil; the second, sixty-five per cent of beef tallow, fifteen per cent of lard and twenty per cent of coconut oil; the third, seventy per cent of bleached palm oil, fifteen per cent of sulphonated olive oil and fifteen per cent of coconut oil; the fourth, sixty-five to seventy per cent of beef tallow, ten to fifteen per cent of castor oil and twenty per cent of coconut oil; the fifth, sixty per cent of bleached palm oil, twenty per cent of beef tallow and twenty per cent of coconut oil.

In making soap bases of second quality good grades of fat refuse are used in large quantities and also palm kernel oil in the place of coconut oil. These raw materials can be converted into well-saponified soaps and of good keeping quality, but only when great care is paid to the details of the process. However, the soap base that is made in this manner cannot be perfumed satisfactorily.

The oldest and mostly used process for the manufacture of excellent soap bases is first to saponify the tallow, lard, palm oil, castor oil and the like and to salt-out the same once or several times. Then the coconut oil is added and the saponification continued and the soap salted out until a niger is obtained. This process has been improved by beginning the saponification of each batch of stock in a different kettle and after the batch has been completely saponified, the salted-out curd soap from a previous saponification is added. It is claimed that this method makes for technically complete saponification of the stock in a more easily and safely attained manner.

A third method of boiling the soap does not involve the addition of any salt. It has been used in various toilet soap works and has been found satisfactory over a period of years. The salting out of the curd from the previous boil as well as of the soap from the boil to which the curd soap has been added is accomplished with concentrated sodium hydroxide lye. The graining of the finished soap is also accomplished with dilute sodium hydroxide solution and not with salt water. The curd soap that is obtained after standing for thirty-six hours in the kettle is quite alkaline. However, the alkalinity of the soap disappears as the latter is dried. The result is that a product is finally obtained which can be readily milled into a perfectly neutral and stable toilet soap. This process has demonstrated its usefulness as it has been employed in practical operations for quite some years.

Half-Boil Process

A fourth process for the manufacture of soap base consists in complete saponification of the fatty mixture (neutral fats) only by the half-boil process. The soap is then comminuted to chips and these are dried in the usual manner as in all the soap making processes and thereafter milled. Toilet soaps that are manufactured by this process contain in excess of eight per cent glycerin. Hence it is evident that the soap is sufficiently plastic and easily millable. A long series of experiments has also proven that the soap is absolutely stable. Naturally a most important prerequisite of this soap making process is that the raw materials used must be absolutely pure and free from any odor as well as free from albumens. If the raw materials received into the plant are not of this quality, they must be purified by suitable means before being used in the kettles. Only when the temperature varies very markedly and when the humidity of the air is very high, close to 100 per cent, do soaps made in this manner become wet. On the other hand, soaps made by other processes of saponification as well as after-treatment become wet much more readily under considerably less severe conditions.

Some toilet soap manufacturers convert the soap base into toilet soap by the following process. The raw materials, consisting of tallow, lard and the like, are completely saponified in a large tank, provided with an agitating apparatus and situated close to the kettle. Saponification is carried out according to the emulsification-saponification process by the half-boil method using a small excess of lye. Then immediately after saponification the mass is added to the curd soap which has been subjected to several changes, the soap obtained from a previous boil. When the entire mixture has been saponified, then the soap is salted out, salt being used in making two changes. The soap is then finished in the usual manner. The emulsification and saponification of the stock, which is carried out in a single operation, gives a soap which is completely saponified. This process is therefore of considerable advantage.

Rose Soap

a.	White Tallow Soap	10,000 g.
	Cinnabar, Moistened	60–80 g.
b.	Rose Essence	25 g.
	Geranium Essence	60 g.
	Clove Essence	15 g.
	Chinese Cinnamon Essence	10 g.

Palm Soap

a.	Pure Palm Soap	5000 g.
	Half Palm Soap	5000 g.
b.	Bergamot Essence	60 g.
	Chinese Cinnamon Essence	25 g.
	Clove Essence	15 g.
	Essence of Fine Lavender	30 g.

Althaea (Marshmallow) Soap

a.	White Tallow Soap	5000 g.
	Pure Palm Soap	5000 g.
b.	Yellow Ochre	30 g.
	Paris Red	30 g.
c.	Essence of Fine Lavender	15 g.
	Essence of Pressed Lemon Peel	16 g.
	Essence of Neroli Petitgrain	16 g.
	Essence of Verbena	10 g.
	Essence of English Mint	3 g.

Bouquet Soap

a.	Soap, White Tallow	10,000 g.
	Brown Ochre	100 g.
b.	Essence of Bergamot	80 g.
	Essence of Cloves	15 g.
	Essence of Neroli	15 g.
	Essence of Sassafras	10 g.
	Essence of Thyme	10 g.
or also:		
b.	Essence of Fine Lavender	20 g.
	Essence of English Mint	20 g.
	Essence of Pressed Lemon Peel	25 g.
	Essence of Sage	20 g.
	Essence of Thyme	10 g.

Cosmetic "Oxygen" Soap

Coconut Oil	15 g.
Castor Oil	7 g.
Tallow	77 g.
Cimol-Neutral	2 g.
Sodium Cholate	.5 g.
Sodium Perborate	5 g.
Preservative	.3 g.
Magnesium stearate	1 g.

Powdered Hand Toilet Soaps

Formula:	No. 1 Bathroom Travel and Home Use	No. 2 Factory and Garage Use	No. 3 Office and Dispenser General	No. 4
Dry Yellow Powdered Soap, 92% plus c.p.s.,* S.N.† to be over 210 titre,‡ 25 to 35° C.	75 lb.	———	40 lb.	60 lb.
Cocoanut soap-powder, 30% Anhydrous Soap Contents, S. N. to be over 210 titre, 30 to 35° C.	———	60 lb.	25 lb.	20 lb.
"Wyo-Jel" No. 719 (Colloidal Bentonite), 200 mesh	24 lb.	33 lb.	30 lb.	20 lb.
Tri-Sodium Phosphate, tech. grade powdered	1 lb.	7 lb.	5 lb.	———
Perfume				
"Citrene"	0.2 lb.	———	———	———
"Girella"	———	———	0.1 lb.	0.1 lb.
Camphory Sassafras Oil	———	0.7 lb.	———	———

* c.p.s. = Chemically Pure Soap.
† S.N. = Saponification Number.
‡ Titre = Melting Point of Fats.

The ingredients are weighed into a clean and dry mixer and intensely mixed for 15 to 20 minutes. The perfume should be sprayed or sprinkled over the powdered soap or soap-powder to avoid caking. As none of the ingredients are hygroscopic it is not necessary to pack the finished product air tight.

For starting production, a clean open-head steel drum rolled and shaken on the floor is satisfactory for mixing, providing some wooden weights are laid inside to assure agitation. However, for big scale production, use one big horizontal mixer, 2000 lb. capacity, cylinder driven from both end countershafts and equipped with a double action agitator which moves toward the 6″ x 8″ outlet in the middle and which is driven by a 15 h.p. motor. A slip ring motor, or a compensator allows this mixer to be started with a full load, thus avoiding accidents and dusting.

The most ideal process to make powdered hand toilet soaps is by making them wet-processed, and if other soaps are also manufactured, it is easy and much more preferable to do so. In the case of Formula 1, the Wyo-Jel is crutched into the hot molten soap stock before cooling and drying and the perfume is added immediately before grinding down of the dried soap flakes. In case of Nos. 2 and 3, paste soap, regular soap-powder is hot mixed with all the ingredients added at once to a bakery-type dough mixer. In case of hot processing much more Wyo-Jel can be used and the final structure will be more uniform and much harder to duplicate.

Glycerin Soaps

Formula No. 1

Tallow	30 kg.
Coconut Oil	30 kg.
Castor Oil	20 kg.
Caustic Soda, (38° Bé)	40 kg.
Glycerin	20 kg.
Alcohol	30 kg.
Water, Distilled	12 kg.
Sugar	8 kg.

Formula No. 2

Tallow	30 kg.
Stearic Acid	10 kg.
Coconut Oil	40 kg.
Castor Oil	40 kg.
Caustic Soda, (38° Bé)	60 kg.
Alcohol	40 kg.
Sugar	20 kg.
Glycerin	20 kg.
Water, Distilled	40 kg.

Formula No. 3
(No Alcohol)

Coconut Oil	75 kg.
Tallow	60 kg.
Castor Oil	60 kg.
Caustic Soda, (38° Bé)	100 kg.
Potassium Nitrate	4 kg.
Water, Distilled	15 kg.
Sugar	60 kg.
Water, Distilled	60 kg.
Glycerin	10 kg.
Fillers *	25 kg.

Soap Filler

* The filler is composed of

Potassium Chloride	4 kg.
Potash Carbonate	4 kg.
Sodium Carbonate	4 kg.
Salt	8 kg.
Water	64 kg.

Dyes for these soaps:

Uranine Yellow
Brillant Orange
Soap Yellow

Use 0.5–1 g. per 100 kg. soap
Perfumes (600–800 g./100 kg. soap) such as

Rose

Geranium Oil	400 g.
Lavender Oil	190 g.
Rose, Special	10 g.
Patchouli Oil	5 g.

Violet

Bergamot Oil	400 g.
Geranium Oil	40 g.
Neroli Oil, Synthetic	20 g.
Iris Oil	10 g.

Lavender

Bergamot Oil	400 g.
Palmarosa Oil	60 g.
Lavender Oil	100 g.

Special Procedure for the Manufacture of Glycerin Soaps

Melt fats in a jacketed-kettle, add all other ingredients one at a time, take up to boil.

The kettle should be big enough to allow the boiling material to "rise" quite a good deal. If the danger of boiling over is too great, add some buckets full of cold water into the outer jacket of the kettle, and go on boiling.

The finished saponification thus yields a clear soap. Now cover the kettle, turn off heat.

Dye, perfume are added at lowest possible temperatures. Cool quickly, pour into molds.

Transparent Glycerin Soaps

	Formula No. 1	No. 2	No. 3
Coconut Oil, Cochin	20	26	30 kg.
Tallow	18	24	20 kg.
Castor Oil	12	10	15 kg.
Caustic Potash,			
40° Bé.	25	—	— kg.
36° Bé.	—	32	— kg.
39° Bé.	—	—	35 kg.
Glycerin	10	13	10 kg.
Sugar	10	40	42 kg.
Water (60° C.)	15	30	38 kg.
"Fillers"	—	30	35 kg.

To this soap-base add *distilled water* in small portions to about 15 (kg.), and to the resulting clear, but very soft, soap add a *hardening solution* (of 15° Bé.), made up of:

Potassium Carbonate	1 kg.
Sal Soda	1 kg.
Salt	1 kg.

Add water to get 15° Bé. Warm to 75° C.

Add enough to get samples of sufficiently hard soap. Let stand covered for an hour, and test result.

Should not be of too high viscosity when spread on a glass-sheet. If too viscous or too foamy add water.

Add perfume at 50° C., sift in dye, stir and pour into molds.

Transparent Soap (Without Glycerin)

Tallow, Cochin	24 kg.
Coconut Oil	24 kg.
Castor Oil	16 kg.

Heat to 50–60° C.

Add in thin jet:

Caustic Soda (39° Bé.) 33 kg.

Stir until soap swims on top, then cover. Stir slowly over water bath. Add

Alcohol 1–2 kg.

then

Water (60° C.)	22 kg.
Sugar	20 kg.

Again

Alcohol 18–19 kg.

Cover. Keep at 75° C. for an hour.

Soap should be dark and clear; foam light. Soap should remain "knife-thick" on a glass-sheet.

If opaque, try (before in test-tube) to add slowly hot water, or caustic soda (20° Bé.).

At 50–60° C. add perfume and the last 3–4 kg. of above alcohol.

Transparent Soft Soaps

For Fall and Spring:

Formula No. 1

Bean Oil	400 kg.
Linseed Oil	300 kg.
Sesame Oil	150 kg.
Rosin	150 kg.
Water	150 kg.
Caustic Soda	30 kg.

Formula No. 2

Bean Oil	500 kg.
Linseed Oil	400 kg.
Pig Fat, Light	100 kg.
Water	150 kg.
Caustic Soda 36° Bé	30 kg.

Formula No. 3

Soya Bean Oil	800 kg.
Colza Oil	50 kg.
Rosin	50 kg.
Beef Fat	50 kg.
Pig Fat, Light	50 kg.
Water	150 kg.
Caustic Soda 25° Bé	50 kg.

"Silver Soaps"

(Fat-Bases)

Formula No. 1

Cottonseed Oil	800 kg.
Tallow	200 kg.

Formula No. 2

Cottonseed Oil	700 kg.
Tallow	250 kg.
Palm Kernel Oil	50 kg.

Formula No. 3

Peanut Oil	600 kg.
Pig Fat	340 kg.
Palm Kernel Oil	60 kg.

Formula No. 4

Cottonseed Oil	500 kg.
Hard Fat	300 kg.
Bone Fat	150 kg.
Coconut Oil Waste	50 kg.

For the saponification, only a part of the alkali used should be caustic. In summer, 18–20% should be potash carbonate or 12–13% sodium carbonate; in winter, up to 22% potash carbonate or up to 17% sodium carbonate should be used.

The test for the correct consistency of these "silver soaps" is made by taking a sample.

This should solidify very quickly, but not so much that it can be moved on the glass (soap too strong).

If the sample is cloudy and gray in the center, the soap is too weak.

Soap Filler Solutions

Formula No. 1

Potash Carbonate Solution (15° Bé)	40 kg.
Borax	1 kg.
Potato Flour	20 kg.
Potassium Silicate (16° Bé)	7–21 kg.

Formula No. 2

Potash Carbonate (10° Bé)	10 kg.
Potato Flour	5 kg.
Potash Silicate (28–30° Bé)	10 kg.

The waterglass is added to the alkaline starch dispersion, or separately later on to the soap.

"Cold Cream" Soaps

(Lanolin & Petrolatum Soaps)

The following fat mixtures are suitable as a base for making both lanolin and petrolatum soaps:

Formula No.

1. 90 kg. of tallow, 10 kg. of coconut oil.
2. 80 kg. tallow, 18 kg. coconut oil, 2 kg. castor oil.
3. 55 kg. tallow, 10 kg. lard, 30 kg. coconut oil, 5 kg. castor oil.
4. 90 kg. palm oil, 8 kg. coconut oil, 2 kg. castor oil.
5. 50 kg. palm oil, 20 kg. olive oil, 25 kg. coconut oil, 5 kg. castor oil.

Various superfatted soaps to meet the different demands can be made according to the following directions, using soaps made from the above mixtures:

A. Petrolatum soaps which leave a protective layer on the skin after washing, creamy but low in lathering power. Mix thoroughly 95 kg. of soap base number 1 with 5 kg. of white petrolatum. If the price permits, use specially treated high grade petrolatum. This is made for use in cosmetic creams. For the cheaper grades of soap, yellow petrolatum serves the purpose. Increased skin protection and a creamy type of lather, are obtained with soaps made from tallow only, or tallow and lard, or lard and olive oil, or vegetable fats other than coconut oil. Such soaps are exceptionally mild but are suitable only for those who do not object to slow lathering, with only a small amount of lather, particularly in cold water. With the omission of emulsifying agents, the pure petroleum soaps must be worked up on cylinders which are not cooled or only slightly cooled, particularly in the beginning. Soaps which do not contain coconut oil require longer working than the others.

It is possible to obtain pure white soaps containing petroleum jelly. The degree of whiteness can be increased by the use of about 1 per cent of zinc oxide or titanium oxide. Strong perfume is not ordinarily used with these soaps. Lavender or rose or other ethereal oils compatible with use on the skin, are suitable.

B. High-content petrolatum soaps, with moderate lathering power. Mix 90 kg. of soap base number 1 with a nearly cooled melt of 8.5 kg. of white petrolatum jelly, 1 kg. of wool fat, and 0.5 kg. of cetyl alcohol. Working these together takes about the same time as in *A*.

C. High-content petrolatum soaps, with good lathering power. Mix 90 kg. of soap base number 2 with an almost cooled melt of 8 kg. of white petrolatum, 1 kg. of wool fat and 1 kg. of lanette wax (sold in America as Brilliant Avirol). The time required for working up this mixture is much less than that for *A* and *B*.

D. High-content petrolatum soaps, with relatively very good lathering power. Mix 90 kg. of soap base number 3 or 5 for about 5 minutes with 2 kg. of casein solution. Mix in an almost cooled melt of 6 kg. of petroleum jelly, 1 kg. of wool fat, and 1 kg. of Brilliant Avirol. The time for working together this mixture is about half as long as for *A* or *B* but longer than for *C*. This type of soap leaves less of a protective layer after washing, but still permits action on the skin by the fat during washing.

Toilet soaps which approach petrolatum soaps in appearance, hardness and foaming power can be produced with 2 to 3 per cent less petroleum jelly, but the cosmetic effect is less striking. The casein solution mentioned is prepared as follows: Let 1 kg. of alkali-soluble casein swell for 2 hours in 2 kg. of cold water. Dissolve 130 grams of borax in 2 kg. of hot water and stir this solution into the casein mixture. Warm until solution is complete. Let partially cool, stir in 100 grams of triethanolamine and after 5 minutes, 200 grams of castor oil fatty acids.

Lanolin soaps are prepared similarly to the petrolatum soaps. Cold process coconut oil soaps are not used. Lanolin combines with soaps more easily than petroleum jelly, decreases lathering power less, and penetrates the skin more readily in washing. The addition of 5 per cent of lanolin has no marked effect on lathering power or stability, and introduces scarcely any odor.

E. Lanolin soaps with a thick, rich lather. Mix 95 kg. of soap base number 1, 2, or 4 with 5 kg. of wool fat. To avoid loss, the perfume is added at the end of the mixing period.

F. High-content lanolin soaps with moderate lathering power, exceptionally mild. Work up 92 kg. of soap base number 1 or 4 with a luke-warm melt of 7 kg. of wool fat, 0.5 kg. of wool wax and 0.5 kg. of Brilliant Avirol.

G. High-content lanolin soaps with good lathering power. Mix 90 kg. of soap base number 3 or 5 with 2 kg. of casein solution for about 5 minutes and work in a luke-warm melt of 7 kg. of wool fat and 1 kg. of Brilliant Avirol.

High-content lanolin soaps with free cholesterol can also be prepared. Such soaps as those given above should improve the condition of the skin. There is considerable difference between the cosmetic action of these soaps and that of ordinary toilet soap with no additions of petrolatum or lanolin. Small amounts of proteins, glycerin, etc., also have a beneficial action. The production of special superfatted soaps may be of importance in counteracting the increasing tendency to replace toilet soap with cleansing creams.

Liquid Soaps (French)

Formula No. 1

Olive Oil Soap

a.	Caustic Potash	227 kg.
	Water minimum possible for solution	
b.	Olive Oil	182 kg.
	Palm Oil	362 kg.
	Coconut Oil	362 kg.

Heat to 49° C., add to *a.*

c. Alcohol 170 l.

Boil the whole under reflux (82° C.). When saponified, cool, and add

d. Water 5.6 l.

Formula No. 2

Coconut Oil Soap

a.	Soda Ash	1 kg.
	Water	10 l.
b.	Wood Ashes	15 kg.
	Water	10 l.

Extract through a tin can with holes, pouring through water 3 to 5 times.

c. Caustic Soda 50 %

1. Boil 10 to 15 min.:

a.	1 part by volume
b.	4 parts by volume
c.	6 parts by volume

Add Coconut Oil 10 parts by volume during the boiling in small parts, stir slowly. Then diminish heat, stir continuously, take off, stir, then pour into wooden forms.

2. Or: Boil 10–15 minutes:

b.	4 parts by volume
c.	6 parts by volume
Sodium Sulphate (10%)	1 part by volume
Salt	½ part by volume

Add:

Coconut Oil 9 parts by volume

and after:

Tallow 1 part by volume

Method as in No. 1. Gentle boiling, thorough stirring, dry.

Formula No. 3

Liquid Coconut Oil Soap

a.	Water	20 l.
	Caustic Potash (Solid)	6 kg.

Add *a* to

b.	Coconut Oil (49° C.)	20 kg.
c.	Alcohol	2.5 l.

Warm the whole to 82° C. under reflux as in 1. Let cool 24 hours, then add:

d.	Water	80 l.
	Sugar	very little
	Potassium Chloride	very little
	Glycerin	optional

Formula No. 4

Liquid Glycerin Soap

Soft Soap, Good	35 g.
Glycerin	21 g.
Water	7 g.
Alcohol	14 g.
Talc or Pumice	5 g.

Let stand for several days; take care to eliminate excessive alkali by adding oleic acid. Filter.

Formula No. 5

Coconut Oil	10 kg.
Oleic Acid	6 kg.
Caustic Potash (50° Bé)	7.7 kg.
Potassium Carbonate	0.3 kg.
Water, Distilled	76 kg.

Formula No. 6

Coconut or Palm Kernel Oil	12 lb.
Peanut Oil, Light	2 lb.
Castor Oil	2 lb.
Caustic Potash (50° Bé)	8 lb.
Water, Soft or Distilled	76 lb.
Perfume	0.5–1 %

If a more viscous liquid soap is wanted, use a 2% sugar solution instead of the water.

Emollient Cosmetic Wash

Triethanolamine	10.0 g.
Stearin	15.0 g.
Paraffin Oil	10.0 g.
Distilled Water	65.0 g.

Heat to 150° F. and mix vigorously.

Cleaners

Hand Cleaning Preparations

The following formulas make preparations for cleaning the hands by just using it and wiping off with a towel:

Liquid

Castor Oil	25 oz.
Caustic Potash (50%)	10 oz.
Alcohol	60 oz.

Petrol (Gasoline)	10 oz.
Water	20 oz.

Neutralize with oleic acid.

Solid

Oleic Acid	4 oz.
Turpentine Substitute	1 oz.
Alcohol	2 oz.
Castor Oil	1 oz.

Neutralize with a solution of caustic potash (1–1). Add water 2 oz. to form a paste, incorporate 15 per cent borax powder.

Hand Cleanser Paste

(Mechanics' Hand Paste)

Soft Soap	100 kg.
Ammonia, (sp. g. 0.91)	6 kg.
Tripoli, Pumice, or Other Abrasive	30 kg.
Sawdust	to desired
Turpentine	consistency

Add the ammonia to the soft soap, mixing thoroughly. Add the abrasive, the saw-dust, and finally the turpentine to obtain a paste of the desired consistency.

Water Soluble Dyes for Soap

These can be used for coloring milled, cold, semi-boiled soaps, liquid soaps and bases, shampoos, toilet waters, bath salts and emulsions.

Pink	—Rhodamine B Extra
Salmon Pink	—Rhodamine 6G Extra
Green	—Cyanine Green
Golden Yellow	—Metanil
Blue	—Alizarine Blue
Red	—Cloth Red
Amber	—Bismarck Brown
Lemon	—Fluorescein
Canary Yellow	—Tartrazine
Heliotrope	—Violamine
Violet	—Alizarine Violet

CHAPTER IX

BATH PREPARATIONS

Pine Needle Bathing Preparations

Pine needle bath milk is prepared as follows: In one process the milky consistency and appearance is secured by emulsification with soap, gum tragacanth and the like. In a second process the same effect is secured with tincture of benzoin. Other directions call for lanolin as an aid in procuring the emulsified condition.

Formula No. 1

The simplest formula calls for 2 g. eucalyptus oil, 2 g. lemon oil, 18 g. oil of silver pine, 15 g. of pine oil, 400 g. of tincture of benzoin, 8,000 g. alcohol and 3,000 g. water.

Formula No. 2

Dissolve 6 g. sodium soap in 100 g. alcohol. Triturate 10 g. of this solution with ½ g. tragacanth. To the resulting soft paste add 4 g. of pine oil plus 1 g. of juniper berry oil or any other suitable perfume compound and mix well with 12.5 g. alcohol. Emulsify with 15 g. of water and later add an additional 50–60 g. water.

Formula No. 3

Mixing equal parts of pine needle oil with sodium sulfo-ricinoleate, gives a fine concentrate to be added to the bath. The product so made is completely dispersed in the bath water. To thin it out, add either water or similar diluent.

Formula No. 4

Turkey Red Oil Neutralized with Caustic Potash	200 g.
Perfume Mixture	350 g.
Add:	
Potassium Carbonate Solution (20° Bé.)	50 g.
Clear Liquid Soap (10%)	400 g.

A higher content of etheric oils necessitates more turkey red oil and potash, and eventually terpineol.

For a thicker balm: Use only 100 g. Turkey Red, but add 100–150 g. oleic acid, and saponify the whole with caustic.

The milky character is bettered by addition of potassium stearate, triethanolamine stearate (or oleate).

Formula No. 5

Turkey Red Oil	10 oz.
Fluorescein	1/10 oz.
Pine Oil	3 oz.
Water	3 oz.

Dissolve the fluorescein in the turkey red oil; add the pine oil and when well mixed add the water, stirring until a uniform liquid results. Strain if necessary.

Formula No. 6

Potassium linseed oil soap (44% fatty acid) 30 oz.; perfume 40 oz.; alcohol 95% 30 oz.

Formula No. 7

Pine needle oil 40 oz.; sodium sulforicinoleate 40 oz.; water 20 oz. Color with fluorescein as required. Mix the perfume oil with the emulsifying agent and add the water very slowly, preferably in an emulsifying machine. More water may be added if desired and pine needle oil replaced by other perfume.

Formula No. 8

Pine needle oil or perfume 70 oz.; triethanolamine oleate 18 oz.; distilled water 160 parts. Dissolve the triethanolamine oleate in the warm perfume and add the water very slowly at the lowest possible temperature in an emulsifying machine.

Many pine needle oil preparations now marketed, do not take into account that when they are put into water the oil floats on top and only makes contact with a very small portion of the body. By using the following formula the oil is emulsified and spreads uniformly through the bath, giving the entire body the benefit of the pine needle oil.

Formula No. 9

1.	Pine Needle Oil	10 lb.
2.	Sodium Sulforicinoleate	10 lb.
3.	Water	5 lb.
4.	Fluorescein	to suit

Mix 1 and 2 until dissolved. Add 3 slowly with stirring. Add 4 and stir until dissolved.

The above formula when thrown into water disperses uniformly to give a milky green solution. Other oils may be substituted for Pine Needle Oil. If a lower cost is desired, part of the pine oil may be replaced by mineral, olive or cottonseed oil and a larger amount of water may be added.

Formula No. 10

Mineral Oil	10 g.
Pine Needle Oil	1 g.
Harcol	10 g.
Water	50–100 cc.

Mix the first three ingredients and then add the water slowly with stirring. A beautiful milk results which diffuses readily in the bath.

Formula No. 11

25 parts of pulverized borax, 25 parts of common salt, 12 parts of calcined soda, 0.05 part of fluorescein and 1½ parts of oil of silver fir. Another formula calls for 5 parts of fluorescein, 10 parts of ammonia, 25 parts of oil of pine, 25 parts of oil of silver fir, 935 parts of 95% alcohol. Uranine may be used in the place of fluorescein with the result that a greener shade is obtained.

Formula No. 12

20 parts of bath chamomille, 40 parts of peppermint leaves, 100 parts of calamus root, 60 parts of woodruff herb and 80 parts of eucalyptus leaves, the entire mixture cut up into proper form, is treated with 4,800 parts of 96% alcohol and macerated for 14 days. Mixture is filtered and residue pressed. The filtrate is mixed with 120 parts of aromatic tincture, 50 parts of oil of Siberian fir needles free from terpenes, 20 parts of pine oil, 20 parts of juniper oil, 15 parts of eau de cologne and 275 parts of pure glycerin of 28° Bé. Residue after filtration may be digested with 4,000 parts of boiling water and filtered. The two extracts are united and colored green with chlorophyll.

The use of herbs for the manufacture of bathing preparations gives excellent results. The herb extract may be made from a number of different botanicals, such as peppermint leaves, sage leaves, rosemary leaves, thyme and chamomille, which may be used in the proportion of 100 g. each. The botanicals must be used free from dust and are treated with 250 g. of 90% alcohol.

Production of this preparation is simpler and less troublesome, if a pine needle milk is prepared for direct use. The first step in the process is to prepare a 5% solution of 80% soda soap in 95% alcohol. Five g. of the finest pulverized white gum tragacanth are triturated with 100 g. of soap solution. Then 45 g. of pine needle oil and 5 g. of juniper oil dissolved in 125 g. of 95% alcohol are mixed with paste. Thereafter 550 g. of water at 30° C. are added and the mixture is agitated for long time. A thick emulsion is formed, resembling a cod liver oil emulsion. This emulsion is ready for use and can be added directly to the bath. Astringent substances such as oak bark extract may be added to the emulsion, but this must be done during the manufacturing process.

Pine Needle Balsam

Pine needle balsam is prepared as follows: 3 parts of lavender oil are mixed with 20 parts of pine needle oil, 25 parts of knee pine oil, 1,000 parts of alcohol and enough chlorophyll to give desired green color. Following formula is for pine needle balsam with approximately 50% alcohol content: 100 parts of tincture of nutgalls, are mixed with 50 parts of aromatic tincture, 50 parts of sweet spirit of niter, 20 parts of ethyl acetate, 25 parts of pine needle oil, 50 parts of knee pine oil, 5,000 parts of 95% alcohol and 5,000 parts of distilled water. Sugar color or chlorophyll may be added to color the mixture.

Pine Needle Bath Tablets

A good formula for the production of pine needle extract bath tablets is as follows: 65 g. common salt, 15 g. of borax, 17 g. true pine needle extract, 3 g. pine needle perfume oil, such as pine needle oil, bornyl acetate, oil of silver pine, oil of knee pine, rounded off with lavender oil, oil of sage, and strengthened with eucalyptus oil. About 10 to 15 g. of fluorescein are used for color.

Pine Needle Bathing Salt

Formula No. 1

a. Salt	100 kg.
b. Water, Containing 5% Uranin (Fluorescein-Sodium)	2.5 kg.
c. Sodium Carbonate, Anhydrous	2.0 kg.
d. Magnesium Carbonate	0.2 kg.
e. Pine Needle Essence	2–3 kg.

Mix *a* with *b* homogeneously, dry on a shelf and sift through a sieve, mix then with *c* and *d*, in a drum, add *e*, mix again thoroughly, fill into sealed cans.

Formula No. 2

Sodium Bicarbonate	10 g.
Starch Powder	1 g.
Tartaric Acid, Powdered	7.5 g.
Fluorescein or Uranin	0.1–0.2 g.

Formula No. 3

Sodium Chloride	70 g.
Pine Needle Extract, Genuine	18 g.
Ammonium Carbonate	10 g.
Perfume (Pine-Needle)	2 g.

Perfumed Bath Milks

A bath liquid made according to this formula will not foam. If this is desired liquid palm kernel soap should be added. Bath milk may be made as follows: Triethanolamine oleate 250 g.; glycerin 120 g.; turkey red oil 270 g.; diethylenglycol 250 g.; rose water 200 g.; color 10 g.; perfume compound 30 g. Lanolin anhydrous 64 g.; glycerin 80 g.; water 120 g.; tincture, gum benzoin 40 g.; mucilage of gum arabic 40 g. (1 g. gum arabic to 2 g. water); perfume compound 10 g.

Aromatic Bath Salts

Potassium Bromide	1 g.
Calcium Carbonate	1 g.
Sodium Sulphate	5 g.
Sodium Phosphate	8 g.
Sodium Carbonate (exsicc.)	300 g.
Lavender Oil	1 g.
Rosemary Oil	1 g.
Thyme Oil	1 g.

Use about 300 grams in each bath.

Methyl Salicylate Bath Preparations

The problem in using methyl salicylate in making bath essences and the like is to obtain the latter in such form that it is readily soluble in water and the methyl salicylate itself in a very fine dispersed emulsion. Turkey red oil, that is sulphonated castor oil, is found to be suitable for this purpose. It is used with the addition of glycerin and potassium carbonate and is obtained thereby in clear solution in water. This solution emulsifies with water without any difficulty. Eucalyptol and menthol may also be used in the place of methyl salicylate or mixed with it in various proportions. An example of a composition is as follows:

Sulphonated Castor Oil	150 g.
Methyl Salicylate	150 g.
Eucalyptol	45 g.
Menthol	5 g.
Potassium Carbonate	50 g.
Glycerin	100 g.
Water	500 g.

Effervescing Bath Salts

Another important class of bath preparations contains oxygenated salts, which release oxygen gas during the bath. Preparations that develop carbon dioxide during the bathing process are closely allied to the former and the two may be grouped together in the class of effervescent bath salts. These are the preparations that have been recommended for attaining slimness of figure.

The simplest carbon dioxide releasing preparation contains sodium acid sulphate and sodium bicarbonate. While this preparation is effective, it is by no means so effective as the mixture which contains tartaric acid or potassium bitartrate. These chemicals increase the cost of the preparation, but they are well worth while adding. They are used in the place of the sodium acid sulphate.

Formula No. 1

If 900 g. of sodium bicarbonate are used, then about 750 g. of pulverized tartaric acid or 1,200 g. of potassium acid tartrate are required. It is essential that this preparation should not react to produce carbon dioxide before it is actually used, and in order to prevent the reaction from taking place prematurely it is sufficient to add to it a water-absorbing salt, such as sodium sulphate, and about 200 g. are enough to give good results. Instead of the sodium sulphate, the same proportion of starch may be used. It is also useful to add a foaming agent so that the carbon dioxide is released in the bath in very fine bubbles. Such an agent is pulverized soap or dry crude quillaia bark extract or else a solution of casein in lye. These preparations may be used in connection with pine needle compositions as well.

Formula No. 2

A new formula for the preparation of bath salts that evolves carbon dioxide is the following: 90 g. of sodium carbonate, 75 g. of tartaric acid, 120 g. of starch, 15 g. of lemon oil and 5 drops of ionone. The oil and starch are mixed and other ingredients added and kneaded into a paste with ether. Approximately 1 g. of gum benzoin is mixed with 30 g. of ether and used for the above purpose. Mixture can be pressed into tablets which are stable due to the starch contained in them.

Formula No. 3

An effervescent pine needle bath salt preparation is made as follows: 300 g. of sodium bicarbonate, 275 g. of pulverized sodium bisulphate, 12 g. silver fir oil. Uranine is added until color is yellow. Tablets may be pressed from this mixture.

Bath salts, which evolve oxygen, are generally made with the aid of sodium perborate. A catalyst must be used in making the preparation. Thus for 1,000 g. of sodium perborate, there is required 1.4 g. of manganese dioxide or 6.7 g. of cobalt carbonate, or 40 g. of gypsum or 26.7 g. of magnesium fluoride.

Formula No. 4

An effective bath salt of this type contains 300 g. of sodium perborate and a catalyst composed of 6 g. of manganese sulphate and 9 g. of potassium bitartrate.

Formula No. 5

3 g. of sodium perborate, 4 g. of manganese sulphate, 11 g. of sodium tartrate. Pressed residues from sweet and bitter almonds can be used to good advantage as catalysts. These residues may be mixed with the dry oxygenated salts. They possess the additional property of creating a lather when the composition is dissolved in water.

Formula No. 6

400 g. of pulverized sodium biborate, 200 g. of sodium sulphate, 300 g. of sodium bicarbonate, 225 g. of tartaric acid, 50 g. of lactose, 25 g. of talc and 15 g. of oleum pinus silvertris and oleum pinus pumilio. Ingredients are mixed 2 or 3 times and passed through a fine sieve, and then the coloring matter, for example fluorescein, is added. Addition of talc and milk sugar is necessary to be able to prepare tablets possessing a certain strength and stability.

Formula No. 7

A powder of the following composition will soften the bath water and produce a stimulating effect by the evolution of carbon dioxide:—

Sodium Bicarbonate	30.6 g.
Tartaric Acid, Powdered	26.4 g.
Starch, Powdered	42.4 g.
Perfume	0.6 g.

Dry the powders and mix them thoroughly, incorporating the perfume, which may suitably consist of a mixture of essential oils of lavender, lemon, etc.

Formula No. 8

Sodium Bicarbonate	300 g.
Sodium Acid Sulphate	275 g.
Starch	25 g.

Formula No. 9

Saponin, Purified	2 g.
Starch	25 g.
Sodium Bicarbonate	90 g.
Tartaric Acid	70 g.

The stability can be increased by pressing the bicarbonate and acid separately.

Effervescent Tablets with Wetting Agents

(*Slow* Development of Carbon Dioxide)

Formula No. 10

Starch	10 g.
Sodium Lauryl Sulphonate	10 g.
Sodium Bicarbonate	46 g.
Tartaric Acid	34 g.

Formula No. 11

Sodium Bicarbonate	57 g.
Tartaric Acid	38 g.
Saponin, Purified	5 g.
Stearin, Powder	5 g.

Carbon Dioxide Baths

Formula No. 12

Ammonium Carbonate	35 g.
Sodium Bicarbonate	20 g.
Tartaric Acid	30 g.
Sodium Perborate	10 g.
Sodium Thiosulphate	3 g.
Disodium Phosphate	2 g.

Formula No. 13

Sodium Bicarbonate	42 g.
Sodium Acid Sulphate	21 g.
Starch	5 g.
Sodium Chloride, Powder	30 g.

Formula No. 14

Ammonium Carbonate	25 g.
Sodium Bicarbonate	20 g.
Tartaric Acid	25 g.
Sodium Perborate	10 g.
Rice Starch	20 g.
Manganese Nitrate	1/10 g.

Mix all components—except the perborate—dry and perfume, then add the perborate. Press in tablets.

Formula No. 15

Sodium Acid Carbonate	40 g.
Starch, Wheat	50 g.
Sodium Carbonate	10 g.
Tartaric Acid	30 g.
Kaolin, Colloidal	20 g.
Soap Powder, Concentrated	45 g.
Saponin	5 g.

Keep completely dry and sealed from air to avoid decomposition. 1–2% perfume (Lavender, Pine Needle, Eau de Cologne, Fancy), is added.

Oxygen Bathing Salt

Formula No. 1

Ammonium Carbonate, Dried	500 g.
Hydrogen Peroxide (3%)	100 g.
Urea	5 g.

Formula No. 2

Urea Hydrogen Peroxide	50–100 g.
Sodium Pyrophosphate	10 g.

Formula No. 3 (Tablets)

Sodium Perborate	800 g.
Starch	100 g.
Ammonium Carbonate	100 g.

Water-Softening "Beauty-Water"

Sodium Metaphosphate, 10% Solution	70 g.
Borax	1.5 g.
Glycerin	13.5 g.
Alcohol	14 g.
Perfume Oil	1 g.

If cloudy, filter through magnesium carbonate.

Bath Salts and Water Softeners

The most widely sold bath salts are products that are based on sodium-sesqui-carbonate. Sodium Bicarbonate and Sodium Chloride are also used.

Formula No. 1

To 100 lb. of sodium sesqui-carbonate is added a mixture of

Dye Stuff (to give desired shade)	1 oz.
Perfume Oil	12 oz.
Alcohol	1 pt.

The entire mass is mixed until the color and perfume are thoroughly dispersed.

Other bases are as follows:

2. Sodium Bicarbonate	100 lb.
3. Sodium Bicarbonate	50 lb.
or Sodium-Sesqui-Carbonate	50 lb.
4. Sodium Chloride	100 lb.

All of the above bases are colored and perfumed. Care should be taken in the selection of the crystals as regards crystal size, appearance and uniformity. In securing dye stuffs, it is necessary that the type base for which they are intended be specified.

Perfuming Bath Salts

The perfume should be diluted with 50% alcohol and sprayed uniformly over the crystals which should then be mixed to facilitate penetration and evaporation of the solvent.

Coloring Bath Salts

The requisites for colors for bath salts are fastness to alkali and light. There are two ways of coloring bath salts. One is to get the color and odor combined and use the proportions recommended by the manufacturer, generally a pound to one hundred to two hundred pounds of bath salts. For the small manufacturer this is the most practical and most convenient method. The other method is to use water or alcohol soluble colors, and add the perfume afterwards. When water soluble colors are used, the solution is made as concentrated as possible. Color some of the salt very heavily and then mix this up with the rest of the salt. This will minimize the water used. Add the perfume and then tumble or mix. The colors recommended are:

Auramine—Yellow
Tartrazine—Lemon
Acridine Orange—Orange
Chrysoidine—Tangerine
Phenylene Brown—Terra Cotta
Methylene Blue—Blue
Rhodamine—Pink
Methyl Violet—Purple
Basic Green—Green
Rose Bengale—Cerise

In mixing and packaging bath salts it is essential that it be carried out in dry air to prevent "caking."

Borated Bathing Solution

Boric Acid	10 g.
Alum, Powdered	2.5 g.
Camphor	1.5 g.
Alcohol	120.0 cc.
Water, enough to make	500.0 cc.

Bath Preparations
Liquid Toilet Ammonia
(For Bath)

Ammonium Stearate (Paste)	8 oz.
Ammonia (28°)	6 oz.
Water	50 oz.
Glycerin	2 oz.

Perfume to suit, avoiding the use of aldehydes and unstable esters.

Violet Ammonia

Ammonia Water	12 pt.
Distilled Water	28 pt.
Perfume	1 oz.
Color	enough

Perfume for the Foregoing

Anisic Aldehyde	½ dr.
Benzyl Acetate	½ dr.
Ionone	1 dr.
Coumarin	1 gr.
Bergamot Oil	15 min.
Neroli Oil	10 min.
Tincture of Musk	4 oz.

Stimulating Bathing Salt

Sodium Chloride, Powder	950 g.
Sodium Bicarbonate	50 g.
Thyme Oil	2 cc.
Bergamot Oil Terpenes	5 cc.
Orange Peel Terpenes	1 cc.
Bergamot Oil	1 cc.
Terpineol	1.5 cc.
Methyl Naphthyl Ketone	0.5 cc.

Medical Bathing Salts
Carlsbad Well

Sodium Sulphate	44 g.
Potassium Sulphate	2 g.
Sodium Chloride	18 g.
Sodium Bicarbonate	36 g.

Friedrichshall

Sodium Chloride	37.7 g.
Sodium Bromide	0.3 g.
Potassium Chloride	5 g.
Calcium Chloride	19 g.
Magnesium Chloride	37 g.
Calcium Sulphate, Precipitated	1 g.

Hallein Well

Sodium Chloride	69.3 g.
Magnesium Chloride	27 g.
Sodium Bromide	0.42 g.
Calcium Sulphate, Precipitated	10 g.
Sodium Sulphate	2.28 g.

Kreuznach

Sodium Chloride	63 g.
Potassium Chloride	75 g.
Calcium Chloride	750 g.
Magnesium Chloride	110 g.
Sodium Bromide	2 g.

Reichenhall

Potassium Chloride	6 g.
Magnesium Chloride	72 g.
Lithium Chloride	0.15 g.
Sodium Chloride	14 g.
Sodium Bromide	0.85 g.
Magnesium Sulphate	7 g.

"Saltrate Rodell"

Sodium Chloride, Powder	0.1 g.
Magnesium Carbonate	0.5 g.
Potassium Carbonate	0.1 g.
Lithium Carbonate	0.05 g.
Calcium Sulphate, Powder	0.25 g.
Borax, Powdered	10 g.
Sodium Bicarbonate	30.5 g.
Ammonium Carbonate	52.5 g.
Sodium Thiosulphate	2.5 g.
Sodium Perborate	3 g.

Vichy

Lithium Carbonate	0.01 g.
Ferrous Sulphate	0.05 g.
Manganese Sulphate	0.01 g.
Sodium Chloride	1.73 g.
Sodium Sulphate	6.2 g.
Magnesium Sulphate	2.6 g.
Calcium Chloride	6.0 g.
Sodium Bicarbonate	83.4 g.

Sulphur Baths

Formula No. 1

Potassium Sulphide	50 g.
Eau de Cologne	50 g.
Distilled Water	950 cc.

Formula No. 2

Soft Soap	250 g.
Glycerin	50 g.
Potassium Sulphide	25 g.

Formula No. 3

Sodium Thiosulphate plus Acid Bath-Water

Formula No. 4

a.	Sulphur Sublimed	50–100 g.
	Ammonium Carbonate	950–900 g.
b.	Distilled Water, Warm	650 cc.
	Potassium Chromate, Neutral	25–50 g.

Mix *a*, dissolve *b*, mix both and stir several hours, until solid. Press and grind; 120 g. used for a bath.

Formula No. 5

(Bain de la Parisienne)

Sodium Bicarbonate	870 g.
Magnesium Carbonate	10 g.
Sulphur Flowers, Ground	100 g.
Sulphur, Precipitated	20 g.
Selenic Acid	0.1 g.

Preparations for Sulphur Baths

Powder

Sulphur, Colloidal	18 g.
Glauber's Salt	20 g.
Sodium Carbonate	50 g.
Starch	8 g.
Turpentine	4 g.

Liquid

Liver of Sulphur *	28 g.
Glycerin	8 g.
Alcohol	50 g.
Turpentine	10 g.
Pine Needle Perfume	4 g.

* Made by melting potassium carbonate with sulphur; yields colloidal sulphur with acid.

Ocean-Water, Artificial

Dry mixture of

Sodium Chloride	75 g.
Potassium Chloride	4 g.
Magnesium Chloride	10 g.
Calcium Sulphate	5 g.
Magnesium Sulphate	6 g.

Make up a 3.5% solution of this mixture in water.

Ocean Bathing Salt

(1000 g. per Bath)

Potassium Iodide	1 g.
Potassium Bromide	0.55 g.
Lithium Carbonate	0.05 g.
Manganese Sulphate	0.01 g.
Ferrous Sulphate	0.01 g.
Potassium Chloride	15 g.

Calcium Chloride	40	g.
Magnesium Sulphate	66.38	g.
Magnesium Chloride	96	g.
Sodium Chloride	781	g.

Perfumed Artificial Sea Salt

Potassium Chloride	1	oz.
Magnesium Chloride	6	oz.
Calcium Sulphate	1	oz.
Sodium Chloride	2	dr.
Coumarin	1	dr.
Alcohol	6	dr.

Sulphur in proper physical state in toilet waters is claimed to be highly useful for keeping skin in good condition and also for treatment of acne and other common skin troubles. To obtain sulphur in proper condition in such preparations, mix:

Borax	5	g.
Water	850	g.

add:

Sodium Thiosulphate	50	g.
Glycerin	50	g.

then add:

Eau de Cologne	50	g.

Sulphur is said to be present in nascent state. When used, the sulphur is precipitated on skin and its action is most effective under such circumstances.

Steel (Iron) Baths

Formula No. 1

Iron Tartrate	100	g.
Distilled Water	900	cc.

Formula No. 2

Iron Sulphate, Pure	30–60	g.
Potassium Carbonate, Pure	120	g.

Formula No. 3

Iron Sulphate	30	g.
Salt	60	g.
Sodium Bicarbonate	20	g.

Mud Bath Salt

Ferrous Sulphate	900	g.
Calcium Sulphate, Precipitated	20	g.
Magnesium Sulphate	20	g.
Sodium Sulphate	40	g.
Ammonium Sulphate	20	g.

Optional, Dry Mud Earth.

Bath Powders

Formula No. 1

Use a mixture of equal parts of sodium bicarbonate and borax.

Formula No. 2

Powdered Borax	1	lb.
Ammonium Chloride	2	oz.
Synthetic Violet	2	dr.
Synthetic Heliotrope	2	dr.

Colloidal Bath

Sodium Bicarbonate	125	g.
Corn Starch	125	g.
Water, at about 96° F.	75,000	cc.

Use about one cupful of soda and starch to a tubful water.

Low-Priced Oxygen Foot-Bathing Powder

Formula No. 1

Soda Ash	50	kg.
Sodium Bicarbonate	30	kg.
Soap, Powdered	10	kg.
Sodium Perborate	10	kg.

High-Quality Oxygen Foot-Bathing Powder

Formula No. 2

Powdered Soap	25	kg.
Borax	15	kg.
Sodium Bicarbonate	30	kg.
Sodium Perborate	30	kg.

Perfume: per 1 kg. of powder use

Pine Needle Oil, Siberian	5	g.
Pinus Montana Oil	4	g.
Bergamot Oil	1	g.
Lemon Oil	1	g.
Eucalyptus Oil	0.5	g.
Coumarin	0.5	g.

For the cheap powder use the same amount of perfume for 2 kg.

Foot-Bath Powders (or Tablets) with Perborate

	Formula No. 1	Formula No. 2
Sodium Perborate	170 g.	180 g.
Boric Acid, Powder	70 g.	60 g.
Borax, Powder	50 g.	—
Sodium Acid Carbonate	250 g.	200 g.
Perfume	5–10 g.	—

Tablet or powder doses for each bath should weigh 10–20 g.

CHAPTER X

HAIR PREPARATIONS

Shampoos

SHAMPOOS are used to clean the hair and leave it in a pleasing and workable condition. Most shampoos consist chiefly of coconut oil soap with or without other minor ingredients. Soapless shampoos are divided into two classes. The first is based on neutralized sulphonated vegetable oils. They are not truly soapless but because they do not lather they are termed "soapless." The second consists of neutralized sulphated higher fatty alcohols or glyceryl or glycol esters of fatty acids.

Shampoo

Formula No. 1

Castile Soap, Powdered	50 g.
Potassium Carbonate	10 g.
Bay Oil	5–8 drops
Hot (Distilled) Water	300 cc.
Alcohol	100 cc.
Water (Distilled) enough to make	500 cc.

Dissolve the potassium carbonate and soap in the hot water, add the alcohol in which the oil has been dissolved. Shake well and make up to 500 cc. with distilled water. Filter when cold and color with chlorophyll or Butter Color.

Formula No. 2

Oleic Acid	55 lb.
Cocoanut Fatty Acids	40 lb.
Triethanolamine	50 lb.
"Carbitol"	55 lb.
Perfume	1 lb.

The product prepared in this way is a liquid soap of a clear red color, which can be diluted with water to any desired consistency or concentration. Glycerin and/or alcohol may replace in whole or in part the "Carbitol."

Formula No. 3

90 kg. castor oil are mixed at 50 to 60° C. with 5 kg. castor oil fatty acids, followed, after complete incorporation, by 1·8 to 2 kg. of triethanolamine. Addition of alcohol reduces the viscosity of the preparation, but this is not advisable with other oils.

Formula No. 4

Coconut Oil, Cochin	25 g.
Castor Oil	25 g.
Caustic Potash (35° Bé)	36 g.
Alcohol	5 g.
Glycerin	25 g.
Sugar	5 g.
Water	100 g.

Melt the coconut oil in a steam-jacketed kettle, add the castor oil. When the mass is about 70° C., add at once the potash and the glycerin, stir thoroughly, and add the water in *small portions.* At the same time, heat gently. The water should be added in small quantities, stopping the addition every time until the emulsification is completed.

When all water has been added, keep stirring and take up to a boil. At this point shut the steam off and stop the stirring (precautions are necessary to prevent boiling over.)

When the boil is over again try to heat. If there is no tendency to rise in the kettle, the saponification is over. Test pH (if necessary, make neutral by adding some boric acid), when cooled. Alcohol and sugar should be added then.

Finish by adding anthrasol (1–2%)

or chamomile extract (2–3%). Filter after some days.

Formula No. 5

Coconut Oil	21 kg.
Castor Oil	10 kg.
Caustic Potash (50° Bé)	15 kg.
Water	140 kg.
Sugar	15 kg.
Perfume	to suit
Alcohol, if desired	about 5 %

Work as in formula No. 4. If the soap is too sharp, one can use Turkey Red oil in water (1:2) instead of boric acid.

Formula No. 6

Potash Soft Soap	50 g.
Potassium Carbonate	5 g.
Glycerin	7 g.
Benzaldehyde	0.25 g.
Distilled Water	938 cc.

The procedure is to dissolve the soft soap, with gentle heating, in half the water. The potash, glycerin and benzaldehyde are incorporated in the rest of the water. After the two solutions have been well mixed by stirring, the finished product is left for a week before decanting, filtering and bottling. At first the perfume will be found to disappear, owing to the splitting up of the benzaldehyde into sodium benzoate and benzyl alcohol—but after the lapse of some days the characteristic almond odor will reappear, owing to the oxidation of the alcohol back to the aldehyde.

In the above formula, the soap content may naturally be increased if desired—also a proportion of alcohol may be added. Instead of the almond perfume imparted above, a stable fougère or similar compound can be employed. Likewise pine tar, or a 10% solution of henna, may be incorporated in the case of antiseptic or liquid henna shampoos respectively. Novel ingredients for imparting a pleasantly "medicated" odor include iso-thymol.

In the manufacture of liquid soap shampoos, careful control at all points is essential. Turbidity must at all costs be avoided, and for this reason distilled water only should be used and the soap itself completely saponified. Unless proper facilities are available for saponification on the premises, it is better to purchase a ready-made soft soap base (carefully standarized examples of which are now on the market).

Shampoos should, in certain cases, be aged for even longer than a week (e.g., 15 to 30 days), then decanted into a tank fitted with a refrigerating coil, chilled to a low temperature and finally filtered through asbestos. It has been suggested that the period of aging can be radically reduced by first running the shampoo through a colloid mill or homogenizer.

Olive Oil Shampoo

Formula No. 1

Olive Oil	4 lb.
Oleic Acid	8 lb.
Cocoanut Oil	8 lb.
Caustic Potash	5 lb.
Alcohol	3 pt.
Water to Make	10 gal.

Dissolve the caustic potash in water. Mix and heat the oils to 120° F. Pour in the alkali solution and stir until saponified. Add two pints of the alcohol and heat to 180° F. Meanwhile prepare the following mixture and add foregoing

Glycerin	16 oz.
Borax	16 oz.
Potassium Carbonate	8 oz.
Oleic Acid	1 oz.

Dissolve the oleic acid in one pint of alcohol. Dissolve borax and potassium carbonate in glycerin with heat, mix thoroughly and add oleic solution. Add this mixture to soap base while still quite hot. Transfer to a refrigerating tank the day after soap has been finished, refrigerate to 40° F., filter and fill at once.

Olive Oil Shampoo (Hot Process)

Formula No. 2

Olive Oil	9.6 g.
Palm Kernel oil	5.4 g.
Coconut Oil	8.0 g.
Caustic Potash, (85%)	4.8 g.
Caustic Soda, (85%)	1.2 g.
Alcohol	2.8 g.
Water	67.2 g.
Perfume	1.0 g.

Dissolve alkalies in one-third of the water. Heat the oils to 130° F. Pour in alkali solution in a thin cream, and continue mixing until the temperature reaches 160° F. Remove from heat and allow to stand overnight. Add the alcohol, perfume, and rest of the water. Age, chill to 32° F., and filter.

Almond Oil Shampoo (Hot Process)

Almond Oil	5 g.
Palm Kernel oil	13 g.
Sesame Oil	12 g.
Caustic Potash, (85%)	6 g.
Caustic Soda, (85%)	1 g.
Alcohol	5 g.
Water	57 g.
Perfume	1 g.

Melt the almond and sesame at 120° F., shut off the heat and mix in palm kernel oil. Dissolve the alkalies in boiling water, half the total amount, and allow to cool until lukewarm. Pour alkalies into oils and stir until saponified. Add the alcohol and perfume, stir until mixed. Allow to stand overnight, and add the rest of the water. Age, chill to 32° F., and filter.

Coconut Oil Shampoo

Coconut Oil	8 lb.
Olive Oil	2 lb.
{Caustic potash	2 lb.
{Water	2 lb.
Water	8 lb.

Shampoo Lotion

Saponin	2 g.
Alcohol	15 cc.
Water sufficient to make	100 cc.
Perfume and colouring matter	to suit

Pine Tar Shampoo

Pine Tar Shampoo can be made by adding a small proportion of solution of coal tar and pine oil to a good shampoo liquid. The following formula serves as a base for the shampoo liquid:

Formula No. 1

Potassium Carbonate	12 oz.
Water	320 oz.
Alcohol	480 oz.
Dry Extract of Quassia	1 oz.
Saponin	2 dr.

Formula No. 2

Pine Tar	25 oz.
Yellow Soft Soap	300 oz.
Industrial Spirit	200 oz.
Water	475 oz.

Non-Alkaline Tar-Shampoo

Wood Tar	7.5 oz.
Triethanolamine	30.0 oz.
Oleic Acid	60.0 oz.
Alcohol, Denatured	15.0 oz.
Water	185.0 oz.

Egg Shampoo

Prepare just before use.

Separate the yolks and whites of four or more eggs in separate bowls. To the yolks add a tablespoonful of cold water and beat until uniform with an egg-beater. Wash off the beater and beat the whites until fluffy and firm. Add the beaten yolks to the whites and fold the former into the latter. The hair is washed and rinsed with lukewarm water. Then work the egg shampoo, a little at a time, into the scalp and hair. Finally wash and rinse the hair with a strong spray of tepid (not hot) water.

Bay Rum Shampoo

White Castile Soap	½ oz.
Rose Water	1 oz.
Solution of Ammonia	1 oz.
Bay Rum	2 oz.
Distilled Water to make	2 pt.

Dissolve the soap in 30 oz. of water by heating; cool to about 100° F., and add the rest of the ingredients.

Hair Washes

Formula No. 1—Soap Paste

Soap, Good Quality	225 g.
Water	340 g.
Glycerin	120 g.
Perfume	to suit

Dissolve the soap in the (hot) water with cautious stirring (to avoid foaming). When homogeneous, add glycerin and perfume. Let stand. Before filling into containers mix the paste thoroughly.

Instead of perfume, menthol, colloidal sulphur, anthrasol (purified tar), or chamomile extract is often employed.

Formula No. 2—Soap Paste

Soap	750 g.
Water	1500 g.
Borax	150 g.
Potash Carbonate	100 g.
Glycerin	150 g.

Prepare the alkali-solution 24 hours beforehand, let stand and allow to settle. The clear solution is heated, and the soap (powder or a toilet soap which is still warm) is dissolved in it. Glycerin is added to the smooth soap solution.

Perfume: Lavender, Eau de Cologne.

Hair Wash

Liquid Soap	90–95 oz.
Triethanolamine Laurate	10–5 oz.
Alcohol	10–5 oz.

Hair Washing Soaps

Formula No. 1 (for Oily Scalp)

Coconut Oil	11,000 g.
Castor Oil	4,750 g.
Caustic Potash (50%)	about 7,515 g.
Distilled or Softened Water	76,000 cc.
Perfume, or Chamomile Extract, or Wood Tar, Pure, or Better Perfume Blended with Extract	500– 2,000 cc.

Formula No. 2

Coconut Oil	11,000 g.
Olive Oil	4,750 g.
Caustic Potash (50%)	about 7,520 g.
Distilled or Softened Water	76,000 cc.
Perfume or Extract	500– 2,000 cc.

Formula No. 3 (for Dry Scalp)

Coconut Oil	15,000 g.
Olive Oil	6,000 g.
Caustic Potash (50%)	10,200 g.
Glycerin	10,000 g.
Alcohol	6,000 cc.
Distilled or Softened Water	53,000 cc.
Perfume or Extract	500– 2,000 cc.

Milky Hair Wash (Kerosene)

Formula No. 1

1. Trihydroxyethylamine Stearate	10 lb.
2. Kerosene	150 lb.
3. Pine Oil	6 lb.
4. Water	250 lb.

Heat Nos. 1 and 2 to 140° F. and stir until dissolved; then stir in No. 3. Now allow No. 4 to run in slowly while stirring. If the pine oil is objectionable, however, any other oil may be substituted for it. It may be colored beautifully by means of any water-soluble dye free from salt.

Formula No. 2

1. Savolin	10 lb.
2. Kerosene	150 lb.
3. Pine Oil	6 lb.
4. Water	250 lb.

Heat Nos. 1 and 2 to 140° F and stir until dissolved; then stir in No. 3. Now allow No. 4 to run in slowly while stirring. If the pine oil is objectionable, however, any other oil may be substituted for it. It may be colored beautifully by means of any water-soluble dye free from salt.

"Oil-Hair Wash"

Formula No. 1

Diethylaminoethyloleyl Citrate	15 g.
Chamomile Extract	1 cc.
Lemon Juice	2 cc.
Water, Distilled, or Alcohol (50%)	81.5 cc.

Formula No. 2

Rape Seed Oil	50 cc.
Hazelnut Oil	30 cc.
Spike Lavender Oil	5 cc.

Hair Wash for Dry Hair

Formula No. 1

An ethanol amine-stearic acid emulsion of castor oil is used with the sulphonated alcohol soap to prevent excessive drying of the hair.

Formula No. 2

Glyceryl Oleate	15 oz.
Deodorized Kerosene	35 oz.
Perfume	to suit

Mix together and add slowly with stirring

Water	50 oz.

"Crudol" Hair Wash

Crude Petroleum (Pennsylvania)	900 g.
Oleic Acid	50 g.

Mix and neutralize with ammonium carbonate.

Powdered Shampoo Mixtures

Powdered shampoos can be prepared by drying soap stock and mixing to a fine powder with other ingredients, according to the formulas.

Formula No. 1

Soap Powder	60 g.
Coconut Oil Soap Powder	10 g.
Disodium Phosphate	10 g.
Sodium Bicarbonate	10 g.
Borax	10 g.

Formula No. 2

Soap Powder	50 g.
Sodium Lauryl Sulphate	15 g.
Sodium Bicarbonate	5 g.
Borax	30 g.

Formula No. 3

Soap Powder	65 g.
Sodium Cetyl Sulphonate	5 g.
Borax	10 g.
Sodium Bicarbonate	15 g.
Trisodium Phosphate (powd.)	5 g.

A second method of preparation is to add the ingredients to the soap mixture before it is sent to the cooling press, as with the following:

Formula No. 4

Soap from the Kettle	75 g.
Protein or Gall Soap	3 g.
Borax	12 g.
Sodium Bicarbonate	10 g.

Formula No. 5

Soap	60 g.
Sodium Lauryl Sulphate	10 g.
Sodium Bicarbonate	20 g.
Borax	10 g.

Formula No. 6

Castile Soap, Powdered	35 g.
Coconut Oil Soap, Powdered	10 g.
Sodium Sesquicarbonate	45 g.
Borax	10 g.
Perfume	to suit

If, as is frequently the case, the materials are purchased in powdered form manufacture reduces itself to the two simple operations of perfuming and mixing. The perfume is best incorporated by the process of rubbing it down with part of the borax. A mixing machine does the rest. The powder may be sifted, if this is thought advisable, though it is not actually imperative.

Formula No. 7

Sodium sesquicarbonate, a compound intermediate in character between sodium carbonate and sodium bicarbonate, is the alkali par excellence for incorporation in shampoo powders. It may be used in quite large proportions. Forty per cent of soap, 50 per cent of sodium sesquicarbonate, and 10 per cent of borax form a good combination.

Shampoo Powder

Formula No. 8

Castile Soap, Powdered	35 g.
Coconut Oil Soap, Powdered	8 g.
Sulphonated Lorol	22 g.
Sodium Sesquicarbonate	35 g.
Perfume	to suit

Formula No. 9

Sulphonated Alcohol or Wetanol	40 g.
Borax	40 g.
Sodium Sesquicarbonate	20 g.

This gives an excellent lather.

Many such additions will suggest themselves to those who wish to experiment. Some include a specially prepared saponin, 2 to 5%, to help the lather-producing properties.

Formula No. 10

Cocoanut Oil Soap Powder	30 g.
Sodium Carbonate Monohydrated	45 g.
Borax	25 g.
Henna Leaves, Powdered	trace
Aniline Yellow	trace
Perfume	to suit

Mix together and sift. Keep in closed containers.

Henna Shampoo Powder

Castile Soap	33 g.
Coconut Oil Soap	7 g.
Sulphated Fatty Alcohol	20 g.
Sodium Sesquicarbonate	33 g.
Egyptian Henna Powder	7 g.
Perfume	0.5 g.

As the sulphated alcohol is most effective, it is also possible to make good shampoo powders containing about 20 or 30 per cent of this constituent plus a filler. Alternatively sulphated alcohol may be used alone, save for perfume, and, if desired, chamomile or henna powder. For example, the following simple formula yields a chamomile shampoo powder of superlative quality:

Chamomile Shampoo Powder

German Chamomile, Powdered	20 g.
Sulphated Fatty Alcohol	80 g.
Perfume	1 g.

In using this powder, the quantity should be reduced to about one-third of that generally employed with a shampoo powder of the ordinary type.

Perfume for Chamomile Shampoos

Chamomile Oil	100 g.
Lemon Oil	200 g.
Bergamot Oil	200 g.

Use 250–350 g. of this composition for 100 kg. soap. Use terpeneless oils.

Soapless Shampoo

Formula No. 1

75% Sulphonated Castor Oil	50 oz.
Warm water	50 oz.
Perfume to suit.	

Formula No. 2

75% Sulphonated Castor Oil	45 oz.
Sulphated Higher Alcohol	5 oz.
Water	50 oz.
Perfume to suit.	

This will lather to a limited extent. Warm the water and dissolve the alcohol before adding the sulphonated oil.

Formula No. 3

75% Sulphonated Olive Oil	40 oz.
White Mineral Oil	20 oz.
Water	40 oz.
Oleic acid to clear	
Perfume to suit.	

Mix the sulphonated olive oil and mineral oil when warm, add water, stir thoroughly and if not clear add oleic acid slowly until it clears. This can also be varied by using less mineral oil and thus eliminate the oleic acid.

Formula No. 4

75% Sulphonated Castor Oil		75 cc.
75% Sulphonated Olive Oil		25 cc.
White Mineral Oil		20 cc.
Water		100 cc.
Oleic acid	to clear	to 3 cc.

Mix and agitate thoroughly while warm.

Formula No. 5

Sapamine Acetate	20 g.
Boric Acid	0.5 g.
Perfume	0.5 g.
Water	79 cc.

Enzymes are supposed to have a certain emulsifying and purifying action. Shampoos containing enzymes are as follows:

Formula No. 6

Soap Powder	80 g.
Sodium Bicarbonate	10 g.
Borax	8 g.
Pancreatin	2 g.

(Maximal enzyme action at 40° C. and pH 7.8–8.0)

Formula No. 7

Sodium Lauryl Sulphate	63 g.
Sodium Phosphate	5 g.
Sodium Bicarbonate	20 g.
Powdered Borax	10 g.
Pancreatic Lipase	2 g.

These preparations are quite stable in dry form, but enzyme activity causes deterioration in solution. Dry shampoos may be rubbed into the hair and then brushed out, without the use of water. They consist largely of starch, as in the following:

Formula No. 7

Rice Starch (defatted)	94 g.
Sodium Bicarbonate	1 g.
Powdered Borax	5 g.

Formula No. 8

Powdered Silica Gel	10 g.
Defatted Starch	85 g.
Powdered Trisodium Phosphate	5 g.

Formula No. 9

Deodorized Kerosene	100 oz.
Diglycol Laurate (neutral)	80 oz.
"Carbitol"	20 oz.
Mineral Oil	100 oz.

This gives a waterless, concentrated, truly soapless shampoo free from alkali. Because it is so concentrated it must be used as follows: pour a little water into the palm of the hand and then rub in a little of the above liquid until it turns to a milky liquid. Wash hair in usual way, first wetting it thoroughly. No foam or lather will be formed but the cleaning efficiency is far superior to all shampoos tested. In addition it leaves the hair glossy and does not produce brittleness like most shampoos.

Formula No. 10

1. Turkey Red Oil	10 lb.
2. Mineral Oil	10 lb.
3. White Oleic Acid	10 lb.
4. Alcohol	2–10 lb.
5. Perfume	4 oz.

Formula No. 11

1. Sulfo Turk "A"	10 lb.
2. Mineral Oil	10 lb.
3. White Oleic Acid	10 lb.
4. Alcohol	2–10 lb.

Mix the above materials in the order given. If desired, the cast can be reduced further by adding an additional amount of water. The water should be added carefully with stirring. The addition of water should be stopped just before a cloudiness appears.

These shampoos are used by pouring a little into the hand and rubbing to a creamy consistency with water and then applying to the hair which must be wet.

Formula No. 12

Sulfonated Olive Oil, concentrated	40 g.
Sulfonated Castor Oil, concentrated	10 g.
White Mineral Oil	15 cc.
Water	35 g.
25% Solution of Caustic Soda to Clear	

Mix all the ingredients with the exception of the caustic soda, warm to 45–50° C. and add enough of the caustic soda solution (1 or 2%) until the mixture turns bright. Perfume as desired.

Formula No. 13

Saponin	10
Water	900
Alcohol	100
Perfume	15

Formula No. 14

"Wetanol" (Wetting Out Agent)	450 g.
Mineral Oil	50 g.
Alcohol	300 g.
Water	to make 1 l.

Formula No. 15

Saponin	2 g.
Rose Water (Diluted)	80 g.
Perfume	1 g.
Alcohol	15 g.
Water (Distilled) to make	100 cc.

To prepare this lotion, the saponin should be dissolved in the rose water, the alcohol containing the perfume added, and the mixture made up to the requisite volume with distilled water. It may be tinted yellow with a trace of tartrazine. Distilled water can be substituted for rose water, and a little phenyl ethyl alcohol added.

Soapless Shampoo Powder

Borax	25 oz.
Sodium Bicarbonate	25 oz.
Soda Ash	48 oz.
Saponin	2 oz.

Non-Lathering Hair Cleanser

Ammonium Stearate (Paste)	30 oz.
Water	2 oz.
Perfume	to suit

This is made cold by simple mixing until homogeneous and until most of ammonia has evaporated.

Hair Tonics

Hair tonics are used not because they will grow hair but because of their stimulating and exhilirating effects. Some are also used because of their odor and hair grooming properties.

Hair Tonics

Formula No. 1

Deodorized Castor Oil	10 oz.
Alcohol (Specially Denatured)	90 oz.
Perfume to suit (flower type)	

Dissolve the oil in the alcohol and add the perfume.

Formula No. 2

Alcohol	10 gal.
Castor Oil	7 gal.
Quinine Ricinoleate	1 lb.
Perfume Oil	1 lb.

Formula No. 3

Tannic Acid	0.5 g.
Salicylic Acid	1.0 g.
Castor Oil	24.5 g.
Resorcinol Monoacetate	5.0 g.
Alcohol	69.0 g.
Perfume	sufficient

Formula No. 4

Quinine	1 g.
Resorcin	3 g.
Glycerin	15 cc.
Alcohol	450 cc.
Distilled Water	450 cc.
Bay Oil	5 drops

Dissolve quinine, resorcin and oil in the alcohol. Add the water with the glycerin. Mix and filter through diatomaceous earth and color with 1 cc. congo red solution.

Formula No. 5

Salicylic Acid	8 g.
Castor Oil	4 cc.
Alcohol	300 cc.

Color with 1 or 2 drops of a saturated aqueous solution of basic fuchsin.

Hair Tonic—Dry Scalp

Castor Oil	1 gal.
Crude Carbolic Acid 30%	8 oz.
Cresol U. S. P.	3 oz.
Lignol	1 gal.
Soya Bean Oil	2 gal.
Precipitated Sulphur	2 oz.

Procedure: Mix the soya bean oil, the castor oil heat to 100° F. and add the lignol. Take a small quantity of this mixture and rub up precipitated sulphur into a smooth paste. Mix with rest of oils. Add carbolic and cresol.

Dry scalp is often a diseased condition, accompanied by dandruff. Often it is caused by poor circulation of blood. Above preparation should be rubbed into scalp at night, and, because odor is obnoxious, shampooed out in morning. Label should contain a statement to the effect that the longer the preparation is left on the better will results be.

Hair Tonic—Oily Scalp

Water	15 gal.
Glycerin	2 gal.
Alcohol	30 gal.
Menthol	7 lb.
Resorcin Monoacetate	8 oz.
Perfume	sufficient

Dissolve menthol and perfume in alcohol, mixing rapidly. Add glycerin and 10 gallons of water. Dissolve resorcin monoacetate in rest of water, add to the above and mix for three hours. Allow to stand overnight and filter.

Bay Rum

(High Grade)

Bay Oil	5 cc.
Pimento Oil	1 cc.
Orange Oil	1 cc.
Alcohol	400 cc.
Water	400 cc.
West India (Santa Cruz) Rum	200 cc.

Dissolve the oils in the alcohol, add the rum, then the water, and, after a few hours, filter. No coloring is needed.

If a "stronger" article is wanted, the amount of bay oil may be increased to 6 cc.; and if the price of Santa Cruz rum is too high, one-half the amount directed may be replaced by diluted alcohol.

Hair Tonic, Foaming

Carbonate of Potash	½ oz.
Borax	½ oz.
Dissolve in water	2 gal.
Then add:	
Glycerin	1 pt.
Ethyl Alcohol	1⅞ gal.
Hair Tonic Perfume Oil	1 oz.
Tint to suit.	

Quinine Hair Tonic

Formula No. 1

Glycerin	1.00 g.
Borax	0.20 g.
Tincture Cantharides	0.40 g.
Quinine Bisulphate	0.10 g.
Alcohol	25.00 cc.
Water	73.30 cc.
Perfume, Color	to suit

Formula No. 2

Eau De Quinine	1	oz.
Tincture of Cantharides	1	oz.
Alcohol	.7	gal.
Red Vegetable Color	24	min. or to suit
Water		to make one gal.

Eau de Quinine Hair Tonic

Formula No. 1

Quinine Hydrochloride	30	g.
Salicylic Acid	.25	oz.
Glycerin	4	oz.
Resorcin	4	oz.
Alcohol	52	oz.
Perfume and Color		
Water to make	1	gal.

Formula No. 2

Tincture of Cantharidin	6	oz.
Quinine Hydrochloride	1	oz.
Tincture of Capsicum	2	oz.
Glycerin	3	oz.
Bay Rum	6	gal.
Tincture of Cudbear		sufficient to color

Formula No. 3

Alcohol	600	g.
Water	400	g.
Quinine Sulphate	5	g.
Saponin	1	g.
Saffron Tincture	2	g.
Orseille (Red Dye)	0.2	g.
Rose Oil	2	g.
Musk, Tincture	1	g.
Lemon Oil	1	g.

Hair Tonic, Cholesterol

Formula No. 1

Alcohol	75	g.
Glycerin	5	g.
Cholosterol	1	g.
Lecithin	1	g.
Distilled Water	12	cc.
Perfume	1	g.
Chloroform	5	g.

Dissolve lecithin in chloroform, add cholosterol and one gallon of alcohol. Mix the perfume with the alcohol, add the glycerin, add the lecithin-cholosterol mixture, agitate for one hour add the water and agitate for two hours. Allow to stand over night and filter.

Formula No. 2

Cholesterol	10	g.
Mineral Oil	50	g.

Heat to 130° F.

Sodium Choleate	5	g.
Glycerin	50	g.

Heat to 130° F. and add to above slowly with agitation.

Then add slowly with agitation a solution of

Borax	5	parts
Water	1000	parts

That has been heated to 130° F. Stir until cold.

Formula No. 3

A much more stable lotion results by replacing the mineral oil in Formula No. 2 with

Lanolin	10	g.
Peanut Oil	10	g.
Cocoa Butter	30	g.
Preservative	1	g.

Castor Oil Hair Tonic

Mercuric Chloride	1	g.
Spirit of Formic Acid	200	cc.
Bergamot Oil	4	cc.
Resorcinol Mono Acetate	50	cc.
Castor Oil	50	cc.
Alcohol	to make 1000	cc.

Hair Tonic, Honey and Flower

Orange Oil	2	oz.
Lemon Oil	1	oz.
Bergamot Oil	½	oz.
Castor Oil	10	oz.
Honey	1	oz.
Clove Oil	1	dr.
Lavender	2	dr.
Geraniol	2	dr.
Coumarin	1	dr.
Synthetic Musk	½	dr.
Mineral Oil	1	gal.
Industrial Methylated Spirit	2	gal.

Hair Lotion

Formula No. 1

Diglycol Laurate	20 oz.
Isohol (or Specially Denatured Alcohol)	80 oz.
Perfume	as required
Spirit Soluble Dye	as required

Dissolve the diglycol laurate in the isohol or alcohol. Add perfume. If color is to be added, dissolve in the isohol first.

This product will wash off completely in cold water. It makes the hair lustrous and REDUCES BRITTLENESS.

Formula No. 2

Mercuric Chloride	1 oz.
Salicylic Acid	5 oz.
Chloral Hydrate	5 oz.
Glycerin	25 oz.
Acetone	10 oz.
Alcohol	200 oz.
Water	825 oz.
Perfume	to suit

Formula No. 3

One part cholesterin, 0.3 part lecithin in 200 parts of 96% alcohol and mixed with 3 parts castor oil.

Formula No. 4

0.5 part oxyquinoline sulfate and 0.2 part salicylic acid in 75 parts 96% alcohol is added and mixture made up to 300 parts by weight.

Cholesterol Hair Lotion

Alcohol	89 cc.
Cholesterol	0.5 g.
Glycerin	3 g.
Water, Distilled	6.5 cc.
Perfume	to suit

Hair Lotion for Baldness

Tannic Acid	2 g.
Alcohol (70%)	150 g.
Glycerin	50 g.
Eau de Cologne	10 g.

For scurf and falling of the hair. Apply daily by means of a sponge.

Martindale's Formula

Pilocarpine Nitrate	2 gr.
Quinine Hydrochloride	8 gr.
Glycerin	2 dr.
Rose Water	6 dr.

If required, tincture of cantharidin (1 dr.) may be added.

Children's Hair Lotion

Stavesacre Seed	1 dr.
Quinine Sulphate	1 gr.
Dilute Acetic Acid	24 min.
Glycerin	24 min.
Sassafras Oil	1 min.
Distilled Water	to 1 gr.

Boil the seed with the acid and 1 oz. of water for an hour, cool, strain, add remaining ingredients and make up to 1 oz.

Powdered Pyrethrum Flowers	11 oz.
Quassia (No. 40 Powder)	1 lb.
Powdered Stavesacre Seed	3 oz.
Glacial Acetic Acid	16 oz.
Lemon Oil	2 dr.
Industrial Methylated Spirit	to 1 gal.

Mix the powders and then macerate with the acetic acid and some of the spirit for 24 hours. Transfer to a percolator and percolate with sufficient industrial spirit to make 1 gal.

Chypre Head Lotion

Geraniol, C.P.	1.4 cc.
Cedar Wood Oil, Rectified	0.25 cc.
Benzyl Acetate, Chlorine-Free	0.6 cc.
Hydroxycitronellal, C.P. (100%)	0.7 cc.
Storax Oil	0.25 cc.
Geranium Oil, Réunion	0.6 cc.
Benzyl Benzoate	2.5 cc.
Linalyl Acetate	0.8 cc.
Linalool, Extra	1.2 cc.
Anise Aldehyde	0.1 cc.
Iris Oil, Genuine, Concrete	0.05 cc.
Coumarin	0.15 g.
Civet, Genuine (100%)	0.02 g.
Patchouli Oil, Genuine	0.2 cc.
Musk, Artificial, Ambrette	0.2 g.
Musk, Artificial, Ketone	0.05 g.
Labdanum Extract	0.15 cc.
Vanillin	0.13 g.
Phenylethyl Alcohol	0.6 cc.
Rosemary Oil	0.05 cc.
Alcohol	670 cc.
Distilled Water	320 cc.

Scalp Tonics

Formula No. 1

Resorcinol Mono Acetate	1 dr.
Cologne Water	2 dr.
Alcohol	2½ oz.
Distilled Water	to make 4 oz.

Formula No. 2

Resorcinol Mono Acetate	1½ dr.
Salicylic Acid	½ dr.
Tincture of Cantharides	1 dr.
Castor Oil	1½ dr.
Alcohol (85%)	to make 4 oz.

Formula No. 3

Resorcinol Mono Acetate	2 dr.
Bichloride of Mercury	2 gr.
Castor Oil	2 gr.
Alcohol (85%)	to make 8 oz.

Formula No. 4

Resorcinol Mono Acetate	1 dr.
White Petrolatum	1 oz.

Dandruff Treatment

This complaint requires for its treatment and cure external medications in the form of ointments, shampoos and hair tonics, and these should contain antiseptics, parasiticides and stimulants. The following formulas indicate the type of preparation:

Scalp Tonic

Resorcin	10 g.
Chloral Hydrate	5 g.
Camphor	0.2 g.
Tincture of Cantharides	10 g.
Alcohol	50 g.
Geranium Oil	
Bergamot Oil	
Lavender Oil	
Bitter Almond Oil	
of each	0.25 g.
Glycerin	2 g.
Distilled Water to make	1,000 g.

Color with trace of aniline dye. Filter perfectly clear and bright.

Apply to scalp three or four times a week and rub in thoroughly.

Hair Tonic for Dandruff

Alcohol (Specially Denatured)	90 g.
Glycerin	10 g.
Capsicum, Tincture	15 g.
Red Rose Oil	2 g.

Add in the above order.

Any perfume may be used. Color green with chlorophyll.

Scalp Tonic

Tannic Acid	0.5 g.
Salicylic Acid	1.0 g.
Castor Oil	24.5 g.
Resorcinol Monoacetate	5.0 g.
Alcohol	69.0 g.
Perfume	sufficient

Alcoholic Sulphur Hair Lotion

Sulphur Glycerin Solution (24%)	5 g.
Water	20 cc.
Salicylic Acid	0.5 g.
Menthol	0.3 g.
Alcohol (24%)	70 cc.
Perfume	to suit

Lotion for Dry Dandruff

Tannic Acid	10 oz.
Chloral Hydrate	16 oz.
Witch Hazel	200 oz.
Castor Oil	5 oz.
Soya Bean Oil	50 oz.
Alcohol	800 oz.

Perfume to suit.

Dissolve the tannic and the chloral in the alcohol, add the witch hazel and the oils and mix thoroughly.

Lotion for Oily Dandruff

Zinc Sulphate	2 oz.
Phenol	1 oz.
Menthol	2 oz.
Glycerin	50 oz.
Water	120 oz.
Formalin	2 oz.
Alcohol	40 oz.

Perfume to suit.

Dissolve the zinc sulphate in some of the water. Dissolve the phenol and the menthol in the alcohol, add the glycerin, the formalin and the remainder of the water. Mix thoroughly and filter.

Other chemicals used in the manufacture of dandruff preparations include: crude oil, precipitated sulphur, oil of tar rectified, oil of camphor white, turkey red oil, oil of thyme, soya bean oil, thuja, cresol, lignol, sulphonated bitumen, lanolin, betanaphthol, croton oil, bismuth subcarbonate, mercuric salicylate, arsenic iodide.

Dandruff Lotion

Formula No. 1

Salicylic Acid	2 oz.
Sulphur, Precipitated	4 oz.

Castor Oil	10	oz.
Gum Tragacanth	1	oz.
Glycerin	1	oz.
Perfume	0.5	oz.
Water	82	oz.

Formula No. 2

Chloral Hydrate	1	dr.
Glycerin	4	dr.
Bay Rum	8	oz.

Mix.

Formula No. 3

Mercury Bichloride	0.5	g.
Resorcinol	5	g.
Alcohol	125	cc.
Water	125	cc.

Dissolve the bichloride and the resorcinol in the water. Then add alcohol. Apply on the dry scalp and rub thoroughly—then shampoo the hair. One treatment a week is usually sufficient for a complete absence of dandruff.

Formula No. 4

Mineral Oil	5	gal.
Turkey Brown Oil	5	gal.
Medicated Perfume	1	lb.

Formula No. 5

Ammonium Carbonate	5	oz.
Alcohol	30	oz.
Glycerin	20	oz.
Rose Water	200	oz.

Dandruff Ointment

Formula No. 1

Dandruff ointment is usually a powerfully antiseptic salve, the following formula being typical of the class:

Precipitated Sulphur	8	lb.
Oxyquinoline Sulphate	1	lb.
Lanolin	10	lb.
Petrolatum	61	lb.
Castor Oil	15	lb.
Tincture Fish Berries	1	lb.
Balsam Peru	2	lb.
Carbolic Acid 85%	2	lb.

Procedure: Mix the sulphur with the castor oil rubbing thoroughly until lumps have disappeared. Mix the oxyquinoline sulphate with ten pounds of petrolatum, run through an ointment mill or milling rolls three times, add the sulphur castor oil mixture, mix thoroughly and run through the mill again. Melt the lanolin, and the rest of the petrolatum, add the remainder of the castor oil, mix thoroughly and then mix in the oxysulphur mass. Mix thoroughly, add the balsam of Peru, continue mixing for thirty minutes, add the tincture fish berries and the carbolic acid and mix again for twenty or thirty minutes. The machine best suited for this ointment is a pony mixer.

Formula No. 2

Mineral Oil	46 g.
Lanolin	26 g.
Beeswax	23 g.
Sulphur, Colloidal	4 g.
Perfume	to suit

Formula No. 3

Lanolin	12	oz.
Water	15	oz.
Silver Lacate	3	oz.
Tincture Fish Berries	5	oz.
Sulphur Iodide	3	oz.
Balsam of Peru	15	oz.
Cocoa Butter	20	oz.
Petrolatum	60	oz.
Glycerin	10	oz.

Perfume to suit.

Dissolve the silver lactate in water and the sulphur iodide in glycerin. Melt the petrolatum, the lanolin and the cocoa butter, stir in the silver lactate solution, add the sulphur iodide solution and finally the balsam of Peru and the fish berries.

Formula No. 4

Salicylic Acid	10	gr.
Precipitated Sulphur	15	gr.
White Petrolatum	1	oz.
Geranium Oil		
Bergamot Oil	of each 2	min.

Apply once or twice a week. Follow with shampoo the next morning.

Hair Treatments

Formula No. 1

Resorcinol	.8	g.
Beta Naphthol	.8	g.
Chloral Hydrate	1.5	g.
Tincture of Capsicum	4.0	g.
Castor Oil	2.0	g.
Alcohol	90.0	cc.
Nutmeg Oil	.9	g.

Dissolve the chloral hydrate in the castor oil. Dissolve the resorcinol in part of the alcohol, the beta naphthol in the remainder of the alcohol. Add the oil of nutmeg to this solution, then the tincture of capsicum, the castor oil mixture and finally the resorcinol. Mix well and filter.

Formula No. 2

Quinine Sulphate	.25 g.
Pilocarpine Hydrochloride	.05 g.
Chloral Hydrate	1.00 g.
Castor Oil	4.00 g.
Chloroform	7.00 g.
Spirits of Formic Acid	12.50 g.
Alcohol	74.95 cc.
Perfume	.25 g.

Dissolve the chloral hydrate in the castor oil. Dissolve the pilocarpine in the formic spirits. Mix the chloroform with about one-half its weight of alcohol and dissolve the quinine sulphate in it. Add the formic spirit solution, mix and add the formic spirit solution. Mix again. Finally add the perfume. Mix well and filter.

Formula No. 3

Resorcinol	.28 g.
Soft Soap	.46 g.
Pine Tar Oil Rectified	2.70 g.
Potassium Sulphide	3.00 g.
Water	93.31 cc.
Perfume	.25 g.

Dissolve the potassium sulphide in half of the water. Dissolve the resorcinol in the remainder of the water. Mix the perfume and pine tar oil with the soft soap and then rapidly mix this with the resorcinol solution. Finally add the potassium sulphide solution.

Formula No. 4

Resorcinol Monoacetate	3.00 g.
Castor Oil	7.00 g.
Spirits of Formic Acid	20.00 g.
Alcohol	69.75 g.
Perfume	.25 g.

Dissolve the resorcinol monoacetate in the formic spirits, the castor oil in the alcohol. Mix the two solutions and add the perfume. Filter.

Formula No. 5

Colloidal Sulphur	5.00 g.
Pulverized Camphor	.40 g.
Tincture of Cantharides	5.00 g.
Resorcinol Monoacetate	1.00 g.
Nutmeg Oil	.50 g.
Alcohol	72.85 cc.
Glycerin	15.00 g.
Perfume	.25 g.

Rub off the sulphur with the glycerin until a smooth mixture is obtained. Dissolve the resorcinol in the alcohol. Mix the pulverized camphor with the tincture of cantharides. Add this to the alcohol mixture and finally add the sulphur mixture. Mix thoroughly and add the perfume. Do not filter.

Preparation for Head Massage

German Patent 616,362

Lauryl Sulphonate	25 g.
Buckwheat Flour	30 g.
Henna	10 g.
Salicylic Acid	5 g.
Sulphur	5 g.
Castor Oil	5 cc.

Scalp Stimulant

Deodorized Kerosene	80 oz.
Resorcinol Monoacetate	3 oz.
Lanolin	10 oz.
Diglycol Laurate	7 oz.

This preparation will clean the scalp thoroughly if rubbed in vigorously and wiped off. It is also an excellent stimulant.

Preparations for Baldness
Ointment

Pilocarpine Hydrochloride	20 oz.
Precipitated Sulphur	120 oz.
Parachol (Absorption Base)	60 oz.
Balsam of Peru	60 oz.
Resorcinol Monoacetate	30 oz.
Petrolatum	900 oz.
Water	60 oz.
Perfume to suit.	

Dissolve the pilocarpine in water and mix with absorption base. Mill the sulphur and the monoacetate with part of the petrolatum. Melt the rest and stir in the absorption base and add finally the sulphur mass. Mix thoroughly.

"Falling Hair" Ointment

Salicylic Acid	1.0 g.
Resorcinol Monoacetate	1.5 g.
Precipitated Sulphur	1.5 g.
Ointment of Rose Water to make	30.0 g.

Rub into the scalp vigorously once a day.

"Lime Juice" and Glycerin (for Hair)

White Wax	500 g.
Oil of Sweet Almonds 2 kg.,	500 cc.

are melted together in a water-bath and added to:

Glycerin	300 g.
Citric Acid	30 g.

dissolved in a liter of rose water. Finally, there are added with stirring in an automatic mixer:

Alcohol	150 g.
Lemon Oil	75 g.
Bitter Almond Oil	10 g.

Quinine Hair Dressing

Quinine, Sulphate	20 g.
Castor Oil	1 oz.
Tincture Cantharides	½ oz.
Jasmine Extract	3 dr.
Eau de Cologne	3 oz.
Bitter Almond Oil	5 drops
Bergamot Oil	½ dr.
Alcohol	8 oz.

Mix and color with tincture of alkanet if desired.

Hair Milk

1. Mineral Oil, White	144 g.
2. Trihydroxyethylamine Stearate	29 g.
3. Water, Warm	320 g.
4. Perfume	3 g.

While stirring heat (1) and (2) until melted together. Add (3) slowly with stirring until uniform. Allow to stand overnight, stir moderately and package.

This preparation corrects dry scalp and hair and imparts a gloss to the latter and keeps it in place. It replaces old fashioned greasy hair oils and brilliantines.

"Ice Water" (for the Scalp)

Alcohol	650 g.
Water, Distilled	350 g.
Menthol	7 g.
Eau de Cologne Oil	3 g.

Lemon Rinse

1. "Lemonone"	3 oz.
2. "Isohol" (or Alcohol)	14 lb.
3. Citric Acid	3½ lb.
4. Tartaric Acid	4½ lb.
5. Water	16 lb.

Dissolve 1 in 2 and add to it slowly with stirring 3 and 4 which have been dissolved in 5.

Hair Luster Powder

Formula No. 1

Alum	60 g.
Tartaric Acid, Powdered	30 g.
Adipic Acid	10 g.

Perfume as desired.

Formula No. 2

Hexamethylene-tetramine	9 g.
Adipic Acid	40 g.

Warm until ester forms. Then add:

Tartaric Acid	50 g.
Perfume	1 g.

Then grind.

Hair Oil

Formula No. 1

Alcohol, Ethyl	400 cc.
Glycerin	200 cc.
Perfume, as desired, about	1 cc.
Salicylic Acid	2 g.
Water	400 cc.

Formula No. 2

Alcohol, Ethyl	400 cc.
Glycerin	300 cc.
Perfume, as desired, about	1 cc.
Salicylic Acid	2 g.
Water	300 cc.

Lavender coloration may be effected by the addition of traces of ferric chloride. The preparation is completely water soluble, hence readily removed by washing, yet it serves as an excellent "stay-comb."

Hair Brightening Oil

A brightening oil for blonde hair. Mix equal parts of hydrogen peroxide and a light mineral oil. Perfume with a stable compound. The product will separate in layers. It is to be shaken before use, at which time a few drops of ammonia water, is to be added to the amount used.

Nursery Hair Oil

Benzoin	½ oz.
Alkannin	½ oz.

Stavesacre Oil	1 oz.
Almond Oil	1 pt.

Macerate for a week, shaking daily, filter, and add

Perfume	½ dr.

Mix.

Baby Scalp Oil

Stavesacre Seed Oil	30 oz.
Olive Oil	70 oz.

The product is simply mixed and filtered. It may be lightly perfumed. This preparation may be converted into an ointment by adding benzoinated lard and a suitable amount of white beeswax to give it proper body and spreading qualities. The stavesacre oil is said to prevent scabies, and scurf.

Scalp Oil

Sesame Oil	80 g.
Parachol (Absorption Base)	10 g.
Tincture of Benzoin	10 g.
Perfume	to suit

Hair Dyes

Hair dyes are based on vegetable, mineral or organic dyes or pigments. The first type is comparatively innocuous. The latter two types should only be applied by experts after testing the individual's reaction to the products to be used.

Before applying a hair dye the hair should be washed thoroughly to remove grease and dirt or uneven coloring will result. This should be followed by drying. Extreme care should be taken that the dyes do not get on the skin or in the eyes.

Hair Dye

Formula No. 1

Neutral Bismuth Solution

An improved bismuth solution is made by precipitating bismuth nitrate (or chloride) solution with ammonia, washing, and then adding the precipitate to glycerin in a solution of Rochelle salt. This mixture is stirred and sodium or potassium hydroxide is added until solution takes place. A saturated solution of tartaric acid is then added until the solution is neutral.

The second solution is made up of glycerin 50–60 oz.; water 30–40 oz.; and sodium thiosulphate 10–20 oz. This is mixed with the bismuth solution just before using. Perfume as desired.

Formula No. 2

German Patent 605,461

Brown; A. Ammoniacal Solution of Hydrogen Peroxide with
B. 4-Aminophenylglycine

Reddish; A. and 2-Hydroxyphenylglycine

Yellow; A. and 4-Nitrophenylglycine

note; Phenylenediamine may be substituted for "B" and a dark color obtained.

Formula No. 3

Good results have been obtained by a combined silver-nickel-cobalt dye prepared according to the following formula:

Silver Nitrate	3.5 g.
Cobalt Nitrate	1.5 g.
Nickel Nitrate	3.0 g.
Ammonia (0.880 sp. gr.)	Sufficient
Water, sufficient to make	100 cc.

After application of the solution of metallic nitrates the color in the hair is developed by means of a 3 to 4 per cent of pyrogallol dissolved in water.

Formula No. 4

Boil for ½ hour 50 g. bismuth subnitrate, 100 g. cream of tartar and 500 g. of water. Decant the supernatant liquid and again boil the residue with 400 g. of water. Unite the two solutions and add enough caustic soda solution to produce a weakly alkaline reaction. Rub to a smooth paste a mixture of 25 g. of precipitated sulfur and 60 g. of glycerin, adding the paste to the bismuth solution. Add water to make 1000 cc.

Formula No. 5

Consists of two solutions, the first consisting of bismuth subnitrate 50 g., rose water 200 g., distilled water 50 g., alcohol 700 g. and sufficient ammonia. The second solution contains 60 g. of sodium thiosulfate and 200 g. of water. The hair is first brushed with the first solution and then with the second.

Formula No. 6

First, 50 parts of bismuth nitrate are dissolved in 250 parts water and 700 parts alcohol and sufficient ammonia is added to form solution number 1; second solution contains 100 parts sodium thiosulfate in one liter of water.

Formula No. 7

50 parts bismuth citrate are dissolved in 33 parts alcohol, 200 parts rose water, 300 parts water and sufficient ammonia to give solution number 1, while second solution contains 120 grams sodium thiosulfate dissolved in 400 grams water.

Formula No. 8

12 parts bismuth subnitrate are mixed with 58 parts water and mixture poured into porcelain mortar and 18 parts nitric acid are gradually added until solution takes place. This solution is then poured into solution of 9 parts tartaric acid, 8.5 parts sodium bicarbonate dissolved in 900 parts water. Precipitate is collected on filter cloth, washed well with water and dissolved in sufficiently strong ammonia solution. Then 6 parts sodium thiosulfate, 30 parts glycerin are added as well as sufficient water to obtain total of 240 parts.

"White Henna"

Formula No. 1

"White henna" is non-existent. The material so-called is nothing more than magnesia, which is made into a paste with hydrogen peroxide. It would be possible to compound suitable white mixtures which would evolve some hydrogen peroxide when treated with water.

Magnesium Carbonate	60 g.
Sodium Perborate	37 g.
Mineral Oil	3 g.

This is made into a paste with water and hydrogen peroxide and applied to the hair. Sometimes magnesium carbonate alone is used.

Formula No. 2

Sodium perborate, 18 g.; henna leaves, 2 g.

Formula No. 3

Magnesium Carbonate	68 g.
Sodium Perborate	32 g.

Make into a paste a 50–50 mixture of hydrogen peroxide and water before use.

Formula No. 4

Sodium Perborate	18 lb.
Henna Leaves	2 lb.

Hair Whitener

Aniline Blue	2 oz.
Distilled Water	15 gal.

Dissolve blue in one half the water by allowing it to stand over night. Mix thoroughly add the rest of the water and filter. It is undesirable to run this preparation through a mechanical filter because the stain is almost impossible to remove. It is better to filter in five gallon bottles reserved for this purpose.

Walnut Hair Dye

Green Walnut Shells	2 oz.
Alum	2 dr.
Olive Oil	4 oz.

Heat all in water bath until all water has been expelled. Express, filter and perfume.

Hair Bleach Paste

Chamomile Flower Powder	5 g.
Tragacanth or Pectin	0.5–1 g.
Sodium Bicarbonate	2 g.

Mix this powder shortly before use with hydrogen peroxide, 6–10% to form a paste of desired consistency.

Brilliantines

Brilliantines are favorite sellers, the liquid being the better seller of the two. Although some chemists insist that brilliantines should be made from vegetable oils, the danger of rancidity in cases where the hair is not shampooed frequently is great and it seems advisable therefore to adhere to light mineral oil.

The purpose of a brilliantine is to brighten the hair, to help hold it in place and to perfume it.

Brilliantine

Formula No. 1

Bitter Almond Oil	1.5 cc.
Clove Oil	3 cc.
Bergamot Oil	6 cc.
Castor Oil	50 cc.
Glyceryl Monoricinoleate	50 g.
Suet	50 g.

Formula No. 2

Light Mineral Oil	99 cc.
Perfume (Usually Flower Type)	1 cc.

Procedure: Mix and filter.

Formula No. 3

Mineral Oil	100 g.
Chlorophyll (Oil Soluble)	to suit
Perfume	to suit

Formula No. 4

Light Mineral Oil	99 cc.
Perfume (Flower Type)	1 cc.

Mix and filter.

Formula No. 5

Mineral Oil (Heavy)	3.5 gal.
Peanut Oil	1.5 gal.
Perfume Oil	5 oz.
Color	to suit

This formula is best used with coloring material, as it looks slightly yellowish when uncolored.

Formula No. 6

(Solid)

Petrolatum Yellow	20 lb.
Ceresin Wax	3 lb.
Mineral Oil (Heavy)	4 pt.

Color and perfume to suit.

It is stated that the product made from this formula has a smooth texture and a fine luster and will never turn rancid.

Formula No. 7

(Solid for Hot Countries)

Ceresin Wax	2 lb.
White Wax	0.1 lb.
Mineral Oil, Light	20.0 lb.
Lemon Oil	0.32 oz.
Geranium Oil	0.16 oz.
Bergamot Oil	0.64 oz.
Color	Sufficient

Formula No. 8

Solid

Petrolatum	100 lb.
Chlorophyll	2 oz.
Perfume Oil	8 oz.

Brilliantine

Formula No. 9

Castor Oil	49 cc.
Alcohol	50 cc.
Perfume Oil	1 cc.

Brilliantine

Formula No. 10

Almond Oil	49 cc.
Alcohol	50 cc.
Perfume	1 cc.

Greaseless Brilliantines for Men

There is a slight difference between the composition of such preparations used by men and those used by women. Those applied to the man's hair are merely required to keep it in place without giving it a greasy appearance. A very satisfactory product is obtained by using the following formula:

Formula No. 1

Gum Tragacanth (in Ribbons)	2 lb.
Sodium Benzoate	1 lb.
Water	55 gal.
Perfume Oil	6 oz.

Yellow, water-soluble dye sufficient to obtain an intensive yellow color.

Take a small vessel (10 gallon capacity); place into it the gum tragacanth in ribbons and 5 gallons of the water required; soak the gum overnight; next morning place the "jelly" in a kettle with a high-speed mixer and let it run for five minutes; then add the balance of the water (cold—50 gallons) slowly while the mixer is still in motion.

After the water is all mixed, add the sodium benzoate, the color, and the perfume. Strain before using through a wide-meshed cheesecloth.

Formula No. 2

Glycerin	59 cc.
Alcohol	50 cc.
Perfume	1 cc.

Formula No. 3

Diglycol Laurate	40 cc.
Alcohol	60 cc.
Perfume and Color	to suit

Formula No. 4

Soft Soap, 100%, White	2	g.
Dextrin, Yellow	6	g.
Water, Hot	12	g.
Glycerin	4	g.
Japan Wax, melted	2	g.
Perfume *	0.8–1.2	g.
* Bergamot Oil	.015	g.
Grape Fruit Oil	.005	g.
Vanillin	.005	g.
Heliotropin	.001	g.

Cream Brilliantine with Cholesterol

Beeswax, White	9.0 g.
Spermaceti	11.0 g.
Peanut Oil	35.0 g.
Cholesterol	1.5 g.
Water	102 g.

Melt cholesterol and waxes on the waterbath, and stir in water, adding it in small portions.

Jelly Brilliantine

Spermaceti	14 lb.
Beeswax	6 lb.
Mineral Oil	100 lb.
Perfume	1 lb.

Color to suit.

Procedure: Melt the waxes in the mineral oil. Strain and allow to cool to about 115° F. Add perfume; stir until cold.

In addition to the hair tonics for the two primary scalp conditions, dry and oily, there are a multitude of others for which various claims are made. This group is so various that it would be impossible to give an adequate outline.

Bay Rum and Quinine Brilliantine

Quinine Hydrochloride	2.0 g.
Bay Oil	1.8 cc.
Pimento Oil	0.5 cc.
Ethyl Acetate	0.2 cc.
Alcohol	200.0 cc.
Peanut Oil to make	1,000.0 cc.

Henna Brilliantine

Macerate ½ drachm of powdered henna with 3½ ounces of oil at 120° F. for three hours, and then filter. This can then be used as an addition to any of the usual types of brilliantine, e.g.,

Castor Oil	2 dr.
Henna Oil as above	4 oz.
Rose Geranium Oil	15 drops
Isopropyl Alcohol	to 6 oz.

Pomades

Yellow Pomade

Yellow Petrolatum	1000 g.
Bergamot Oil or Terpineol	5 g.

White Pomade

Snow White Petrolatum	1000 g.
Perfume	5 g.

Quinine Pomade

Snow White Petrolatum	1000 g.
Quinine Sulphate	5 g.
Terpineol or Bergamot Oil	5 g.

Red Pomade

Amber Petrolatum	1000 g.
Eosin	2 g.
Terpineol	5 g.

Directions: Melt petrolatum and add perfume and color when required.

Hair-Darkening Pomade

Silver Nitrate	1.0 g.
Ammonium Carbonate	1.5 g.
Rose Water	20 drops
Pomade	30.0 g.

Apply twice a week.

Hair Pomade and Straightener

Yellow Petrolatum	6 oz.
Yellow Beeswax	1 oz.
Peanut Oil (Refined)	2 oz.
Perfume Oil	Sufficient

Melt the petrolatum in double boiler and add the other ingredients. The perfume should not be added until the mixture begins to solidify around the edges. This is an amber product. If a water white product is desired use white petrolatum and white beeswax and substitute equal parts of deodorized castor oil and mineral oil for the peanut oil. By adding more wax and less of the oils a product can be obtained that will straighten the most unruly hair.

"Kinky" Hair Straightener

Formula No. 1

Beef Suet	16 oz.
Yellow Beeswax	2 oz.
Castor Oil	2 oz.
Benzoic Acid	10 gr.
Perfume	sufficient

Melt the suet and wax, add the castor oil and acid, allow to cool, and add perfume.

Formula No. 2

Ceraflux	40 lb.
Glyco Wax A	10 lb.
Petrolatum, White or Yellow	100 lb.
Rosin	40 lb.

Melt together until clear and stir until uniform. Pour into jars while melted.

Formula No. 3

Beeswax	10 lb.
Petrolatum, Yellow or White	100 lb.
Ceraflux	40 lb.
Rosin	36 lb.
Rosin Oil	4 lb.

Method as given for formula 2. Formula 2 will give a very light colored product if white petrolatum, and FF rosin is used. Harder or softer product may be gotten by slight variation of the above.

Hair Fixatives

Formula No. 1

Fixative jellies for the hair may be prepared by mixing tragacanth (5 parts), with alcohol (5 to 10 parts) and glycerin (5 to 10 parts), coloring and perfuming the mixture and then adding, all at once, 75 to 85 parts of water. Alternatively, the jellies may be made without the use of alcohol, but the process is more troublesome, and the use of a mechanical mortar is recommended, in order to get a perfect mixture of the glycerin and the gum. The addition of a preservative is desirable, especially if the jelly does not contain alcohol. Sodium benzoate is often employed, but sodium fluoride and esters of para-hydroxy-benzoic acid are more efficient. The use of perfumes containing clove oil or eugenol are also recommended.

Formula No. 2

Tincture Benzoin	7 g.
Tincture Quillaja Bark	15 g.
Water	up to 60 g.

Formula No. 3

Alcohol	200 g.
Locust Bean Gum	50 g.
Water, Distilled	9100 cc.
Polyglycol	50 g.
Preservative	to suit
Perfume	to suit

Formula No. 4

Tragacanth Mucilage (0.3–0.4%)	90 g.
Glycerin	7 g.
{ Alcohol	3 g.
{ Perfume	to suit

Formula No. 5

Water	20 gal.
Gum Tragacanth	1 lb.
Boric Acid	1 lb.
Preservative	2 oz.

Allow to stand over night and stir until uniform; then stir in

Perfume Oil	4 oz.
Color	to suit

Formula No. 6

Liquid Hair Fixative

Tragacanth, Powdered	0.2–0.5 g.
Glycerin	5–10 g.
Alcohol	1 g.
Distilled Water	93.8–88.5 cc.

Dissolve gum in hot water, adding it together with the glycerin (ground together previously), filter; perfume with water soluble essential oils, or use orange flower (rose flower) water instead of distilled water, then dye pale green.

If paste is wanted for collapsible tubes, use 3–4 g. of gum tragacanth.

Hair Fixative Creams

The simplest type of fixative cream is a tragacanth mucilage containing up to 25% of liquid paraffin, more or less emulsified. Such creams require vigorous shaking, as the oil separates on standing. Permanent creams which now enjoy tremendous popularity, thanks to good advertising and their own inherent good qualities, are of two types:—oil-in-water emulsions and water-in-oil emulsions, the oil in both cases being mainly liquid paraffin. The most popular of these new fixatives is of the second type, a water-in-oil emulsion. It is not, as it is often supposed, a triethanolamine emulsion, but resembles a semi-liquid cold cream. A formula for this type of cream, which has been published and widely quoted, is as follows:

Formula No. 1

Liquid Paraffin	3000 cc.
White Beeswax	100 g.
Borax	6 g.
Water	150 cc.

Formula No. 2

Liquid Paraffin	45 cc.
Stearic Acid	5 g.
Water	49 cc.
Triethanolamine	1 cc.
Perfume	to suit

Add the liquid paraffin and stearin heated to about 65° C. to the solution of triethanolamine in water at the same temperature, and stir until it thickens. When nearly cold add the perfume. Avoid too vigorous stirring which causes frothing.

This formula gives a very thick cream which can easily be thinned by diluting with water if desired.

Formula No. 3

1.	Stearin	180 g.
	Water	400 g.
2.	Potassium Carbonate	18 g.
	Water	400 g.
3.	Lanolin, Anhydrous	40 g.
4.	Beeswax, White	10 g.
5.	Glycerin	300 g.
6.	Water	800 g.
7.	Perfume, Alkali-Proof	20–40 g.

Melt up 1 on water-bath, saponify with 2 at same temperature. Add 3, and 4, stir until homogeneous, add 5, 6, and finally 7.

Stir until cold, let stand 24 hours, and "work through" again thoroughly. Fill into jars or collapsible tubes which seal tightly.

Formula No. 4

Diglycol Stearate	14 oz.
Coconut Oil	12 oz.
Mineral Oil	12 oz.
Glyceryl Monostearate	2 oz.
Water	60 oz.

Formula No. 5
(Without Oil)

Gum Tragacanth	1.5 g.
Castor Oil	8.0 g.
Glucose	8.0 g.
Alcohol	14.0 g.
Sodium Benzoate	0.2 g.
Formaldehyde	0.4 g.
Water to	160.0 cc.
Perfume	sufficient

Formula No. 6
(With Oil)

Gum Tragacanth	1.5 g.
Castor Oil	4.0 g.
Glycerin	8.0 g.
Alcohol	14.0 g.
Sodium Benzoate	0.2 g.
Formaldehyde	0.4 g.
Water to	160.0 cc.
Perfume	sufficient
Mineral Oil	48.0 g.

The best method of compounding is to place together the tragacanth, castor oil, spirit, and perfume, stir well and briskly, add the glycerin, again stir, and slowly add 16 parts of water (the cream will not thicken at this stage). Then continually and briskly stirring, run in the remainder of the water at a fairly fast rate. Should the cream show any sign of not being homogeneous (in other words, being lumpy) at any time during the operation, cease the flow of water until the cream rectifies itself. Finally complete the formula.

Tincture of benzoin as an aid to an opaque cream has not been overlooked, but in this formula it is not required. It has been remarked that most men prefer a fugitive odor, and this can only be obtained by the use of essential oils. Lavender and eau de Cologne are the most popular, but offer nothing to distinguish one cream from another. At the same time, there is little to choose when using essential oils; from the following a choice can be made for experiment:

Suggested Perfume Combinations

	A	B	C	D	E
Lavender	4	2	1	—	—
Bergamot	4	4	6	6	10
Geranium	2	2	1	2	1
Petitgrain	—	—	2	1	3
Bois de rose	1	—	1	—	—
Lemon	—	—	1	1	1
Orange	—	—	½	½	½

Formula No. 7

White Wax	10 g.
Liquid Paraffin	125 g.
Borax	1 g.
Distilled Water	14 cc.

Allow the wax to dissolve in 60 parts of liquid paraffin, then stir in the remainder of the liquid paraffin. Dissolve the borax in the distilled water, add to the previous solution, and stir the cream so formed very thoroughly.

Formula No. 8

French Patent 787,918

Henna	4 kg.
Sulphur	15 kg.
Quinine	1½ kg.
Camphor	5 kg.
Castor Oil	1 kg.
Formaldehyde	4½ kg.
Alcohol	1000 l.
Perfume	to suit

Formula No. 9

Flaxseed (Whole)	1 lb.
Boric Acid	2 oz.
Glycerin	12 oz.
Water	1 gal.

Color and perfume to suit.

Boil the flaxseed with the water until syrupy; filter by squeezing through a linen bag. Discard the residue. Add the boric acid and glycerin (above) to the liquid.

Hair Dressing Lacquers

Formula No. 1

Tincture Benzoin	200 g.
Alcohol	120 g.
Turpentine, Larch	5 g.
Perfume *	to suit

Formula No. 2

(a) Benzoin, Siam	5 g.
Alcohol	80 g.
(b) Water	about 20 g.

Digest the benzoin in alcohol for a week, pour off the clear solution. Add to this slowly, the water; stop as soon as cloudiness appears; clear by adding alcohol.

Formula No. 3

Turpentine, Larch	5 g.
Tincture of Benzoin, Sumatra	200 g.

Formula No. 4

Rosin	50 g.
Alcohol	500 g.
Perfume Composition *	to suit
* Vanillin	5 g.
Aubépine	5 g.
Geranium Oil	15 g.
Rose, Artificial	25 g.

Formula No. 5

(a) Shellac, Bleached	150 g.
Borax	25 g.
Water	1000 cc.
(b) Alcohol	200 g.
Water	300 cc.
Dye, Water Soluble, Non-Toxic	to suit

Formula No. 6

Benzoin, Siam	5 g.
Alcohol	100 g.

Formula No. 7

Benzoin, Gum	5 g.
Turpentine	0.5–1 g.
Alcohol	100 g.

Formula No. 8

1. Shellac, Bleached	10 g.
2. Water, Hot	68 g.
3. Borax	2 g.
4. Eau de Cologne	30 g.
5. Dye	to suit

Dissolve the shellac in the hot borax solution, cool, and add the eau de Cologne.

Hair Fixative Perfumes

The popular ingredients include the citrus oils (orange, lemon, bergamot and lime), lavender, rosemary, geranium, petitgrain and coumarin; about 1% of perfume is sufficient. The following table will serve as a guide:

Formula	No. 1	No. 2	No. 3	No. 4	No. 5	No. 6
Bergamot Oil	55 cc.	20 cc.	45 cc.	40 cc.	50 cc.	40 cc.
Lavender Oil	10 cc.	50 cc.	—	50 cc.	—	40 cc.
Lemon Oil	3 cc.	—	20 cc.	—	—	—
Orange Oil	5 cc.	—	5 cc.	—	15 cc.	—
Lime Oil	5 cc.	—	5 cc.	—	—	—
Petitgrain Oil	15 cc.	15 cc.	25 cc.	—	10 cc.	—
Rosemary Oil	5 cc.	5 cc.	—	—	5 cc.	—
Geranium Oil	2 cc.	—	—	—	15 cc.	20 cc.
Coumarin	—	10 g.	—	10 g.	5 g.	—

Hair Setting Lotions

Hair setting lotions are known as "Finger" waving lotions, known also as "wave sets" or "setting lotions." Although commonly used in beauty parlor practice, they have a much wider sale to the private consumer, for use in "home treatments." The total volume of sales and the low cost of production combine to make the setting lotion a very attractive line, in the eyes of the manufacturer.

Basically, they may be said to consist of (*a*) vegetable mucilage; (*b*) alkali; (*c*) alcohol; (*d*) perfume and (*e*) colour. This constitution varies considerably, for sometimes both alkali and alcohol are omitted.

The fundamentals upon which the development of setting lotions is based are: first, that a vegetable mucilage is harmless to the hair, while holding the latter in shape during the drying process, which actually produces the wave. The second is, the addition of alkali enhances the value of such a preparation by softening the cuticle and making the cortex of the hair shaft bend more readily, so as to make a better wave prior to drying.

Vegetable mucilages have long proven their merit. As no material is desirable for this purpose, which leaves a noticeable residual film on the hair, many products of an otherwise attractive character (e.g., some of the modern cellulose derivatives) are automatically ruled out of consideration.

Karaya and quince seed mucilages are the most popular in America. Tragacanth and quince seed appear to be the most widely used in England. One advantage of gum karaya over tragacanth is that it gives a really clear solution over a wide range of strengths. Both karaya and tragacanth mucilages are best made without heat by soaking overnight, but a quicker method is to use them in powder form, moisten with the minimum quantity of industrial spirit, and then add gradually, with constant vigorous stirring, to the full volume of water.

The usual alkaline ingredients of a setting lotion (when such are incorporated) are borax, sodium carbonate and potassium carbonate. Alcohol is not an essential ingredient but a desirable one, owing to the fact that it facilitates rapid drying. Up to 40 per cent is commonly employed in typical wave sets. Isopropyl alcohol is useful, provided that it is not incorporated in quantities high enough to render its unpleasant odour too pronounced.

All of these materials undergo decomposition in water solutions over a period of time even when preserved. The use of a good preservative is essential to avoid gas and malodorous products. The best preservatives are formaldehyde and preservatives of the moldex (*p.*-hydroxybenzoic acid ester) type. These are used in the proportion of 18 oz. per 100 gal. of finished product.

To speed up the drying rate of these preparations many add alcohol to them. Too large an amount of alcohol will cause the gums to precipitate; smaller amounts do not appreciably increase rates of drying.

Many small manufacturers of hair waving fluid, made from quince seed, do not wash the seed in cold water previous to extracting the mucilage. This procedure cleans the seed of clay, dirt or sand, as well as wormy seeds. Then, to get a clean fluid of light color, the extraction of the mucilage should be made with cold water too. About 3% of seed gives a thick slime, of sufficient viscosity to be used along with 2% borax and an aromatic agent of some type. Dissolve the borax in a little water, then add to the quince slime. Hot water produces a turbid mixture, use cold water throughout.

Formula No. 1

Gum Tragacanth, Powdered	2.0 oz.
Potassium Carbonate	4.0 oz.
Preservative	0.2 oz.
Alcohol	15.8 oz.
Distilled Water	78.0 oz.

In such a formula as the above, the preservative (methyl ester of parahydroxybenzoic acid) is dissolved in the spirit, the potassium carbonate being dissolved in the water. The gum is then moistened with the spirit as previously described and added with vigorous stirring to the aqueous solution. Perfuming and colouring present no special problems, except that water-soluble perfumes must be employed in non-alcoholic lotions, or else simply aromatic waters such as rosewater, orange-flower water, etc.

Formula No. 2

Clear Setting Lotion, White

Quince Seed Mucilage Base*	2 gal.
Alcohol	1.25 gal.
Water	6.75 gal.
Perfume	0.5 oz.

Up to 1 oz. tincture of benzoin, added to the above, increases the whiteness.

Formula No. 3

Pink Finger Waving Lotion

Quince Seed Mucilage Base	6 gal.
Alcohol	2 gal.
Water	2 gal.
Perfume	1.5 oz.
Rhodamine Solution (1.5 per cent)	12 cc.

It should be noted that amber, pink, blue and green lotions have all been placed on the market with varying success. Hair curling or waving products in powder form are also worth attention. These latter consist essentially of the powdered gum base (such as gum acacia) sprayed over with an alcoholic solution of the desired perfume and colour, allowed to dry, and then packed in envelopes with a fairly high percentage of preservative (about 5 per cent has been recommended), and about an equal quantity of anhydrous sodium carbonate to make 7 or 8 grams. The consumer is directed, on the label, to mix the powder in a pint of warm water.

QUINCE SEED MUCILAGE BASE

* The "quince seed mucilage base" is a heavy stock base made up of 12 lb. of quince seeds (carefully cleaned and free from mould) dissolved in 30 Imperial gals. of distilled water, the resulting mucilage being pressed free from the seeds in a fruit juice press, presumably of the Seitz type. Sodium benzoate (1 lb.) is used as the preservative, but this might well be replaced by 0.2 per cent of the methyl ester of parahydroxybenzoic acid.

Formula No. 4

("Stringy")

Ondulum is a newly developed edible gum which produces in water a clear transparent liquid with exceptional "stringiness" or length. This length can be reduced by the addition of small amounts of acids. Ondulum produces thick solutions in water and is of interest as a suspending medium for pigments, colors, abrasives and other insoluble materials in water.

As a hair waving medium, its clarity and stringiness make it of considerable importance.

The following formula is suggested:

Ondulum	6 oz.
Glycerin	3–4 oz.
Alcohol	2 oz.
Water	50–600 oz.

The Ondulum is first thoroughly wetted by the Glycerin-Alcohol mixture. Then the water, preferably warm, is added slowly, stirring thoroughly until the material is completely dispersed. If less water is used, a jelly is formed which can be marketed as a concentrate.

In all cases the addition of a preservative such as Moldex in the portions of 18 ozs. to 100 gals. of finished product is suggested. The Moldex can be dissolved by heating in the water.

Formula No. 5

(Dries quickly and leaves no visible residue.)

1.	Glycomel	5 g.
	Isohol (or Alcohol)	20 g.
	Karaya Gum, White	5 g.
	Formaldehyde	1 g.
	Lilac Oil	3 g.
2.	Water	454 g.
3.	Water	454 g.

Mix together ingredients in (1). This is then poured slowly into (2) while stirring thoroughly until all particles are dispersed. This gives a concentrate. To make a finished product for use on the hair, this mixture is stirred into (3).

If a colored product is desired a little spirit soluble aniline green is dissolved in (1).

In making concentrated hair wave sets where Gum Karaya is used the latter is first ground with an equal amount of Aquaresin G.M.C. and then suspended in alcohol. By doing this, caking or lumping is avoided.

Formula No. 6

Gum Karaya	1 oz.
Aquaresin G.M.C.	2 oz.
Alcohol	16 oz.
Perfume and color to suit	

The above formula is a concentrated product which can be poured slowly into water with stirring without lumping to form a good bodied product which will leave no visible residue in the hair and impart a soft feel and glossy sheen to the hair.

Formula No. 7

(a)	Water	700 g.
	Glycerin	30 g.
	Borax, Powdered	25 g.
(b)	Benzoin, Tincture of	235 g.
	Perfume Composition	10 g.

To the solution (a) add (b) in a thin jet while agitating continuously and quickly. Mix thoroughly; allow to stand for a couple of days. Filter.

Formula No. 8

(a)	Borax, Powdered	20 g.
	Water, Distilled, Hot	700 g.
(b)	Shellac, Bleached	100 g.
(c)	Perfume Composition	10 g.
	Alcohol	170 g.

Dissolve (a) hot, and stir in (b) on the waterbath. Agitate until smoothly dispersed, cool to 50° C.; add (c), stir until cold. Let stand, filter.

Formula No. 9

Benzoin, Tincture of	970 g.
Perfume Composition	10 g.
Turpentine, Venice	20 g.

Formula No. 10

Rosin, Pale	90 g.
Alcohol	900 g.
Perfume Composition	10 g.

Formula No. 11

Isopropyl Alcohol	10.0 g.
Terpineol	0.25 g.
Water, Distilled, or Rose	to 100.0 cc.
Emulsone B, in Powder	0.1 g.

Thoroughly mix the Emulsone B with 0.2 of isopropyl alcohol in a perfectly dry, capacious bottle. Add 8 of water all at once, and shake violently. Dilute with water, adding the rest of the isopropyl alcohol in which the terpineol has been previously dissolved, towards the end.

After standing, it is desirable to filter the lotion, or to decant it from the sediment, if a perfectly clear product is required, and perfectly clear lotions make a much stronger appeal than cloudy ones. As is well known, terpineol has a lilac-like odor, and, especially if made with rose water, this lotion smells quite well. The terpineol, however, may be replaced by any water-soluble perfume, a number of which, already compounded, are now on the market. A bare trace of carmoisine gives the lotion a pretty tint, or any other innocuous water-soluble dye can be employed.

Formula No. 12

Powdered Gum Karaya	0.75 g.
Glycerin	2.5 g.
Alcohol	18.0 g.
Preservative	0.1 g.
Perfume	0.25 g.
Colour	to suit
Water to make	100 cc.

Perfume, glycerin and preservative are dissolved in and the gum suspended in the alcohol and the whole is run into the coloured water in a thin stream with vigorous agitation. It is allowed to stand three days before bottling.

Formula No. 13

High Grade Quince Seed	3.00 g.
Borax	3.00 g.
Formaldehyde	.15 g.
Water	93.85 cc.

Boil half the water, add the quince seed, soak 10 to 12 hours and strain. Dissolve the borax in the rest of the water, filter and add to the mucilage. Mix well, add formaldehyde and perfume.

Formula No. 14

Quince Seed	30 oz.
Water	10 gal.
Borax Powdered	20 oz.
Perfume	4 oz.
Benzoic Acid	3 oz.
Alcohol	10 oz.

Boil the water, add the quince seed and allow to stand overnight stirring occasionally. Add the borax solution (made with part of the water). Filter. Add perfume and benzoic acid solution and mix thoroughly.

Formula No. 15

1. Trogeen	4 lb.
2. Polychol	16 lb.
3. Isohol (or Alcohol)	16 lb.
4. Water	128–256 lb.

Wet 1 thoroughly with 2 and 3 and allow to stand (overnight if possible). Stir 4 in slowly a little at a time. The viscosity of thickness of this fluid decreases with the use of more than a certain amount of water. This dries rapidly and does not leave a white deposit on the hair. It requires no preservative and will not spot.

Formula No. 16

Ondulum	6 oz.
Glycerin	10 oz.
Water	200 oz.

The Ondulum is first thoroughly wetted by the Glycerin. Then the water, preferably warm, is added slowly, stirring thoroughly until the material is completely dispersed. If less water is used a jelly is formed which can be marketed as a concentrate.

The addition of a good preservative such as Moldex in the proportions of ⅙ oz. to one gal. of the finished product is necessary. The Moldex can be dissolved by heating in the water.

Ondulum, when used in the above manner, produces a clear liquid with the characteristic stringiness so necessary in a good hair waving lotion.

Formula No. 17

Powdered Pectin	48 oz.
Tartaric Acid	48 oz.
Methyl *p*-Hydroxybenzoate	2 oz.
Perfume	2 oz.
Colour	to suit

¼ oz. of above makes 1 pt. solution.

Formula No. 18

Gum Tragacanth	1 g.
Alcohol	100 cc.
Rose Water	300 cc.
Potassium Carbonate	4 g.
Borax	1 g.
Perfume	2 g.

Formula No. 19

Gum Acacia, Powdered	3 g.
Borax	20 g.
Alcohol	100 cc.
Water	900 cc.

Formula No. 20

Mix:

Madagascar Quince Seed	10 lb.
Water	35 gal.

Keep at 180° F. for 24 hours. Then strain.

Add:

Borax	1 lb.
Alcohol	5 gal.
Perfume	1 pt.

Color as desired.

Formula No. 21

Borax	600 g.
Acacia, Gum	80 g.
Boiling Water	18 l.
When cold add:	
Spirits of Camphor	75 cc.
Perfume	as desired

Formula No. 22

Psyllium Seed	1 oz.
Distilled Water	5 gal.
Water soluble Perfume	

Prepared by boiling for five minutes, straining, cooling and mixing with an equal bulk of alcohol.

Formula No. 23

Potassium Carbonate	40 g.
Borax	10 g.
Mucilage of Tragacanth	100 cc.
Coumarin	5 g.
Methyl Acetophenone	1 cc.
Alcohol	100 cc.
Rose Water to make	1000 cc.

Formula No. 24

Borax	600 g.
Acacia	80 g.
Boiling Water	18 l.
When cold add:	
Spirit of Camphor	75 cc.
Heliotropin	enough for perfume

Formula No. 25

Gum Karaya	12.50 g.
Sodium Benzoate	0.50 g.
Alcohol	10.00 g.
Water	77.00 g.
Color, Perfume	to suit

Concentrated Hair Wave Set Lotion

Formula No. 1

Gum Karaya	9½ lb.
Aquaresin G.M.C.	12 lb.
Isopropyl Alcohol	2 gal.

Put the first two ingredients together in a mortar until the gum is uniformly wetted then work in the alcohol. The Aquaresin prevents the gum from caking and lumping and also renders the hair brilliant and flexible.

Formula No. 2

Gum Karaya White	4½ lb.
Aquaresin G. M.	5–10 lb.
Pectin	½ lb.

Rub together thoroughly and stir in

Isopropyl Alcohol (99%)	20 lb.

Perfume and color to suit.

This concentrate when thrown into water and stirred gives a uniform product whose thickness depends on amount of water used. This product differs from similar preparations in that it gives the hair lustre and does not flake off.

Formula No. 3

Gum Karaya	25 lb.
Alcohol	10 gal.
Liquid Glycol Bori-Borate	¼ gal.
Perfume Oil	8 oz.
Color	to suit

Shake and stir into water for use.

Formula No. 4

Gum Karaya	3 g.
Glycol Bori-Borate (Liquid)	6 g.

Rub together until smooth. Stir in

Alcohol, Anhydrous	48 g.

Formula No. 5

Gum Karaya	12 g.
Glycerin or Glycol	12 g.
Alcohol	30 cc.
Perfume	to suit

The above is added to one pint of water for use.

Formula No. 6

A	Gum Karaya	2 oz.
	Glycerin	5 oz.
B	Sodium Boro-phosphate	25 oz.
	Water	68 oz.

Mix A until uniform; stir B until dissolved: Mix A & B.

Hair Wave Jelly

Formula No. 7

Gum Tragacanth	12 oz.
Alcohol	½ gal.
Water	3 gal.
Borax	8 gr.
Benzoic Acid	8 dr.
Perfume	3 dr.

Put the tragacanth into a vessel, add the water and borax and allow to stand until dissolved, a period which will depend upon whether the tragacanth is powdered in ribbons or lumps. Add alcohol to which perfume and benzoic has been added and mix thoroughly. Squeeze through muslin bag.

Hair Wave Powder

Gum Karaya	100 g.
Sodium Benzoate	2 g.
Perfume Oil	1 g.
Color	to suit

To use put in water to swell and stir till uniform.

Curling Liquid

Quince Seed	30 oz.
Water	10 gal.
Borax, Powdered	20 oz.
Perfume Compound	4 oz.
Benzoic Acid	3 oz.
Alcohol	10 oz.

Boil the water, add the quince seed and allow to stand overnight, stirring occasionally. Add the borax solution (made with part of the water). Filter. Add perfume and benzoic acid solution and mix thoroughly.

Extracting the quince seed hot increases the turbidity of the extract. If margin of profit is great enough it is better to extract the mucilage cold. As an additional precaution the quince seed should be cleaned by blowing. This wastes a little of the mucilage but it also removes clay and sand which the seed is apt to contain.

PERMANENT HAIR WAVING PREPARATIONS

Permanent waving fluids are strongly alkaline solutions, compounded and chosen for their ability to soften the hair shaft and make it more pliable, without giving rise to noticeable brittleness or other undesirable after-effects. Ammonium hydroxide (known also as "aqua ammonia" or "liquid ammonia") is the most popular and widely used basic ingredient of such solutions. Various salts of ammonia, such as ammonium carbonate, ammonium borate and ammonium phosphate, are also commonly employed, as well as volatile amines.

Ammonia or ammonia-forming lotions do have the advantage of not concentrating or depositing a hair harshening chemical upon the hair, yet they also have two serious disadvantages. They are unpleasant to use, since the evolution of ammonia gas is neither conducive to the comfort of the patron nor to ease of handling by the operator. Moreover, unless tightly stoppered, the ammonia gas volatilises and thus leaves a weaker solution.

Nevertheless, the advantages are generally held to outweigh the disadvantages, for nothing could be worse than a heat concentrated solution of a strongly alkaline chemical fused into the hair (as certain old-fashioned products were wont to do). At the same time, ammonia-containing solutions may be improved upon by the addition of a stabilising agent such as borax, sodium carbonate or potassium carbonate. A typical permanent waving solution of this kind may be compounded as follows:

Formula No. 1

Ammonium Hydroxide	9 oz.
Borax	3 oz.
Water	88 oz.

Formula No. 2

Ammonium Chloride	4 g.
Potassium Carbonate	8 g.
Glycerin	16 cc.
Floral Perfume Extract	32 cc.
Alcohol	60 cc.
Water	1,100 cc.

Formula No. 3

Sodium Carbonate Anhydrous	4 g.
Ammonium Carbonate	1 g.
Powdered Rosin	1 g.
Diethylene Glycol	5 g.
Alcohol	200 g.
Distilled Water	to 1,000 cc.

Non-Ammonia containing types of "perming" solution are still, of course, in use. They usually contain from 5 to

20 per cent of sodium or potassium carbonate, either alone or in association with borax, tribasic sodium phosphate or other suitable alkaline material.

"Oil waving solutions" experience an increasing vogue. The oil content is obviously best added just prior to the waving process, in order to avoid saponification. Sulphonated olive or sulphonated castor oil are the most frequently employed, the method being to supply them in a separate container, when delivering the solution itself to the hairdressing salon or beauty parlour. The operator is then recommended to add not more than 5 per cent of the sulphonated oil to the solution proper, when the latter is ready to be applied to the hair. This milky-looking lotion has some merit and is particularly impressive to the patron receiving the wave. It also has a slight tendency towards reducing the dryness consequent on permanent waving.

Permanent waving sachets consist almost invariably of borax, which in this type of product is quite satisfactory.

Formula No. 4

Ammonia (0.910)	200 cc.
Sodium Sulphite, Crystals	5 g.
Water, Distilled	800 cc.

Formula No. 5

(For dry, weak hair)

Ammonia (0.910)	250 cc.
Glycerin, Water-White	50 g.
Soap, Liquid (20–25% Fatty Acids)	20 g.
Water, Distilled	to make 1 l.

Formula No. 6

(For hair of normal color)

Ammonium Sulphite Solution, (22° Bé)	200 g.
Water	800 cc.

Formula No. 7

Ammonia (0.910)	100 g.
Sodium Sulphite, Crystallized	100 g.
Water	900 cc.

3–5% solutions of Sulphites in water, most frequently ammonium or sodium sulphite are used. Their actions can be made stronger by alkalies, such as ammonia, potash carbonate, caustic potash, borax, etc. and they usually contain materials which help their adaptation to the hair, such as Turkey red oils: for instance.

Formula No. 7

Water, Distilled	1000 g.
Ammonium Sulphite	50 g.
Glycerin	30 g.
Turkey Red Oil	5 g.

Formula No. 8

Crystalline Sodium Carbonate	11.7 g.
Potassium Carbonate	1.9 g.
Ammonium Carbonate	3.8 g.
Dilute Solution of Ammonia	9.5 g.
Water to	100.0 cc.

Formula No. 9

The following is a suitable formula for a permanent waving solution of the non-ammonia type:

Potassium Carbonate	40 g.
Borax	10 g.
Tragacanth Mucilage	100 cc.
Alcohol	100 cc.
Rose Water to make	1000 cc.

Formula No. 10

Permosalt	1 lb.
Water	5 gal.

Allow to stand overnight and filter.

To this add

Sulfoturk C	13 oz.
Ammonium Hydroxide	125 oz.

A milky mixture results.

Formula No. 11

Sodium Sulphite Heptahydrate	25 gr.
Borax	12½ gr.
Sodium Carbonate Decahydrate	2 gr.
Ammonium Carbonate	1 gr.
Water to	1 fl. oz.

Formula No. 12

Sodium Carbonate Anhydrous	4.52 g.
Potassium Bicarbonate Anhydrous	3.32 g.

Sodium Chloride Anhydrous	0.2 g.
Borax	0.34 g.
Glycerin about	2.0 g.
Alcohol, perfume, and coloring matter	traces

Formula No. 13

Ammonia (22° Bé)	50 cc.
Perfume	1 to 2.5 cc.
Glycerin	25 g.
Rosewater	1 l.

Formula No. 14

Borax	10 g.
Sodium Bicarbonate	50 g.
Glycerin	50 g.
Perfume	1 to 2.5 cc.
Distilled Water	1000 cc.

The amount of alkali present in the ordinary setting lotion is too high, the following quantities are maxima per litre: ammonia 10 g., sodium carbonate (anhydrous) 5 g., sodium carbonate hydrated 10 g., sodium bicarbonate 20 g., sodium biborate 20 g. Aromatics and synthetics should not be used if they give a colouration with alkalies, e.g., indol and vanillin—brick red; nitrated musks and cinnamates—bright yellow. Natural essential oils are to be preferred.

When waving is done by electrical machines the following formula is recommended:—

Formula No. 15

Sodium Carbonate, Anhydrous	4 g.
Ammonium Carbonate	1 g.
Colophony	1 g.
Diethylene Glycol	5 g.
Alcohol	200 cc.
Distilled Water	to 1 l.

Diethylene glycol is stated to assist solution of the colophony and essential oils, and does not make the hair sticky as glycerin does.

The following is a solution commonly used in France:—

Formula No. 16

Colophony	5 g.
Alcohol (90%)	420 g.
Potassium Hydroxide	2 g.
Ammonia (0.925)	5 g.
Rosewater	100 g.
Distilled Water	1 l.

This solution is suitable for waving by machine metal curlers, or for use with rubber wavers. With the latter the hair is damped, taking care that the solution does not get into the eyes, curled, and left for at least three to four hours.

Mucilage of gum tragacanth may be used: mix 20 g. powdered tragacanth with 50 g. alcohol, and add 1 litre of perfumed water. The hair should be damped very slightly with this mucilage; if too much is used the hair will have a glittering appearance in sunshine.

Formula No. 17

Permosalt A	20 lb.
Glycerin	1 lb.
Water	100 lb.

Stir the above till dissolved, filter the next day.

The above lotions can be colored by the use of water soluble dyes, stable to alkalies.

Formula No. 18

Permosalt	75 lb.
Ammonia (28°)	72 lb.
Glycerin	7 lb.
Water	800 lb.

Stir the above until dissolved and filter the next day.

Formula No. 19

Borax	3.75 g.
Sodium Bicarbonate	3.50 g.
Linseed Oil	0.17 g.
Starch	0.40 g.
Water	99.00 cc.

Formula No. 20

Hydrazine Hydrochloride	4 g.
Water	96 cc.

Formula No. 21

Borax	3.75 g.
Sodium Bicarbonate	3.50 g.
Linseed Oil	0.17 g.
Starch	0.40 g.
Water	99.00 cc.

Formula No. 22

(Jugoslavian Patent 11,829)

Ammonium Carbonate Powder	49 g.

Sodium Sulfite Anhydrous	49 g.
Boric Acid	1.5 g.
Rose Oil	0.5 g.

For use dilute with water. The material should be sold in the shape of tablets and kept tightly sealed.

Milky Permanent Wave Solution

Sodium Sulfite	6.5 g.
Ammonium Carbonate	2.0 g.
Ammonium Hydroxide (26%)	5.0 g.
Water	86.5 cc.
Carnauba Wax Emulsion	1–2 cc.

Permanent Wave Oil

Rubberseed Oil	25 g.
Walnut Oil	15 g.
Tea Seed Oil	4 g.

The above is used on the hair after it has been baked on waving machine.

Hair Curling Preparations

French Patent 777,906

Formula No. 1

Stearic Acid	1000 g.
Soda	50 g.

Formula No. 2

Stearic Acid	1000 g.
Sodium or Ammonium Sulphoricinoleate	300 g.

Formula No. 3

Sodium Carbonate	15 g.
Sodium Bicarbonate	85 g.

Mix powders thoroughly.

Emulsion for Permanent Waves

British Patent 423,741

Olive Oil	20 cc.
Mineral Oil	20 cc.
Sodium Sulphite	5 g.
Sodium Carbonate	6.2 g.
Sodium Orthoborate	2 g.
Triethanolamine	2.1 g.
Water	60

Other fatty oils may be substituted for olive oil, such as linseed oil, cotton seed oil, maize oil.

There may be used as emulsifiers gelatine, agar-agar, Irish moss. The patent claims furthermore the use of alkali ortho- and metaborates, alkali sulfonates, carbonates, or bicarbonates, alkali hydroxydes, ammonium salts.

Permanent Waving (Without Heating Machinery)

French Patent 790,338

Aluminum Powder	20–60 g.
Sodium Persulfate	50–100 g.
Maleic Acid	50–150 g.
Copper Oxide	40–100 g.
Talc or Other Filler	500–1000 g.

The above is mixed and put into a cloth pad which is wrapped around strands of hair. When wet it generates the necessary heat.

Burns from Permanent Wave Machine

In undertaking to treat burns resulting from this process, one must take two things into consideration: first, that usually the burns are deep (third degree) and, second, that they are frequently infected from the ever present bacteria on the scalp and hair. It is the infection that at times causes considerable trouble, not only because it retards healing but because it is not infrequent to find a persistent furunculosis as a sequela on the neck and back or other parts of the body.

The routine in treating these patients is as follows:

1. The area surrounding the burn is washed well with soap and water.
2. An adequate area is shaved around the burn.
3. A corrosive mercuric chloride (1:3,000) compress is applied and left in place for fifteen minutes every twelve hours.
4. Débris is removed without causing bleeding.
5. The burn is dressed with a piece of gauze that has been saturated with an aqueous solution of tannic acid, 5 per cent. This gauze is held in place with hairpins.
6. If the posterior cervical glands are affected (and this is very frequent) and the patient shows any systemic reaction (fever, leukocytosis), she is put to bed. Ice caps are placed over the inflamed cervical lymph nodes for thirty minutes at intervals of an hour.
7. If furunculosis develops, the patient is treated with an autogenous vaccine.

Cold Permanent Waving

U. S. Patent 2,056,358

This invention relates to the art of waving hair to produce so-called permanent waves and departs from the art as heretofore known in that the method and composition of this invention make possible the production of a permanent wave without resorting, as is ordinarily done, to hazardous, discomfiting temperatures in excess of body tolerance. The invention consists in a method of waving in which a composition having the power to hydrolyze or soften the keratin of hair to a moldable consistency within a few minutes, at room temperature, although not active enough to jellify the hair substance even after several hours of contact, is applied to the hair. Shortly after application, a moldable consistency having been obtained, the hair is molded mechanically to the configuration desired. The desired mold of wave having been attained, the hydrolytic or softening action of the applied composition is arrested and the removal of the composition effected. Upon removal of the composition the hydrolysis or softening of the hair substance reverses to a degree and the natural elastic, nonmoldable properties of the hair return, retaining the molded wave. Additional steps to complete the removal of the composition and to assist the reversal of the hydrolysis or softening are sometimes also employed with beneficial results. All of the above steps may take place at moderate temperatures, usually below a body heat.

Sodium Hydroxide	1 to 3 oz.
Sodium Carbonate	1 to 3 oz.
Sodium Benzoate	½ to 1 oz.
Trypsin	1/10–¼ oz.
Gum Tragacanth	5 to 15 oz.
Sodium Chloride	5 to 30 oz.
Lavender Oil as desired	
Methyl Orange as desired	

A softening solution prepared as outlined above is then applied to the hair and a softening action begins immediately. After a thorough application of the solution the hair is combed and mechanically arranged in the configuration of waves. This may be accomplished by the familiar, well-known manipulation known as wave setting, or separate tresses of the hair may be wound on curlers or the like and tied. By this time the hair has lost its elastic properties to a large extent and becomes of a moldable consistency. When this stage is reached a suitable current of drying air is applied to the hair and the water in the composition removed to a great extent. During this operation the adherent in the composition helps to preserve the contour of the waves which have been set. As drying progresses the alkaline material as well as the enzyme is thrown out of solution and the hydrolytic action upon the hair is arrested. The removal of water from the hair substance itself also actually brings about a reversal of the hydrolysis and a consequent restoration of elastic properties of the hair to a large extent.

When the hair has been quite thoroughly dried the composition, including the adherent and the enzyme, forms a dry, dusty powder which is then combed and brushed from the hair as thoroughly as possible. A very slight residue of the treating material, however, still remains in the hair and as a preferred final step, although not essential, the hair is shampooed in a slightly acid solution, such as is commonly called a lemon rinse or a vinegar rinse. This step assists in more completely reversing the hydrolysis of the hair substance and the hair, although somewhat softened by the water, regains quite completely its normal natural properties. Following the acid wash and a thorough rinsing of the hair with water the waves are remanipulated mechanically into place and the final drying of the hair is completed.

CHAPTER XI

MANICURE PREPARATIONS

Nail Polish

The formulation of a suitable nail polish presents problems peculiar in itself. The properties desired in the finished product are:

1. Ease of application
2. Drying time
3. Appearance of dry film
4. Permanency

Ease of application is essential. If the polish is too thin, it will tend to flow too readily when applied to the nail, and will give difficulty in securing a smooth even coat. If the polish is too thick, a lumpy, streaky finish will result. In other words, the viscosity of the polish should be such that it will allow an even film to be brushed upon the nail. The drying time should be such that when the nails of the second hand are finished, the coat on those of the first hand should be sufficiently dry to permit the second application. Naturally, this applies only to the so-called "2 coat polishes."

The dry film should present an even appearance, any ridges, streaks, or even pinholes being absent. Finally, a good nail polish should remain on the finger nails for at least 5–7 days with little diminution of its original brilliance, and should show no signs of cracking and peeling.

True solvents, such as acetone, butyl acetate, amyl acetate, etc., give free flowing solutions whose viscosity can be influenced by increased concentration of low viscosity cotton, or by the addition of non-solvents, such as toluene, xylene, etc. Commercial nitrocellulose is manufactured in various viscosities, ½ second, 4 seconds, 15–20 seconds, 40 seconds, etc. However, ½ second regular soluble nitrocellulose generally furnishes the basis of nail polishes. This permits the incorporation of a sufficient solid content, whereas the higher viscosity cottons, even in small quantities, give a much too viscous product.

"Regular Soluble Cotton" is nitrocellulose soluble in acetone, amyl acetate, etc., but not in ethyl alcohol. There is another type of nitrocellulose produced, the alcohol soluble type. This type of cotton is sometimes used in formulating nail polishes where a high alcohol content is desired. However, the film of this type of cotton is not as strong as that of an equivalent amount of Regular Soluble Cotton. Where the incorporation of a large percentage of low boiling solvent is desired, the use of R. S. Cotton and ethyl acetate is preferable.

The solvents most commonly used in nail polishes are: ethyl acetate, absolute denatured ethyl alcohol, butyl acetate, normal butyl alcohol, amyl acetate, glycol ethers (cellosolve, cellosolve acetate, butyl and methyl cellosolve) and acetone oil. The non-solvents are toluene, benzol and VMP Naphtha. Most polishes contain little or none of these non-solvents as they have a disagreeable odor which is objectionable in the finished product. The evaporation rate of solvents is related, in most cases, to their boiling points.

In formulating, it is necessary to make sure that at all times there is sufficient true solvent for the cotton present. Otherwise, although the polish may be clear, the resultant film deposited may be cloudy due to the "throwing out" of solution of the nitrocellulose. The presence of resins further complicates this problem, as the solvents must also be balanced to insure sufficient solvents being present to prevent the resins from being thrown out.

The solvents boiling below 100° C. generally constitute 50% more of the total solvents of a nail polish. This insures a sufficiently rapid evaporation rate. If the solvents are very volatile and the air humid, the rapid evaporation cools the air about the film to below the dew point and the condensing moisture whitens and makes the film opaque. This is commonly termed "blushing." A film that has "blushed" quickly peels. This condition is alleviated by incorporation of small amounts of high boiling solvents that have the property of absorbing the condensed moisture, preventing the precipitation of cotton and resins, and causing the water to evaporate with the constituents of the polish. These compounds are the glycol ethers and acetone oil.

The manner in which nitrocellulose is deposited from solution depends upon the solvent used. In many cases, the resultant film is ridged and rippled. Certain solvents have the ability to "flat" the film and markedly alleviate the above condition. Such solvents are: ethyl alcohol, butanol, cellosolve and methyl cellosolve.

Pyroxylin solutions have, to a pronounced degree, the property of contracting upon drying, and this causes it to buckle away from the surface to which it has been applied. To prevent this, substances called "plasticizers" are incorporated. These plasticizers are high boiling organic solvents which very slowly evaporate from the film. But small amounts of these substances are used, as their too liberal use would retard the setting of the film. The commonly used ones are castor oil, tricresyl phosphate, dibutyl phthalate, butyl stearate and camphor. The one that gives more plasticizing value, ounce for ounce, than any of the others is tricresyl phosphate. It tends to discolor and blacken with age, changing the color of the polish.

Castor Oil is widely used, but in slight excess it softens the film. Camphor is objectionable because of its odor and the fact that the luster of polishes containing camphor rapidly diminishes and in some cases the surface of the film soon presents a dull pitted appearance. The best of the lot is dibutyl phthalate, as it gives a good plasticizing effect, is stable and relatively odorless.

A number of resins can be used in pyroxylin lacquers and it is here that the formulator has his evident choice as well as one of his greatest troubles. The resins are two types, natural and synthetic.

Many of the natural resins and gums must be treated before incorporation in pyroxylin lacquers, as they contain waxes and other constituents which are incompatible with nitrocellulose. Each has its own treatment, to remove the insoluble matter.

The synthetic resins need no previous treatment before incorporation in lacquers, but in the main they have the drawback that they are colored compounds, yielding lacquers that are suited only for dark colored polishes.

All resins should be used as stock solutions in appropriate solvents, and the solutions assayed for resin strength from time to time thus insuring the proper percentage of this ingredient in the finished product.

All components should be combined on a weight basis as this alleviates any errors due to expansion or contraction. The total solids (cotton, resin and plasticizers) constitute from 10–30% of the polish, depending upon the desired thickness of final film. Plasticizers are added in the ratios of 20–30% of the weight of dry cotton, or 5% of the resin content. Actual mixing is done in glass or tin lined containers. All motors or shafting should be grounded and adequate ventilation provided.

Caution! Nitrocellulose is explosive when dry and highly inflammable when wet with solvents.

Formula No. 1

½ Sec. R.S. Wet Cotton	24 oz.
Ethyl Acetate	25 oz.
Butanol	5 oz.
Toluene	48 oz.
Damar Solution	19 oz.
"Cellosolve" Acetate	4 oz.
Dibutyl Phthalate	2 oz.
Tricresyl Phosphate	2 oz.
Butyl Acetate	25 oz.

Formula No. 2

Dry Alcohol Soluble Cotton	12 oz.
Shellac	1 oz.
Castor Oil	1 oz.
Alcohol	50 oz.
Ethyl Acetate	20 oz.
Butanol	5 oz.
Amyl Alcohol	6 oz.
Acetone Oil	5 oz.

Coloring Nail Polishes

Either basic dyes soluble in acetone and ethyl acetate are used, or oil soluble dyes. The basic dyes generally used are Rhodamine B (Pink), Safranine Y

(Red). They are used alone or mixed with Auramine (Yellow) or Chrysoidine (Orange) to give all desired shades. The oil reds given below are used, or shaded with oil yellow.

In coloring polishes, it is best to secure dye stuffs for this particular purpose, from dye stuff houses.

Formula No. 3

Part No. 1 (Solids)

Cellulose Nitrate (½ sec.) on Dry Basis (by weight)	65 g.
Dibutyl Phthalate (by weight)	15 g.
Ester Gum (Low Acid Number and Pale) (by weight)	20 g.

Part No. 2 (Solvents)

Acetone (by volume)	15 g.
Methanol	15 g.
Benzol	25 g.
Ethyl Acetate	30 g.
Butanol	5 g.
Butyl Acetate	10 g.

The finished polish contains 15 g. of Part No. 1 to 85 g. of Part No. 2.

The solvents are mixed and the plasticizer added. If the cellulose nitrate is purchased submerged in water, it is carefully dried at low temperatures and added to the above mixture. The ester gum is powdered by beating or in mortar with pestle, or in a coffee grinder or similar mill. This will hasten its passing into solution. If the cellulose nitrate is purchased already in solution, the solvents it contains, will have to be deducted from the above formula.

Formula No. 4

Amyl Acetate	700 g.
Methyl Alcohol	300 g.
Nitrocellulose	50 g.
Benzoin	100 g.
Carmoisine (1% Alcoholic Solution)	50 cc. or to suit

Formula No. 5

Butyl Acetate	250 g.
Ethyl Acetate	150 g.
Ethyl Alcohol	400 g.
Butyl Alcohol	200 g.
Damar	5 g.
Color	to suit

Formula No. 6

Methyl Ethyl Ketone	650 g.
Resorcinol Diacetate	100 g.
Ethyl Lactate	200 g.
Nitrocellulose	100 g.
Sandarac	5 g.
Color	to suit

Sometimes the polish is perfumed with a little ionone or ylang ylang oil, but more often this is not done.

Formula No. 7

Nitrocellulose (Low Viscosity)	225 g.
Damar	75 g.
Butyl Acetate	25 g.
Butyl Alcohol	20 g.
Ethyl Acetate	15 g.
Alcohol	40 g.
Carmine Red	sufficient to color

Formula No. 7

Stock Solution

½ Second Cellulose Nitrate (Damped with Butyl Alcohol)	20 lb.
Amyl Acetate	40 lb.
Ethyl Acetate	40 lb.

Take 10 pounds of the above and add to the following:

Safranine (0.5% Solution in Alcohol)	1 lb.
Ethyl Acetate	10 lb.
Castor Oil	1 lb.

The nitrocellulose is dissolved in the solvents by shaking, and allowed to stand until bright, when the other ingredients are added. The tinting is very important, and dyes are specially prepared by various makers for this purpose—safranine and carmoisine, for example. Castor oil serves as a plasticizing agent and prevents too rapid drying (which gives a streaky finish) and improves the adhesion of the enamel. Butyl alcohol may be added if the enamel is poor in adhesion and flakes off quickly.

Formula No. 8

(a)	Nitrocellulose, Medium Viscosity	10 g.
	Butanol	sufficient to wet
(b)	Amyl Acetate	10 g.
	Ethyl Acetate	10 g.
(c)	Castor Oil	0.5 g.
	Ethyl Acetate	4.5 g.

(d) Solution of Carmoisin,
Rhodamin,
Safranin to dye weakly

To the wetted (a) add (b) to dissolve, (c) to superfat, (d) to dye. Let stand and filter.

Pearl Nail Enamel

High Viscosity Nitrocellulose	20 oz.
Low Viscosity Nitrocellulose	10 oz.
"Cellosolve" Acetate	¼ pt.
Pale Damar Gum	10 oz.
Butyl Acetate	1 qt.
Toluol	3 gal.
Ethyl Acetate	2 gal.
Pearl Essence	18 oz.
Dibutyl Phthalate	1 pt.

Nail Polish (Paste)

A good formula for a nail polish in paste form contains 100 parts of light colored rosin, 60 parts of stearin, 60 parts of yellow beeswax and 200 parts of ceresin wax. These ingredients are melted together on water bath and then 300 parts of white petrolatum are mixed in. Then a well mixed mixture of 200 parts of washed kieselguhr, 140 parts of zinc oxide and 100 parts of tin oxide is mixed with the waxy base. Before mixture is removed from water bath, coloring matter is added, for example alkanna pink, as well as 15 to 20 parts of perfume. These ingredients must be added shortly before mass becomes solid and is poured into containers.

"Amor" Nail Polishing Paste

Ceresin	6 g.
Olein	44 g.
Precipitated Chalk	50 g.

Color and perfume to suit.

Nail Polish Powder

Formula No. 1

Stannic Oxide	1600 g.
Talcum	420 g.
Zinc Oxide	210 g.
Bengal Red	Trace
Perfume	Sufficient

Formula No. 2

Pumice Powder	40 g.
Talc	15 g.
Stannic Oxide	45 g.

Formula No. 3

Titanium Dioxide	65 g.
Talc	10 g.
Pumice Powder	25 g.

Formula No. 4

Putty Powder (Tin Oxide)	40 oz.
Infusorial Earth (325 Mesh)	55 oz.
Stearic Acid (Powdered)	5 oz.
Color (Pigment)	to suit
Perfume	to suit

Formula No. 5

Finest Powdered Silica	800 g.
Talcum (Extra Fine)	180 g.
Starch Rice	70 g.

The powder is tinted with a solution of eosin and perfumed suitably rose or muguet.

Nail Polish Stick

The stick or pencil type polish makes up in convenience what it lacks in efficiency. It is prepared by adding to a gum mucilage (such as tragacanth) an abrasive mixture of 90 per cent stannic oxide, 5 per cent pumice powder, 5 parts zinc oxide, dyed carmine. The mixture is moulded into pencils of the required shape and size, which are then wrapped in tinfoil to prevent excessive drying and cracking. A proportion of magnesium carbonate can also be incorporated in the formula to absorb the gum. If this method is not suitable a little zinc oleate or stearate might be used, or, alternatively, a mixture of fat and wax. Glycerin is another possible binding agent, but the tendency of this product to sweat should always be carefully watched.

Removers, Nail Polish

Formula No. 1

The nail polish remover consists chiefly of the solvent alone. It has been found, however, that butyl stearate has a particularly rapid action on the film, and many modern removers make use of it in conjunction with other solvents. An effective remover can be made by mixing butyl stearate 1 part, amyl acetate 3 parts, and acetone 4 parts. Diglycol laurate is also included to prevent brittleness of nails (about 1–2%).

Formula No. 2

Amyl Acetate	1 oz.
Acetone	1 oz.

Formula No. 3

Amyl Acetate	1 oz.
Alcohol	1 oz.
Acetone	1 oz.
Diglycol Laurate	⅛ oz.

Formula No. 4

"Cellosolve"	2 fl. oz.
Diacetone Alcohol	1 fl. oz.
Acetone	4 fl. oz.
Ethyl Acetate	3 fl. oz.

Formula No. 5

A low priced solvent mixture which is more effective than acetone alone, and useful on a wider variety of polishes is the following, which is stated in parts by volume:

Acetone	30 cc.
Methanol	24 cc.
Benzol	40 cc.

Formula No. 6

Amyl Acetate	20 lb.
Acetone	60 lb.
Ethyl Acetate	20 lb.

This is perfumed as desired.

Nail Bleach

Formula No. 1

Glycerin	420 cc.
Hydrogen Peroxide (20 vol.)	2000 cc.
Rose Water	1500 cc.

Formula No. 2

Hydrogen Peroxide (20 vol.)	130 cc.
Water	68 cc.
Ammonium Hydroxide	0.1 cc.
Alcohol	.1 cc.
Perfume Compound	0.5 cc.

Nail Polish Liquid

Nail polish liquids are essentially of the same composition, plus water and glycerin. The abrasive is kept uniformly suspended in the liquid by a colloidal agent such as china clay. The following is a typical formula:

Stannic Oxide	450 g.
Talc	450 g.
Glycerin	75 cc.
Colloidal China Clay	150 g.
Gum Tragacanth or Gum Arabic	3 g.
Water	1000 cc.
Perfume	sufficient

Nail White

Zinc White, Sifted	5 g.
Chloroform	20 g.
Paraffin Wax	2 g.
Neroli Oil	15 drops

Dissolve the paraffin in the chloroform and add the other ingredients with constant agitation.

Prevention of Brittleness of Finger-Nails

Formula No. 1

Alum	6 g.
Water, Distilled	60 g.
Glycerin	20 g.

Apply with a brush or pieces of cotton. After this use an abrasive polish of

Talc, Very Fine	4 g.
Zinc Oxide, Very Fine	10 g.

Formula No. 2

Alum	3 g.
Water, Distilled	60 g.
Glycerin	40 g.

Apply as in formula No. 1. Use lanolin cream or sweet almond oil over night as softener.

Formula No. 3

The following preparation is recommended for brittle finger nails:

Almond Oil	25 g.
Soft Paraffin	20 g.
Water	35 g.
Glycerin	5 g.
Stearic Acid	5 g.
Triethanolamine	4 g.

This is applied at night and allowed to dry. In the morning the nails are rubbed (polished) with the following powder: Tin oxide 7, talc 2, zinc oxide 1.

Formula No. 4

Diglycol Laurate	1 oz.
Water	4 oz.
Perfume	to suit

Rub into the nails before going to bed. Wipe off the next day. This gives excellent results.

Nail Cream

Anhydrous Lanolin	30	gr.
Soft White Paraffin Wax to	½	oz.

This may be perfumed and coloured, and is to be applied at night in order to keep the cuticle supple.

Cuticle Skin Cream

Petroleum Jelly (Pale Yellow)	1½	oz.
Deodorized Coconut Oil	1	oz.
Hard Paraffin Wax	1	dr.
Stearic Acid	2	dr.
Lanolin, Hydrous	1	dr.
Water	2	dr.
Borax	5	gr.

Cuticle Softener

Formula No. 1

White Petrolatum (Short Fiber)	87.75	oz.
Paraffin Wax (m.-p. 125° F.)	9	oz.
Menthol	3	oz.
Thymol	.25	oz.
Color (Oil Soluble Red)	to suit	

Formula No. 2

Lanolin (Anhydrous)	12	oz.
Water (Distilled)	12	oz.
Lecithin	0.5	oz.
Cream Petrolatum (Short Fiber)	55.5	oz.
Mineral Oil (White)	20	oz.
Perfume	to suit	

Formula No. 3

Light Turbine Oil—color and perfume to suit.

Formula No. 4

Diglycol Laurate	10	oz.
Deodorized Kerosene	10	oz.
Perfume	to suit	

Formula No. 5

Olive Oil	88	oz.
Petroleum Jelly	12	oz.
Red Dye Oil Soluble	to a pink color trace	
Perfume Lilac, enough,	about 0.3	oz.

A lower priced product may be prepared by using a medium bodied white mineral oil. The petroleum jelly should be nearly white. This jelly is melted at a low heat and added to the olive oil. The dye is macerated with a small portion of the oil and this paste is used to tint the entire mass. The perfume is added in amount varying with the strength of the particular product used.

Cuticle Remover

Formula No. 1

Sodium Peroxide	1	g.
Triethanolamine	3	g.
Glycerin	10	g.
Alcohol	10	g.
Water	76	g.

Formula No. 2

Sulphonated Castor Oil	3	oz.
Potassium Hydroxide	2	oz.
Potassium Carbonate	1	oz.
Water	93	oz.
Sulfatate or Other Wetting Agent	½	oz.
Perfume	½	oz.

Mix until uniform

Formula No. 3

Sodium Hydroxide	5	g.
Glycerin	5	g.
Water	95	g.
Diglycol Laurate	2	g.

Formula No. 4

Glycerin	20	oz.
Potassium Hydroxide	4	oz.
Water	76	oz.
Perfume	0.3	oz.
Basic Red Dye	trace	

The potassium hydroxide is dissolved in the water and the glycerol then added. The perfume usually used is a terpeneless lemon oil. Just enough dye is added to give same a pink color in the bottle.

Formula No. 5

Distilled Water	178	lb.
Caustic Potash	4	lb.
Glycerin	10	lb.
Perfume Compound	sufficient	

Formula No. 6

Potassium Hydroxide	2 oz.
Water	1 gal.
Phenyl Ethyl Alcohol	¼ oz.

Fingernail Cleaner

A fingernail stain remover consists of a saturated solution of tartaric acid in water.

Miscellaneous Nail Preparations

Nail bleach consists of 3% borax, 7% glycerin (28° Bé.), 90% perfume water, 2.4% preservative. Bleach of greater potency is made with 65% hydrogen peroxide (3%), 34% distilled water, 1% alcoholic solution of ammonia, 0.5% terpeneless pineneedle oil. Liquor for removing nicotine stains contains 90% hydrogen peroxide (3%), 10% ammonia solution (density 0.96), or bisulfite liquor or sulfur dioxide may be used. Polishing powder contains 40% pumice powder, 15% talc and 45% stannous oxide, or 65% titanium dioxide, 10% talc and 25% pulverized pumice. Nail enamel consists of 7% white carnauba wax, 7% Japan wax, 2.5% spermaceti, 80.5% white petrolatum, 0.25% turpentine, 0.5% acetic acid (80° Bé.), one per cent ethyl alcohol (96 to 98%), 0.25% alcanin and one per cent perfume. Nail paste contains 99% white petrolatum and 0.5 to one per cent of non-poisonous, fat-soluble, scarlet red, or 15% white beeswax, 10% white ceresin, 30% sweet oil of almonds, 35% tartaric acid, 4% citric acid and 6% alum. Liquid cream for after-treating nails contains one per cent white beeswax, 4% glyceryl monostearate, 10% sweet oil of almonds or apricot kernel oil, 5% white petrolatum, 80% distilled water and one per cent preservative.

CHAPTER XII

FACE POWDERS AND TALCS

THE most important consideration in the manufacture of face powders and the various talcum powders is in the selection of the raw materials. First, and most important, is the talc employed which should be judged on the basis of slip and smoothness, grit, color, mica content, fineness, acid soluble materials, and specific gravity both actual and apparent.

These properties should be carefully considered in the selection of the talc and more so after a selection has been made in checking of subsequent shipments from the raw material source. For the better products the Italian and Manchurian talcs are to be recommended. French talcs find their use in the medium grade products, and particularly in compacts. Californian talcs are also suitable for medium grade products, while the various other talcs are employed in low-priced products.

Face Powders

Base I—Medium Weight

Talc	50 oz.
Chalk, Precipitated	15 oz.
Kaolin Bolted	20 oz.
Zinc Oxide	15 oz.
Zinc Stearate	5 oz.
Perfume Oil	12 oz.

Base II—Rice

Talc	45 oz.
Rice Starch	20 oz.
Zinc Oxide	15 oz.
Kaolin	10 oz.
Zinc Stearate	10 oz.
Perfume Oil	8 oz.

Base III—Light

Talc	60 oz.
Chalk, Precipitated Light	15 oz.
Zinc Oxide	10 oz.
Zinc Stearate	10 oz.
Kaolin	5 oz.
Perfume Oil	10 oz.

Base IV—Heavy

Talc	45 oz.
Kaolin	30 oz.
Zinc Oxide	10 oz.
Titanium Oxide	10 oz.
Zinc Stearate	5 oz.
Perfume Oil	10 oz.

Coloring

The raw colors as bought are mixed with talc in the ratio

1 Color
9 Talc

and are either ball milled or screened through fifty mesh wire screen and then bolted through a 120 mesh silk screen. The talc used is figured as part of the formula. These colors are then known as bases.

Geranium Lake Base
Burnt Sienna Base
Persian Orange Base
Yellow Ochre Base
Burnt Amber Base
Purple Lake Base or Violet Lake Base.

Approximate coloring for powders 100 lb. Base.

Face Powders

Formula No. 1—Heavy

Talc	40 oz.
Magnesium Carbonate	5 oz.
Zinc Oxide	10 oz.
Zinc Stearate	5 oz.
Rice Starch	10 oz.
Kaolin	30 oz.
Color—See Coloring	
Perfume	6–14 oz.

Formula No. 2—Medium

Talc	50 oz.
Zinc Oxide	15 oz.
Zinc Stearate	10 oz.
Kaolin	20 oz.
Precipitated Chalk	5 oz.
Color—See Coloring	
Perfume	6–14 oz.

Formula No. 3—Light

Talc	65 oz.
Zinc Oxide	10 oz.
Kaolin	10 oz.
Precipitated Chalk	5 oz.
Color—See Coloring	
Perfume	6–14 oz.

Miscellaneous Face Powders

Formula No. 1

Rice Starch	30.00 g.
Zinc Stearate	4.00 g.
Zinc Oxide	4.00 g.
Talc	62.00 g.
Color } Perfume }	to suit

Formula No. 2

Osmo Kaolin	45 g.
Zinc Oxide	10 g.
Rice Starch	15 g.
Magnesium Carbonate	7 g.
Talc	18 g.
Magnesium Stearate	5 g.
Perfume (Compound)	2 g.
Heliotropine	1 g.

Sift through 120 mesh.

Poudre De Riz, Light

Osmo-Kaolin	47 lb.
Titanium Dioxide (Finely Pulverized)	8 lb.
Italian Talcum	15 lb.
Rice Starch	20 lb.
Magnesium Stearate	5 lb.
Magnesium Carbonate	5 lb.
Perfume Oil	Sufficient
Powdered Color	Sufficient

Add to perfume oil equal amount of alcohol. Then place in a mortar the magnesium stearate and magnesium carbonate, rubbing the perfume into these two ingredients. When thoroughly mixed, if it is found that the powder mixture is still damp, add enough osmo-kaolin until you have a dry mixture.

Place all other ingredients in the mixer and start the mixing machine running. Then add the balance of the ingredients containing perfume. Run mixer for about two hours and after the machine has run for about one hour, add powdered color. Take powder from mixer, putting it into tightly covered galvanized cans and allow to age for one month. Then place powder back in mixer and run for thirty minutes.

Put powder in bolting machine and continue bolting until thoroughly blended. The powder then should be immediately boxed and sealed.

Poudre De Riz, Medium

Best Italian Talcum	600 lb.
Zinc Stearate	130 lb.
Rice Starch	175 lb.
Osmo-Kaolin	50 lb.
China Clay (Pulverized and Bolted)	20 lb.
Magnesium Carbonate	10 lb.
Titanium Oxide (Finely Pulverized)	25 lb.
Perfume Oil	Sufficient
Powdered Color	Sufficient

Add to perfume oil equal amount of alcohol. Then place in a mortar the magnesium stearate and magnesium carbonate, rubbing the perfume into these two ingredients. When thoroughly mixed, if it is found that the powder mixture is still damp, add enough Osmo-Kaolin until you have a dry mixture.

Place all other ingredients in the mixer and start the machine running. Then add the balance of the ingredients containing perfume. Run mixer for about two hours and after the machine has run one hour, add powdered color. Take powder from mixer, putting it into tightly covered galvanized cans and allow to age for one month. Then place powder back in mixer and run for thirty minutes.

Put powder in bolting machine and continue bolting until thoroughly blended. The powder then should be immediately boxed and sealed.

Skin-Colored Powder

Wheat Starch	60 g.
Talc	40 g.
Zinc Stearate	30 g.
Red Bolus, Floated	5 g.

To obtain a deeper shade, umber or English red should be added.

Suntan

Burnt Sienna Base	20 lb.
Talc	180 lb.

Violet or Lavender shades are secured with a Violet Lake Base. Greens with a Green Lake Base. Dullness in shades is secured with Burnt Amber Base.

All materials are brushed through a thirty mesh screen into mixer and color added: Mixed for an hour or until a good distribution is effected. The perfume is rubbed into 2 pounds of Magnesium Carbonate and screened to break particles. The perfume and Magnesium Carbonate is then added to the balance of the ingredients, mixed again and all sifted through a 100 to 150 mesh silk screen.

Face Powder (Heavy for Night Wear)

Osmo Kaolin	30 oz.
Titanium Dioxide	30 oz.
Talc	23 oz.
Magnesium Carbonate	10 oz.
Magnesium Stearate	7 oz.
Perfume	3 oz.
Heliotropine	2 oz.

Sift through 120 mesh.

Poudre Azyade

Rice Starch	10 g.
Talc	40 g.
Basic Bismuth Nitrate	70 g.
Perfume	2 gr.

Compact Powder Base

(Pouring Method)

Talc	40 kg.
Kaolin, Floated or Dialyzed	20 kg.
Magnesium Carbonate	10 kg.
Zinc Oxide or Titanium Dioxide	8 kg.
Alabaster Gypsum, Finest	22 kg.
Water	to paste

Color (per 100 kg. powder)

Pink:	
Carmine Red Nr. 33	2 kg.
Flesh:	
Ochre No. 19	3 kg.
Theater Red No. 41	1 kg.
Sun-Tan:	
Sun tan-Color Nr. 14	10 kg.

Compact Powder Bases for Wet-Pressing Method

Formula No. 1

Zinc Oxide	20 kg.
Rice or Maize Starch	45 kg.
Talcum	30 kg.
Magnesium Stearate*	5 kg.

Formula No. 2

Titanium Oxide	20 kg.
Potato Starch	35 kg.
Wheat Flour	10 kg.
Talcum	25 kg.
Lycopodium Spores	10 kg.

Formula No. 3

Dialyzed Clay	20 kg.
Talcum	30 kg.
Rice or Maize Starch	40 kg.
Magnesium Stearate*	5 kg.
Zinc Stearate**	5 kg.

The procedure for the formulae 1–3: Make a dough with water and press the powder-cake.

Formula No. 4

Talcum	50 kg.
Zinc Oxide	15 kg.
Potato Starch	10 kg.
Magnesium Carbonate	15 kg.
Magnesium Stearate*	10 kg.

Formula No. 5

Titanium Oxide	20 kg.
Talcum	30 kg.
Dialyzed Clay	20 kg.
Magnesium Carbonate	20 kg.
Zinc Stearate	10 kg.

Formula No. 6

Zinc Oxide	25 kg.
Talcum	35 kg.

Dialyzed Clay	20 kg.
Magnesium Carbonate	20 kg.

The procedure for the formulae 4–6: Make a paste with a "*binder*"-solution (tragacanth, agar-agar, or similar mucilages). Caution: It is necessary to avoid too hard powder-cakes (a sign that too much gum used).

*How to Prepare Magnesium Stearate**

Neutralize a hot solution of stearic acid in alcohol by means of hot magnesium acetate. Filter. Wash with hot alcohol, later with water. Dry.

*Zinc Stearate***

Neutralize a hot solution of caustic potash with stearic acid (melted) at 100° C. Temperature should be kept high to avoid lumping.

The hot stearic soap is precipitated with a hot, concentrated solution of zinc chloride or sulphate, decanted, filtered, washed with hot water.

Dry.

Compact Powders

Compact powders are made in the same manner as are compact rouges, except that coloring is done with color bases, the same as are used in face powders. About 50% of the amount of color used in face powders is usually sufficient to give the same intensity of color.

Compact Powder Base (Dry Pressing Method)

The formulas for the wet pressing method can also be used for this method; after being properly dried and powdered, the pastes can be dry-pressed. Other formulae follow:

Formula No. 1

Zinc Oxide	20 kg.
Rice or Maize Starch	30 kg.
Talcum	30 kg.
Dialyzed Clay	5 kg.
Magnesium Stearate	15 kg.

Formula No. 2

Titanium Oxide	15 kg.
Potato Starch	25 kg.
Wheat Flour	10 kg.
Talcum	30 kg.
Zinc Stearate	10 kg.
Lycopodium	10 kg.

Formula No. 3

Zinc Oxide	20 kg.
Starch Wax	30 kg.
Talcum	30 kg.
Magnesium Carbonate	10 kg.
Dialyzed Clay	10 kg.

Formula No. 4

Titanium Oxide	10 kg.
Starch Wax	25 kg.
Talcum	35 kg.
Zinc Stearate	10 kg.
Magnesium Stearate	10 kg.
Dialyzed Clay	10 kg.

Make paste (in all formulae) with water, mix thoroughly, dry, grind. Perfume. Press.

Liquid Face Powder

Liquid face powders are suspension of chalk and zinc oxide in a water, alcohol and glycerin solution. The coloring is done with the color bases that are used in face powders.

Liquid Powder

Formula No. 1

Zinc Oxide	3 lb.
Precipitated Chalk	3 lb.
Diethylene Glycol	1 pt.
Alcohol	4 pt.
Perfume	4 oz.
Water	4 gal.

Color

(See Face Powder)

Rachel—Yellow Ochre Base	1 oz.
Tan—Burnt Sienna Base	1 oz.
Flesh—Geranium Base	1 oz.
Peach—Persian Orange Base	½ oz.

Further ideas for coloring may be had by referring to the various shades and the combinations necessary to secure them.

The zinc oxide may be replaced in whole or in part with titanium oxide.

Diethylene glycol may be used in place of glycerin.

Formula No. 2

Zinc Oxide	3 lb.
Precipitated Chalk	3 lb.
Glycerin	1 pt.
Alcohol	4 pt.
Perfume	4 oz.
Water	4 gal.

Color

(See Face Powder)

Rachel—1 oz. Yellow Ochre Base
Tan—1 oz. Burnt Sienna Base
Flesh—1 oz. Geranium Base
Peach—½ oz. Persian Orange Base

Formula No. 3

Osmo-Kaolin	3½ oz.
Precipitated Chalk	2½ oz.
Glycerin	2½ oz.
Spirit	1 oz.
Water	20 oz. or 25 oz.

If suspension is deemed necessary mucilage of tragacanth 1 oz. may be used, but a portion of the powders must first be rubbed down with a mucilage, otherwise, if the tragacanth is added last, the deposit is much more noticeable. The following are suitable colors:

White, no addition; pearl white, 10 minims of erythrosin solution (1–80); pink, 40 minims of the same solution; naturelle, 20 minims of the above solution and 1 dram of yellow ochre; rachel, 1½ drams of yellow ochre.

Milky Powder Base

1. Glycosterin	10 lb.
2. Water	300 lb.
3. Perfume	to suit

Heat 1 and 2 until melted. Stir while cooling, adding perfume at 105° F. By decreasing the amount of water more viscous products are obtained. By reducing the water to 100 lb. a paste cream is formed. The addition of titanium dioxide to the above forms a liquid powder or *"night-white."*

Powder Cream

Formula No. 1

{ Talc	10 g.
{ Titanium Dioxide	5 g.
Vanishing Cream	75 g.
Perfume and Color	to suit

The talc and titanium dioxide are thoroughly mixed with the perfume and color. Vanishing cream is made in the usual way, preferably with the addition of a little glycerin. The pigments are added to the cream while the latter is still hot, then thoroughly beaten into it by means of a beater-mixer.

Formula No. 2

{ Rice Starch	50 g.
{ Titanium Dioxide	50 g.
{ Talc	50 g.
Glyceryl Monostearate	90 g.
Liquid Paraffin	40 g.
Glycerin	40 g.
Spermaceti	40 g.
Stearic Acid	20 g.
Caustic Potash	1 g.
Perfume and Color	to suit
Water	550 cc.

The procedure in this case is to melt together the glyceryl monostearate, liquid paraffin, spermaceti, stearic acid and glycerin. Dissolve the caustic potash in the water contained in the bowl of the mixing machine. Meanwhile mix and sift the powder materials with the color. Next, add the melted fats, etc., to the caustic potash solution and, with constant stirring, bring to the boil. The mixed powders and color are then added gradually. When this is done, shut off the heat and continue stirring until the mass is cool, adding the perfume also at this time. If thought necessary, the finished product can be run through an ointment mill before filling into containers, ready for despatch.

White Liquid Powder Cream

Zinc Stearate	20 g.
Glycerin	10 g.
Orange Flower Water	25 g.
Rose Water	25 g.

Grind up the stearate and the glycerin and add the rose water. "Shake-before-use" label.

Cream Face Powders

To either a soft or medium vanishing cream there is added (by grinding) 25% colored face powder made as below, to give the new type cream face powders. 1% of Parachol added to the melted stearic acid used gives a very smooth texture and keeps the skin soft and flexible.

Powder for Face Cream Powder

Talc	60 lb.
Zinc Stearate	10 lb.
Titanium Dioxide	10 lb.
Kaolin	20 lb.

Color as desired; mix and sift thru 100 mesh (or finer) silk.

Nose Shine Preventer

Corn Starch	1	lb.
Glycerin	2½	lb.

Rub together.

Water	2	pt.
Turkey Red Oil	1	pt.
Eosin (0.1% solution)	7	oz.

Heat to 85° C. and add to above.

Zinc Oxide	2½	lb.
Zinc Stearate	1	lb.
Clay (Colloidal)	1½	lb.
Sienna (Raw)	1	oz.

Rub together at 30° C. and mix in.

Red Rose Oil	¼	oz.
Lilac Blossom Oil	¼	oz.

Liquid White (for Skin)

A lotion for hands and arms contains 2,500 parts witch hazel extract, 5,000 parts rose water, 1,000 parts alcohol, 1,800 parts glycerin, 100 parts tallow, 100 parts magnesium carbonate, 50 parts magnesium stearate and 1,000 parts antipyrine. First, the antipyrine is dissolved in the witch hazel extract and rose water. Then glycerin is added. The perfume used is absorbed by the magnesium carbonate, magnesium stearate and tallow. Then alcohol is added. This suspension is strongly shaken for two days. The milk is filtered through coarse filter paper. The two preparations are united with vigorous stirring and decanted. This preparation is applied with cotton. The skin is rubbed and the preparation is allowed to dry. The skin remains white the entire evening. The advantage of this preparation over ordinary liquid powder is that a dull white effect is obtained, lasting 4 to 6 hours.

Powder Dyes

"Color Rachel"

For 1 kg. of powder take

Ochre No. 19	80 g.
or Rachel I No. 7	60 g.
or Rachel II No. 8	70 g.

Pink

For 1 kg. of powder take

Carmine Red No. 27	8 g.
or Theater Red No. 41	6 g.
or Rosa I Nr. 2	10 g.
or Rosa II Nr. 3	10 g.
or Rosa III Nr. 4	10 g.

Flesh Color

Ochre No. 19	20 g.
Theater Red No. 41	2.5 g.

---

or Ochre No. 19	25 g.
Theater Red No. 41	2 g.

---

per kg. of powder.

Mix in before wetting the powder, to obtain an even distribution.

Coloring for Face Powders and Talcs

The colors necessary to secure most shades of face powder are yellow ocher, geranimum lake, persian orange lake, orange lake, burnt umber, burnt sienna, ultramarine blue, violet lake and green lake. These colors are diluted to make color bases as follows:

Rachel Color Base

Yellow Ocher	1 lb.
Talc	4 lb.

Flesh Color Base

Geranium Lake	1 lb.
Talc	9 lb.

Peach Color Base

Persian Orange Lake	1 lb.
Talc	3 lb.

Orange Color Base

Orange Lake	1 lb.
Talc	9 lb.

Grey Color Base

Burnt Umber	1 lb.
Talc	5 lb.

Tan Color Base

Burnt Sienna	1 lb.
Talc	3 lb.

Blue Color Base

Ultramarine Blue	1 lb.
Talc	9 lb.

Lavender Color Base

Violet Lake	1 lb.
Talc	10 lb.

Green Color Base

Green Lake	1 lb.
Talc	10 lb.

To secure the various shades of face powder, the following are used in conjunction with the above bases.

Light Cream

Base	100 lb.
Rachel Color Base	24 oz.

Rachel

Base	100 lb.
Rachel Color Base	48 oz.

Rachel or Cream

Yellow Ochre Base	5 lb.

Peach

Persian Orange Base	5 lb.

Brunette

Burnt Sienna Base	4 lb.
Yellow Ochre Base	4 lb.

Flesh

Yellow Base	2 lb.
Geranium Base	1 lb.

Dark Rachel

Yellow Ochre	7 lb.
Burnt Sienna Base	3 lb.
Geranium Base	1 lb.

Medium Rachel

Base	100 lb.
Rachel Color Base	64 oz.
Tan Color Base	8 oz.

Dark Rachel

Base	100 lb.
Rachel Color Base	48 oz.
Tan Color Base	16 oz.
Lavender Color Base	4 oz.
Grey Color Base	8 oz.

Various intermediate shades can be secured by combining two or more of the above formulae, or by increasing or decreasing the components of these formulae, or by the addition or deletion of items from these formulae. The procedure in the manufacture of these powders is: mix the dry materials, including the color base, in a horizontal type enclosed mixer, or else in a pebble mill, until all the materials are thoroughly distributed. The perfume is worked into about twenty (20) times its weight of either magnesium carbonate or powder base, and sifted through a wire screen and then a silk cloth as mentioned under talcum powders. The perfume mass is then added to the dry materials and the entire mixture is brushed through a sixty (60) mesh wire screen and then bolted through at least a one-hundred and twenty (120) mesh silk, with the finer mesh screens being more advisable. If it is so desired, the powder may be ground through a hammer mill or similar apparatus.

In the formulation of the powder, these factors are considered:

Talc is used for slip and its lubricating effect.

Kaolin—there are two (2) types available—the osmo or colloidal kaolin, and the bolted kaolin.

The *osmo kaolin* is much whiter and drier than the bolted, and has its main use in bodying the powder, giving it slip and coverage, and for its powers of absorption, especially in regard to perspiration and moisture.

The *bolted kaolin* is greener and much more moist than the osmo kaolin, and it is used to secure additional slip and a creaminess that can not be secured otherwise.

Rich Starch is used for the smoothness it imparts. Its absorption of moisture or perspiration with a subsequent swelling of the particles, resulting in enlarged pores, is a question of reasonable doubt, and can not be answered with entire satisfaction.

Magnesium Carbonate is used for securing lightness and bulkiness of the powder, and also as an absorbent of perfumes.

Zinc Oxide is used for its tinting covering powers.

Titanium Oxide is used for its covering powers which it possesses to a much greater degree than zinc, oxide, but its tendency to pack and "ball" a powder in which it is used makes it a product not usually found in face powders; zinc oxide still being considered more favorable for securing cover. However, if care is taken in the formulation of a product, excellent powders can be made with titanium oxide as a component of the powder.

Zinc Stearate is used in securing adhesiveness of the powder, as well as softness and lightness.

Magnesium Stearate has properties similar to zinc stearate but it is heavier. It finds its main use to replace zinc stearate where the use of zinc stearate is prohibited.

Precipitated Chalk is used in securing the smoothness that rice starch imparts without running into the difficulties that might be encountered in the use of rice starch by reason of its property of swelling.

Dusting Powders

Formula No. 1

Phenol	1 g.
Camphor	3 g.
Exsiccated Alum	96 g.

Formula No. 2

Salicylic Acid	4 g.
Boric Acid	5 g.
Starch	16 g.
Purified Talc	60 g.

Formula No. 3

Salicylic Acid	10 g.
Bismuth Subnitrate	15 g.
Zinc Stearate	10 g.

Formula No. 4

Salicylic Acid	2 g.
Tannoform	13 g.
Talcum	15 g.

Formula No. 5

Salicylic Acid	2 g.
Tannic Acid	5 g.
Orris Root	33 g.
Alum	60 g.

Formula No. 6

Bismuth Subgallate	5 g.
Boric Acid	15 g.

Formula No. 7

Bismuth Subnitrate	20 g.
Starch	10 g.
Purified Talc	70 g.

Formula No. 8

Mercuric Chloride	0.06 g.
Sodium Salicylate	26 g.
Prepared Chalk	4 g.

Face and Body Powders

Type of Powder	Rice Starch.	Talcum.	Osmokaolin.	Magnesium Carbonate.	Magnesium Stearate.	Zinc Oxide.	Vaseline or Cold Cream.	Miscellaneous Ingredients.
Face powder.........	600	200	—	100	40	60	—	
	450	300	—	50	—	220	—	
	500	300	—	25	—	150	—	70 TiO_2
	500	100	100	250	5	—	—	
Body powder.........	—	900	—	—	—	90	—	10 Salicylic acid
	—	800	—	70	20	10	—	100 Boric acid
	70	850	—	—	—	—	—	60 Boric acid
	80	490	300	—	100	—	—	
Fatted powder........	450	350	—	60	—	—	20	20 Lycopodium
	500	300	—	—	—	150	10	
Infant powder........	—	1,000	—	—	—	—	6	1 Lanolin
Perspiration powder...	—	850	—	—	—	100	—	10 Salicylic acid 20 Boric acid
		800	—	—	—	200	—	100 Boric acid
		750	—	—	—	200	—	350 Kieselguhr
		600	—	—	—	—	—	10 Thymol 0.1 Formaldehyde

Dusting Powder No. 1

Talc	95 lb.
Boric Acid	2 lb.
Magnesium Carbonate	3 lb.
Perfume	4–8 oz.

Dusting Powder No. 2

Talc	85 lb.
Magnesium Carbonate	10 lb.
Boric Acid	2 lb.
Zinc Stearate	3 lb.
Perfume	4–8 oz.

After-Bath Powder No. 1

Talc	80 lb.
Zinc Stearate	10 lb.
Boric Acid	3 lb.
Magnesium Carbonate	7 lb.

After-Bath Powder No. 2

Talc	85 lb.
Magnesium Carbonate	7 lb.
Zinc Stearate	7 lb.
Boric Acid	1 lb.

The zinc stearate is used for the adhesiveness and softness which it imparts to the powder. The boric acid is used for its antiseptic action. The magnesium carbonate is used for securing lightness and fluffiness. Substitutions, such as the use of magnesium stearate in place of zinc stearate, the use of a light precipitated chalk in place of magnesium carbonate can be made. The incorporation of other antiseptic bodies, such as methyl-para-hydroxy-benzoic-acid, tertiary-chlor-butanol, chlor-meta-Xylenol, is effected by melting these materials into the perfume oil (with the addition of a small amount of alcohol if desired). The perfume is incorporated in the usual manner.

The procedure in the manufacture of these talcum products is as follows:

Dry materials are mixed (usually in a horizontal type enclosed mixer) for a period of time. The perfume is added to a quantity of magnesium carbonate or of the mixed powder, equivalent to twenty (20) times the weight of perfume oil, mixed and then brushed through a forty (40) mesh wire screen, and then through at least a ninety (90) mesh silk screen. The perfume mixture is then added to the full batch of dry materials and bolted through a silk screen of at least one-hundred (100) mesh. A mesh of two-hundred (200) should be used for the highest quality product. At times a pebble mill is used for a simultaneous mixing and grinding operation, preparatory to sifting. The powders may be tinted slightly by using the same color as used in a face powder to secure a rachel, peach, flesh or any other desired shade. The amount of color usually used is about 20% that used in the equivalent face powder shade. However, in talcums for men, the colors are about equivalent in intensity to regular face powder shades.

Talcum Powder

Formula No. 1

Venetian Talcum Powder	700 g.
Osmo-Kaolin or Colloidal Clay	200 g.
Magnesium Stearate	100 g.
Benzyl Ethyl Carbinol	3 g.
Alpha Ionone	2 g.
Cyclamen Aldehyde or Cyclosal	1 g.
Ethyl Vanillin Crystallized	0.5 g.
Heliotropin Crystallized	5 g.
Titanium or Zinc Oxide	25 g.

Formula No. 2

Talc	71 g.
Precipitated Chalk	20 g.
Zinc Stearate	3 g.
Boric Acid	5 g.
Perfume	1 g.

"Cooling" Talcum Powder

Menthol	1–4 g.
Alcohol	10 g.

Dissolve the above and add to:

Talcum Powder	100 g.

Mix until uniform.

Mentholated Talcum

Menthol	0.25 g.
Alcohol	5 cc.
Talcum	50 g.

Dust freely on itching part.

Bath Powder

Formula No. 1

Talcum	8 oz.
Boric Acid	1 oz.
Starch	1 oz.

Baby Powder

Talcum	700 g.
Rice Starch	200 g.
Zinc Oxide	50 g.
Zinc or Magnesium Stearate	45 g.
Lanolin	5 g.

Baby Dusting Powder

Benzocaine	2 g.
Picric Acid (20%)	4 g.
Tincture of Benzoin	5 g.
Boric Acid	5 g.
Talc	74 g.
Purified Kaolin	10 g.

This powder is intended for badly chafed skin, diaper scalds, prickly heat and sunburn.

The picric acid is mixed with the kaolin. This is thoroughly dried and sifted. The benzocaine and tincture of benzoin are mixed with a little talc until absorbed. Then all ingredients are mixed together thoroughly and sifted.

Antiseptic Dusting Powder

Formula No. 1

Potato Starch	700	g.
Light Magnesium Carbonate	1750	g.
Precipitated Chalk	350	g.
Talc	350	g.
Quinosol	5.25	g.
Tincture Benzoin	17.5	g.

Formula No. 2

Thymol	2 g.
Boric Acid	50 g.
Precipitated Chalk	100 g.
Zinc Oxide	300 g.
Talc	450 g.
Almond Oil	20 g.

Formula No. 3

Petrolatum Dusting Powder

Yellow Petrolatum	176 g.
Lanolin	44 g.
Rice Starch	1000 g.
Talc	800 g.
Zinc Oxide	400 g.

Rice starch, talc and zinc oxide are first very thoroughly mixed. Petrolatum and lanolin are melted in kettle at moderate temperature, being well stirred with wooden paddle. Powder mixture is gradually introduced into the still hot fat melt with vigorous agitation. Addition of more powder gradually converts mass into pasty condition, and then coarsely grained mass is obtained. Remainder of powder is added and mixture ground in roller mill to convert it into fine granular state. Uniform distribution of fatty particles, which is an important prerequisite, is thus obtained.

Formula No. 4

Bismuth Subnitrate	10 g.
Boric Acid	10 g.
Mercurous Chloride	10 g.

Dose: Apply locally as a dusting powder.

Formula No. 5

Thymol Iodide	5 g.
Acid Boric	5 g.
to make	10 g.

Dose: for use in powder blower.

Thiosulphate Dusting Powder

Sodium Thiosulphate	6 g.
Boric Acid	24 g.

Dusting powder (prophylactic) for ringworm.

"Prickly Heat" Powder

Starch	12½ lb.
Talc	7 lb.
Zinc Stearate	½ lb.
Camphor	2 oz.
Zinc Oxide	5 lb.
Menthol	1 oz.

"Wet White" Body Powder

Zinc Oxide	100 g.
Osmo-Kaolin	50 g.
Bismuth Carbonate	50 g.
Starch	50 g.
Glycerin	150 cc.
Rosewater	600 g.

Body-Powder for the Tropics

Formula No. 1

Boric Acid, Powder	20 g.
Magnesium Stearate	50 g.
Zinc Oxide	100 g.
Perfume of Good Stability	to suit
Magnesium Carbonate	150 g.
Rice Starch Powder	150 g.
Talcum	500 g.

Mix first the first three ingredients thoroughly, perfume, and mix with the last three ingredients (mixed previously). Sift.

Formula No. 2

(a)	Petrolatum, White	50 g.
	Lanolin, Anhydrous	30 g.
	Beeswax, White	20 g.
	Cetyl Alcohol	15 g.
	Water	75 g.
(b)	Magnesium Carbonate	250 g.
	Zinc Oxide	300 g.
(c)	Zinc Oxide	300 g.
	Bismuth Carbonate, Basic	50 g.
	Talcum	1300 g.
(d)	Perfume	

To the emulsion (a) add (b) while warm, stir thoroughly; add (c), ultimately (d). Mill in a ball-mill, sift at least twice.

Formula No. 3

Zinc Stearate	50 g.
Titanium Dioxide	50 g.
Magnesium Carbonate	50 g.
Talcum	150 g.
Rice Starch	150 g.
Colloidal Caolin	500 g.

CHAPTER XIII

PERFUMES AND TOILET WATERS

Perfumes

THE familiar article known as "perfume" carries with it, as it passes over the counter, a great deal of unnecessary mystery. It is true that many of the ingredients used in compounding it are completely unknown to the general public, and their names would be equally meaningless. But perfumes are "mysterious" and alluring: they are made so deliberately by the advertisements of the manufacturers: a little mystery enhances greatly the charm of the odor.

But from the standpoint of the manufacturers there is of course no mystery: and it is our purpose here to enlighten the reader to the extent of dispelling any mystery that may exist in his mind.

In one detail at least, perfumes are very simply constructed. They consist merely of a small proportion of aromatic substance dissolved in 95% ethyl alcohol. No other known substance will satisfactorily replace ethyl alcohol with the exception of methyl alcohol, and methyl alcohol being poisonous is not used. Ethyl alcohol possesses a very mild and unobtrusive odor which blends happily with *all* perfume odors, and which recedes or disappears altogether after the mixture is aged for a sufficiently long period of time. It is non-poisonous, evaporates rapidly, can be obtained readily at small cost, and is an excellent solvent for the aromatic substances constituting the basis of the perfume. For very coarse perfumes used for other than personal purposes, isopropyl alcohol is successfully substituted. The quantity of aromatic material used in perfumes varies somewhat according to the type of odor, and the strength of odor desired, but varies even more according to the selling price of the product. Very cheap perfumes may contain as little as four or five percent of aromatic substance; high grade perfumes may contain as much as 20%. There is no fixed rule however; very fine perfumes of a light delicate odor, such as violet perfume, would be ruined by too great concentration; in this case the proportion of basic perfume substance is reduced in order to emphasize the delicacy of the scent.

Toilet waters are perfumes in which the proportion of aromatic substance is reduced to one to two percent, and as a consequence of this reduction, the concentration of the alcohol can safely be reduced by the addition of water. Generally speaking, a toilet water may be assumed to be composed of two percent of perfume substance and 98% of 80% alcohol.

So far the making of a perfume is very simple; anyone in possession of the desired aromatic substance can produce a perfume from it by merely adding the proper quantity of alcohol, ageing the mixture from a week to a year, according to the quality of the product and the conscience of the maker, filtering until brilliantly clear, and bottling. But it is to the making of that aromatic substance that the perfumer gives his attention. This material, which is a liquid, an "oil" except in very rare instances, is a complex mixture of aromatic substances so blended as to produce the final odor-complex which is recognizable as a "perfume."

The blending of aromatic substances is analogous to the blending of flavors. Very few indeed of the materials used by the perfumer possess a very agreeable odor in themselves; many of them are decidedly unpleasant. But then, salt, pepper, bay leaves, are not pleasant tasting, yet our food would be in a sorry plight without them. It is the business of the perfumer to mix his basic aromatic substances in such proportions, giving due care to their selection, so that the final effect will be a bland even-toned *perfume.* This procedure is a very difficult, but very highly developed art, comparable with the art of producing a beautiful picture by the proper distribution of an original conglomeration of rather messy smears of color on a palette.

If one were to believe the advertisements, one would be quite certain that the perfumer's art consisted chiefly in transferring perfumes from the flowers to the "flacon." As a matter of fact, there does exist a branch of industry devoted to the extraction of perfume substances from certain flowers, but this is a branch of chemistry, and is almost wholly a scientific subject. Furthermore, the number of flowers from which aromatic substances may be obtained is surprisingly small. Many of our most familiar and highly prized flowers yield no aromatic materials whatever. In this class are lilacs, sweet-peas, morning glory, gardenia. The perfumes which are so easily obtainable which so closely resemble these flowers in odor, are composed entirely of substances not a single one of which was derived from the flower that the perfume imitates. Other flowers do indeed yield up their odoriferous substances when properly treated; the "attar of roses," for example, has been known for thousands of years. Further examples of this type of flower are Jasmine, Hyacinth, Carnation, Lily of the Valley, Violet. These last two, however, produce an extract at so great a cost that their corresponding perfumes are invariably the result of the perfumer's art, and owe nothing whatever to the blossom.

So while it is true that flower extracts are used in making perfumes, their use is restricted to the higher priced perfumes, and even in these instances, the proportion of flower extract used is relatively small. The reason for this is more than the greed of the manufacturer who tries to make his product yield as much profit as possible. It is a much more wholesome reason than that, namely, it is impossible to make a *good* perfume, conforming to the modern standards of goodness, without the use of a fairly large proportion of other substances *not* derived from flowers.

In addition to having the charm of a pleasing odor, a perfume of quality must possess several other characteristics. It must be *lasting.*

It must be a *complex* odor; that is to say, it must possess what is known as "body"; it must not be *thin* or simple in its odor value. The separate odor parts of a perfume must blend in one harmonious whole, like a musical chord, and the notes of the chord must be as numerous as possible. The more numerous they are, and the more perfectly they blend, the better the perfume—from the odor standpoint. A high quality perfume must be enduring; it must not fade too rapidly, and further, the character of the odor should not change noticeably after exposure. In former years when it was customary to apply perfume to the clothing, an indispensable characteristic was paleness of color, so that the perfume did not stain the clothing. Nowadays this is not considered important, since it is common practice to apply the perfume to the person. At the same time, a light colored perfume is usually more pleasing to the eye than a dark one, and the public has been educated to suppose that paleness of color was a mark of quality; quite erroneous, of course, but something for the manufacturer to consider, in planning his product.

The substances used by the perfumer are divided naturally into four classes, according to their source. First, there are flower extracts, derived from actual flowers. Second, there are extractive materials derived from plants, which are not derived from the flower part of the plant; such as oil of wintergreen, oil of rose geranium, sandalwood oil, cedarwood oil. A subdivision of this class is represented by that class of bodies which are obtained by fractional distillation or other means, from the type of essential oils just mentioned. Thus from oil of rose geranium is obtained a liquid known as rhodinol, which is the basis of all imitation rose perfumes and which plays an important part in genuine rose perfumes as well as many other types; from oil of citronella is produced another rose-like oil called geraniol, and this is the basis of imitation rose perfumes of the cheaper variety, such as those used in soaps. Third, are aromatic substances of *animal* original, among which are, the well known Musk and Ambergris, and the lesser known Civet and Castoreum. The fourth class, which is probably the least suspected of all, but which is really the most important, since without it there would be no such thing as modern perfumes, is represented by a long list of aromatic substances which exist nowhere in nature, but which are produced synthetically by chemical methods. It is because these substances are available to the perfumer that you can buy such perfumes as Violet, Sweet Pea, Lilac, Gardenia, Lily of the Valley. All of the curious and intriguing perfumes that have assumed so great a popularity in recent years owe their charm to the presence of synthetic substances which nature does not produce. For, while a perfume must be *flowery,* it need not simulate the odor of a flower. It might be further stated, at this point, that without synthetic chemicals to aid the perfumes, the degree of floweriness itself would be sadly lacking for want of materials to produce it. Floweriness, sweetness, and radiance are *effects* imparted to the composition by the proper use of materials nearly all of which are synthetic in their origin.

The perfumer then has a number of things to bear in mind in beginning to concoct his perfume. The final effect may be any one of a thousand types of odor, but the finished odor must be smooth; that is, no single ingredient should predominate in such a way as to be perceptible to the nose; it must have a pleasing floweriness regardless of how remote from any known flower its odor may be; its odor must last *long* and the odor must not change appreciably while it is in use.

To accomplish this end, considerable knowledge of the properties of the many available aromatic materials is indispensable. The perfumer must know not only the odor of all his materials, but the *strength* of the odor, and the probable *effect* of the substance when blended with other substances. A knowledge of this last marks the difference between the experienced perfumer and the amateur. The beginner would suppose, logically and excusably enough, that the effect of mixing two aromatic substances would be some sort of mathematical average of the two odors. This is often the case but very often too it is not the case at all. The addition of citronellol to hydroxycitronellal gives a result which is olfactorily an average of the two ingredients roughly in the proportion of the mixture; on the other hand, the addition of amyl salicylate to hydroxycitronellal yields a totally new odor only remotely related to the odors of the ingredients in the mixture. A further example of this remarkable property of 2 and 2 equaling 6 instead of 4, is the effect of mixing amyl salicylate and anisic aldehyde.

An analogous effect which is out of all proportion to the properties of the substances alone, is the fixative effect which certain materials have upon the whole mixture. It has been noted above that a perfume should be *lasting,* and further, the *original* type of odor should last. When it is understood that most of the ingredients of perfumes are essential oils, which are also "volatile" oils, it will be at once clear that it is the natural tendency of the perfume to evaporate and disappear; and also a natural effect for the more volatile portions of the mixture to evaporate at a faster rate than the lesser volatile portions, with the consequence that after the evaporation of some of the more volatile portions, their odor effect will have ceased to be as powerful as it was at the beginning, and hence the character of the scent will necessarily have changed. To correct this inconvenient inevitability, the perfumer has recourse to certain types of aromatic substances which, because of their peculiar properties, are known as fixatives. They have the power, in a lesser or greater degree, according to their inherent nature and according to the fitness of their associated components, of retarding the evaporation of the more easily volatile substances, and hence delaying the rate of loss of odor, as well as stabilizing the character of the odor.

The most successful fixation occurs when the fixative can combine with one or more of the other ingredients to produce a blended effect, as noted above. Thus hydroxycitronellal is a good fixative, but it is a most extraordinary fixative when combined with amyl salicylate.

The number of bodies sold and used for fixation purposes is much too multitudinous to be referred to here: space permits us to mention but a few. The finest and most potent of all fixatives is musk. Musk is expensive, it is worth more than its weight in gold, and because of this, it can be used only in the finer grades of perfumes; but it does much more than merely fix the perfume—it creates, through the above described "blend effect" a new and most subtle nuance of odor not attainable by any other means. Ambergris has a similar value, but to a decidedly lesser extent. Other fixatives of great value are Vanillin, Labdanum and Oak Moss. In a general way any difficultly volatile substance will act as a fixative, although the actual fixative value derived from this property of non-volatility is grossly exaggerated in the literature. Attempts have been made, with some success, to produce fixative bodies synthetically, the most noteworthy of these being the series of three musks: Musk xylol, musk ambrette and musk ketone. These are crystalline bodies of some value as fixatives, but the term "musk" does not signify that they are to be compared in potency or even in value with the natural musk.

To impart floweriness, the perfumer has recourse to sweeteners and substances which increase the diffusion of the odor. Floweriness must not be confused with resemblance to a flower. The resemblance is merely in delicacy and sweetness, not in character. It is quite possible, as many struggling perfumers have found out to their discomfiture, to create a perfume lacking sadly in floweriness but at the same time emitting an odor that resembles some given flower beyond criticism. Oil of rose geranium itself may be used as an example of this kind. In itself it resembles the rose in odor, especially when diluted, but it lacks floweriness. Oil of cloves possesses neither floweriness in itself nor does it resemble the odor of any flower (Clove oil, or its extractive eugenol, is the basis of carnation perfume, but the gap between the odor of clove oil and the odor of a carnation is *wide*). Yet, clove oil added judiciously to oil of rose geranium creates this much desired quality of floweriness. Vanillin itself is remote from a perfume, yet it is indispensable in many formulas of converting an insipid dull odor into a sweet and pleasing one. The re-created odor does not smell of *vanilla*—it is merely altered—just as the addition of the proper amount of salt will change an insipid food into a pleasing one.

The *type* of perfume is determined by the use of a predominance of odor values *of that type*. Thus Lily of the Valley perfume is produced by the use of a large proportion of hydroxycitronellal with other ingredients to round out the floweriness. Carnation is the result of a much lower proportion of eugenol, isoeugenol, or clove oil, or a selection of these, with a larger proportion of other ingredients. Aside from the distinctive character of a flower odor, the basic odor of all flowers is much alike; thus the use of rose, jasmine and the lily type, is used in nearly all flower compositions. These separate odors are obscured finally by careful blending and fixation and the individuality is imparted by the use of suitable synthetic bodies. Cheap lilac owes its character to Terpineol; the better grade lilacs are based on anisic aldehyde. The peculiar tinge of odor which identifies the Sweet Pea is obtained with Benzylidene Acetone. Orange Blossom is created by the use of Methyl Anthranilate. The basis of Hyacinth is Phenyl Acetic Aldehyde. Jasmine is produced by a generous use of Benzyl Acetate or Amyl Cinnamic Aldehyde.

The compositing of a perfume is a simple mixing operation. The final product is a liquid, because most of the useful ingredients are liquids, and those which are crystalline, or otherwise solid, such as galbanum or benzoin, are readily soluble in the liquid portion. Once the formula is established, or otherwise known, the procedure then consists merely in weighing out the ingredients in the prescribed proportions and mixing them. Warming the mixture will accelerate the solution of the solid ingredients, but the warming must be done *gently:* a water bath is the most convenient means of accomplishing this.

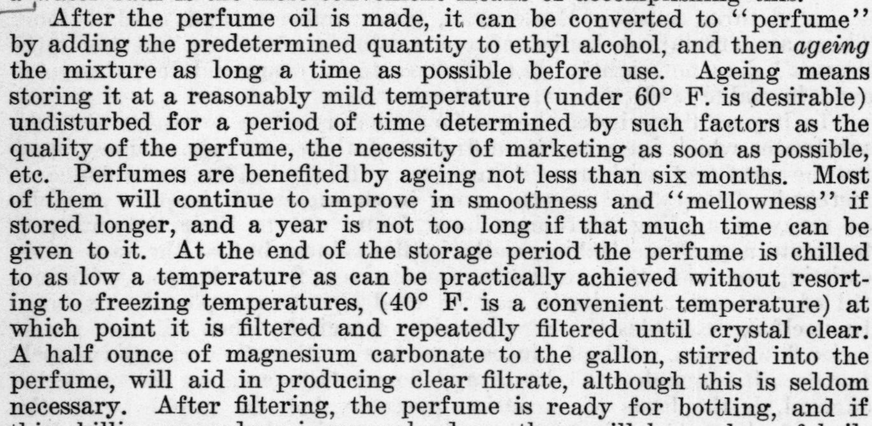

After the perfume oil is made, it can be converted to "perfume" by adding the predetermined quantity to ethyl alcohol, and then *ageing* the mixture as long a time as possible before use. Ageing means storing it at a reasonably mild temperature (under 60° F. is desirable) undisturbed for a period of time determined by such factors as the quality of the perfume, the necessity of marketing as soon as possible, etc. Perfumes are benefited by ageing not less than six months. Most of them will continue to improve in smoothness and "mellowness" if stored longer, and a year is not too long if that much time can be given to it. At the end of the storage period the perfume is chilled to as low a temperature as can be practically achieved without resorting to freezing temperatures, (40° F. is a convenient temperature) at which point it is filtered and repeatedly filtered until crystal clear. A half ounce of magnesium carbonate to the gallon, stirred into the perfume, will aid in producing clear filtrate, although this is seldom necessary. After filtering, the perfume is ready for bottling, and if this chilling procedure is properly done, there will be no loss of brilliance afterward. Perfumes which are not sufficiently aged, or which are filtered warm, are likely to give rise to some precipitation of solid material after standing longer, and when this occurs in a commercial product, it is usually fatal. Hence while the ageing process may seem tedious, and the chilling operation may be inconvenient, the permanence and quality of the finished product will amply repay the trouble.

Perfume Bases

In all of the perfume formulation in this chapter where units of measure are not indicated use grams throughout.

	New Mown Hay	Chypre	Locust
Alpha Ionone	10	—	—
Citronellol	20	—	—
Amyl Salicylate	100	25	5.5
Anisic Aldehyde	20	—	—
Coumarin	5	—	—
Vanillin	5	5	—
Heliotropin	7	—	7
Linalool	10	10	2.5
Petitgrain	10	20	2.5
Jasmine, Artificial	20	25	4
Patchouli Oil	1	25	—
Aldehyde C_{10}, (50%)	1	—	.15
Iso Eugenol	5	—	2.3
Phenyl Ethyl Alcohol	—	25	20
Musk Xylol	—	25	—
Copaiba, Balsam	—	15	—
Birch Tar	—	10	—
Lemon Oil	—	3	—
Bergamot Oil	—	100	—
Rose, Artificial	—	75	—
Cedar Oil	—	15	—
Phenyl Acetic Aldehyde, (50%)	—	—	1
Phenyl Acetic Acid	—	—	.25
Hydroxycitronellol	—	—	12.5
Cinnamic Alcohol	—	—	3.5
Cananga Oil	—	—	3
Methyl Heptine Carbonate, (5%)	—	—	1.0
Geranyl Acetate	—	—	1.3
Amyl Cinnamic Aldehyde	—	—	5

	Flowery Bouquet	Bouquet	Oriental	Oriental A
Rose Gernaium Oil	100	—	—	—
Rose, Artificial	20	—	—	—
Valley Lily, Artificial	500	500	350	100
Terpineol	200	—	110	100
Hydroxycitronellal	200	—	—	—
Bois de Rose	200	—	—	—
Coumarin	30	100	—	—
Anisic Aldehyde	20	—	30	30
Methyl Anthranilate	150	20	—	—
Civet Tincture	50	—	100	60
Hyacinth, Artificial	100	—	—	—

	Flowery Bouquet	Bouquet	Oriental	Oriental A
Benzyl Benzoate	200	200	200	100
Musk Ambrette	50	—	50	30
Opoponax	10	—	200	100
Oak Moss, Liquid	200	—	100	50
Cananga Oil	100	—	—	—
Lavender Oil	—	20	20	10
Bergamot Oil	—	100	—	—
Cassia Oil	—	10	—	—
Tuberose, Artificial	—	100	—	—
Methyl Heptine Carbonate, (5%)	—	100	—	—
Geraniol	—	100	—	—
Vanillin	—	100	—	—
Musk Ketone	—	50	—	—
Orange Blossom, Artificial	—	—	610	100
Jasmine, Artificial	—	—	440	—
Vetivert Oil	—	—	—	100
Jasmine Aldehyde	—	—	—	200
Petitgrain Oil	—	—	—	100
Phenyl Ethyl Alcohol	—	—	—	30
Linalyl Acetate	—	—	—	50
Linalool	—	—	—	50

	Flowery Bouquet A	Bouquet A	Bouquet B
Aldehyde C_9	20	20	20
Oak Moss, Liquid	100	—	—
Jasmine Liquid, Absolute	500	200	200
Rose, Artificial	500	1000	300
Iso Butyl Salicylate	200	100	100
Methyl Ionone	500	—	300
Lilac, Artificial	500	200	300
Musk Ketone	200	—	200
Methyl Heptine Carbonate, (5%)	50	—	—
Valley Lily, Artificial	500	200	—
Bois de Rose	200	200	200
Melittis (Givaudan)	200	—	—
Orange Blossom, Artificial	—	300	300
Methyl Phenyl Acetate	—	40	—
Musk Ambrette	—	100	—
Para Cresyl Phenylacetate	—	50	—
Vanillin	—	30	—
Aldehyde C_{10}, (5%)	—	100	100
Olibanum Gum, 2:1	—	150	—
Terpineol	—	—	200
Hydroxycitronellal	—	—	200
Cananga Oil	—	—	100
Rose Geranium Oil	—	—	100

	Flowery Bouquet A	Bouquet A	Bouquet B
Coumarin	—	—	30
Anisic Aldehyde	—	—	20
Methyl Anthranilate	—	—	100
Civet Tincture	—	—	50
Labdanum	—	—	100
Coriander Oil	—	—	20
Castoreum, 10%	—	—	100
Ambergris Tincture	—	—	100

	Chypre A	Bouquet C	Bouquet D
Jasmine, Artificial	200	500	80
Musk Ketone	400	200	500
Oak Moss, Liquid	500	100	—
Bergamot Oil	1000	—	—
Rose, Absolute	400	—	—
Patchouli Oil	500	—	—
Musk Tincture	200	—	200
Vanillin	100	—	—
Coumarin	200	—	—
Indol, (5%)	100	—	—
Hydroxycitronellal	200	—	—
Lemon Oil, Terpeneless	30	—	—
Phenyl Ethyl Alcohol	—	100	—
Methyl Ionone	—	500	—
Aldehyde C_9, (50%)	—	40	—
Methyl Heptine Carbonate, (10%)	—	50	—
Melittis	—	200	—
Iso Butyl Salicylate	—	200	—
Rhodinol	—	500	150
Lilac, Artificial	—	500	—
Valley Lily, Artificial	—	500	—
Bois de Rose	—	200	—
Cassie, Artificial	—	—	60
Benzyl Benzoate	—	—	1000
Diethyl Anthranilate	—	—	50
Linalyl Acetate	—	—	300
Benzyl Acetate	—	—	300
Tolu, Balsam	—	—	300
Rose, Artificial	—	—	90

	Carnation	Honeysuckle
Eugenol	1600	—
Jasmine, Artificial	400	1500
Heliotropin	400	—
Rose, Artificial	100	—
Phenyl Ethyl Alcohol	50	2000
Orange Blossom, Artificial	100	200
Ocillet	100	—
Orris Liquid. (10%)	150	—
Musk Ketone	100	—
Ambreol	100	—
Benzyl Iso Eugenol	100	—
Bergamot Oil	—	600
Indol, (5%)	—	250
Hydroxycitronellal	—	1000
Benzyl Acetate	—	5000
Benzyl Butyrate	—	500
Benzyl Formate	—	200
Benzyl Propionate	—	2000
Benzyl Benzoate	—	2000
Bois de Rose	—	700
Aurania	—	800
Cananga Oil	—	1000
Amyl Cinnamic Aldehyde	—	500
Para Cresol, (10%)	—	100
Petitgrain Oil	—	500

	Lilac	Rose	Orange Blossom	Heavy Modern Oriental
Citronellol	10	30	3	—
Cananga Oil	20	5	—	—
Amyl Cinnamic Aldehyde	10	—	—	50
Methyl Acetophenone	5	—	—	—
Hydroxycitronellal	10	—	10	—
Phenyl Ethyl Alcohol	11	20	—	—
Linalool	10	5	10	—
Terpineol	20	—	—	—
Methyl Para Cresol	1	—	—	—
Musk Ketone	5	—	—	—
Valley Lily, Artificial	10	—	—	—
Iso Eugenol	5	—	—	—
Aldehyde C_{10}, (5%)	—	5	—	—
Benzyl Acetate	—	10	30	—
Geraniol	—	50	—	—
Ionone	—	5	—	—
Geranyl Acetate	—	10	—	—
Copaiba Balsam	—	10	10	—
Patchouli Oil	—	2	—	—

	Lilac	Rose	Orange Blossom	Heavy Modern Oriental
Phenyl Acetic Acid	—	2	2	—
Linalyl Acetate	—	3	—	—
Petitgrain Oil	—	—	100	—
Methyl Anthranilate	—	—	15	—
Beta Naphthyl Ethyl Ester	—	—	10	50
Amyl Salicylate	—	—	—	30
Ionone	—	—	—	10
Benzylidene Acetone	—	—	—	6
Musk Xylol	—	—	—	5
Vanillin	—	—	—	3

	French Type	French Lilac Type
Oak Moss, Liquid	200	—
Bergamot Oil, Terpeneless	150	—
Linalyl Acetate	50	—
Sweet Orange Oil	200	—
Valley Lily, Artificial	300	—
Narcissus Absolute	100	—
Jasmine, Artificial	400	200
Rhodinol	200	—
Alcohol C_9	70	—
Aldehyde C_9, (5%)	100	30
Linalool	200	—
Geranyl Acetate	200	—
Methyl Phenylacetate	50	—
Alpha Ionone	100	—
Vetivert Oil	100	—
Terpineol	100	100
Coumarin	200	—
Vanillin	100	—
Musk Ketone	100	100
Canada Snake Root Oil	100	—
Hydroxycitronellal	—	2000
Geraniol	—	50
Phenyl Acetic Aldehyde, (50%)	—	50
Phenyl Ethyl Alcohol	—	300
Anisic Aldehyde	—	20
Rose, Artificial	—	30
Labdanum	—	100

	Bouquet E	Violet
Bergamot Oil, Terpeneless	200	—
Linalyl Acetate	100	—
Jasmine, Artificial	500	100
Aldehyde C_9, (5%)	100	—
Vetivert	100	—
Coumarin	400	—
Rose Geranium Oil	200	—
Rose, Artificial	100	—
Bay Oil, Terpeneless	300	—
Eugenol	100	—
Petitgrain Oil	400	—
Bergamot Oil	300	—
Indol, (5%)	150	—
Ambreol	500	—
Lavender	150	—
Raldeine D	300	100
Lemon Oil	20	—
Rhodinol	—	100
Alpha Ionone	—	1000
Hydroxycitronellal	—	300
Cananga Oil	—	100
Aldehyde C_{12}, (5%)	—	100
Methyl Heptin Carbonate, (10%)	—	200
Cassie, Artificial	—	100
Guaiac	—	300
Methyl Ionone	—	100
Orris, Liquid (10%)	—	175

	Jasmine	Sweet Pea	Heavy Oriental
Benzyl Acetate	1500	—	—
Bergamot Oil	150	300	3000
Bois de Rose	150	—	200
Benzyl Alcohol	300	—	—
Phenyl Ethyl Alcohol	300	—	—
Indol, (5%)	50	—	—
Hydroxycitronellal	250	200	200
Orange Blossom, Artificial	250	200	—
Cananga Oil	150	—	200
Jasmine Absolute	300	200	—
Amyl Cinnamic Aldehyde	100	—	—
Benzylidene Acetone	—	150	—
Heliotropin	—	450	100
Musk Ketone	—	50	—
Phenyl Acetic Aldehyde, (50%)	—	100	—
Terpineol	—	1000	—
Iso Butyl Phenylacetate	—	120	—
Rose, Artificial	—	80	—

	Jasmine	Sweet Pea	Heavy Oriental
Tolu	—	150	—
Alcohol C_9	—	60	—
Benzyl Benzoate	—	150	400
Anisic Aldehyde	—	—	100
Lavender Oil	—	—	60
Tolyl Acetate	—	—	100
Vanillin	—	—	200
Oak Moss, Liquid	—	—	400
Aldehyde C_{10}, (5%)	—	—	160
Diethyl Anthranilate	—	—	580
Ambreol	—	—	600

Rose

Formula No. 1

Rose, Otto	150
Rose, Absolute	50
Rhodinol	200
Phenyl Ethyl Alcohol	300
Phenyl Ethyl Propionate	100
Alpha Ionone	50
Vetiverol Acetate	25
Rhodinol Acetate	25
Citronellol Butyrate	25
Phenyl Acetic Aldehyde (50%)	50
Aldehyde C_9 (10%)	15
Alcohol C_{10} (25%)	10

Formula No. 2

Rhodinol	20.0
Nerol	5.0
Geraniol	5.0
Phenyl Ethyl Alcohol	8.0
Citronellol	3.0
Geranyl Acetate	2.0
Phenyl Ethyl, Methyl Ethyl Carbinol	3.0
Terpeneless Rose Geranium	2.0
Guaiacum Wood Oil	1.5
Terpeneless Petitgrain	0.5
Nonyl Aldehyde (1–10)	0.5
Decyl Aldehyde (1–10)	0.2

Build the formula in the order shown, special attention being given to the effect of each addition. Rhodinol, particularly if a natural isolate, has a decided rose odor, but would lack power and body as a scent by itself. Other constituents of a rose-like odour, or that have a decided value in the synthesis, must be added. Nerol is next in importance; note the effect of this addition; repeat with the addition of each item until the terpeneless rose geranium has been included. Up to this stage the compound will not have shown any definite character; the items that follow are included to act as toning agents. Guaiacum wood oil has a slight orris note; this is the reason for the inclusion, but at the same time it can be classed as a fixative. Any ingredient with a slight odor of orris can be used in this formula as a modifier, so the question arises: Why not orris itself? Oil of orris (orris liquid) can be used, of course, but the other serves the purpose well at a greatly reduced cost; and orris concretes need a deal of preparation. However, liquid orris appears in the violet formula, so those who wish to try it must use only 1 gm. Terpeneless petitgrain is also used as a modifier; it greatly helps to impart the somewhat bland note necessary in "rose." The aliphatics are best manipulated in a 10 per cent solution. Benzyl benzoate is the fixing agent. Rhodinol (ex Bourbon geranium), geraniol (ex palmarosa) and citronellol are the isolates to use for the best results. Finally, the addition of 5 per cent pure virgin otto is left to the compounder's discretion.

Formula No. 3

Pelargol	100 g.
Diphenyl Oxide (1:1)	25 g.
Vanillin	10 g.
Geraniol	75 g.
Terpineol	20 g.

Formula No. 4

Phenyl Ethyl Alcohol	70
Rhodinol	15
Phenyl Acetaldehyde	5
Methyl Phenyl Acetate	1
Vetivert Bourbon	2
Geranium Bourbon	2
Methyl Ionone	3
Aldehyde C_{10} (10%)	2

Red Rose

Geraniol	7½
Lilac, White	1½
Jacinth	¾
Benzyl Acetate	1½
Terpenyl Acetate	1½
Benzyl Benzoate	1½
Geranium Oil (Reunion)	1

Carnation

Formula No. 1

Geraniol, Pure	12.0 g.
Rhodinol	2.0 g.
Geraniol (ex Palma Rosa)	2.0 g.
Citronellol	5.0 g.
Otto of Rose, Bulgarian	1.0 g.
Geranyl Acetate	0.5 g.
Phenylethyl Alcohol	12.5 g.
Isoeugenol	10.0 g.
Eugenol	10.0 g.
Amyl Salicylate	10.0 g.

Formula No. 2

(Do not use in Creams or Lipsticks)

Phenyl Ethyl Alcohol	100
Isoeugenol	250
Eugenol	300
Rose Otto	25
Rhodinol	100
Ethyl Vanillin	10
Musk Ketone	50
Benzyl Isoeugenol	50
Methyl Ionone	50
Oppoponax Resin	2
Tolu Resin	8

Wallflower

Formula No. 1

Geraniol	40.0 g.
Benzyl Alcohol	20.0 g.
Anisic Aldehyde	20.0 g.
Ionone (100%)	10.0 g.
Bergamot Oil	10.0 g.
Benzyl Acetate	20.0 g.
Heliotropin	10.0 g.
Rose, Synthetic	15.0 g.
Jasmin, Synthetic	5.0 g.
Coumarin	2.5 g.
Vanillin	2.5 g.

Formula No. 2

(Do not use in creams or lipsticks as it is apt to irritate.)

Isoeugenol	30
Eugenol	30
Rhodinol	10
Phenyl Ethyl Alcohol	10
Vanillin	3
Alpha Ionone	5
Synthetic Rose	7
Benzyl Salicylate	5

Honeysuckle

Formula No. 1

Phenyl Ethyl Alcohol	100
Cinnamyl Alcohol	100
Heliotropin	50
Alpha Ionone	100
Mimosa, Synthetic	50
Jasmin, Synthetic	100
Rose, Synthetic	50
Terpineol	50
Phenyl Acetic Acid	10
Musk Ketone	25
Musk Ambrette	25
Methyl Naphthyl Ketone	50
Para Cresyl Phenyl Acetate	10
Hydrotropic Aldehyde	10
Neroli, Synthetic	50
Phenyl Ethyl Phenyl Acetate	50
Linalool	50
Nerol	50
Hydroxycitronellol	170

Formula No. 2

Hydroxycitronellal	25
Alpha Ionone	10
Terpineol	5
Phenyl Ethyl Alcohol	6
Cinnamyl Alcohol	10
Vanillin	3
Jasmin, Absolute	2
Mimosa, Absolute	5
Neroli, Absolute	1
Musk Ketone	2
Methyl Naphthyl Ketone	5
Linalool	5
Benzyl Acetate	5
Rhodinol	5
Cinnamyl Acetate	5
Heliotropin	5
Phenyl Acetaldehyde (50%)	1

Sweet Pea

Phenyl Ethyl Phenyl Acetate	5
Dimethyl Acetophenone	3
Ethyl Vanillin	1
Benzyl Acetate	5
Musk Ketone	5
Ylang Manila	5
Benzyl Salicylate	10
Synthetic Rose	2
Cinnamyl Alcohol	20
Hydroxycitronellal	20
Linalool	10
Hydrotropic Aldehyde	1
Neroli, Petale	5
Terpineol	8

Gardenia

Formula No. 1

Benzophenone	10
Amylol (Norda)	25
Ylang Ylang Bourbon	60
Linalool	35
Acetophenone	3
Dianthine, Naef	15
Orange Floressence	20
Alpha Ionone	20
Jasmin Floressence	125
Orange Absolute	20
Hydroxycitronellol	30
Rhodinol	15
Phenyl Ethyl Alcohol	20
Aldehyde C_{18}	1
Solution Lauric Aldehyde (10%)	10
Otto Rose, Genuine	25
Musk Ketone	10
Methyl Napthyl Ketone	10
Vanillin	1
Resin, Guaiac Wood	15
Yara Yara	1
Amyl Cinnamic Aldehyde	5
Amyl Salicylate	20
Solution Amyl Acetate (10%)	4

Formula No. 2

Solution Duodecyl Aldehyde (10%)	1
Jasmin from Pomade	2
Orange Floressence	5
Paramethoxy Phenyl Acetaldehyde	10
Eugenol	2
Tuberose Aldehyde (Dodge & Olcott)	3
Musk Ambrette	3
Jasminique Aldehyde (Verley)	2
Phenyl Ethyl Acetate	1
Oil Neroli Petale	1
Benzyl Propionate	5
Jasmin, Artificial	70
Amylol (Norda)	5
Amyl Cinnamic Aldehyde	2
Methyl Ionone	8
Dianthine	2
Solution Aldehyde C_{18} (10%)	3

Orchid

Formula No. 1

Jasmin de Provence	30
Amylol (Norda)	10
Rose Floressence	5
Methyl Naphthyl Ketone	10
Methyl Ionone	5
Orange Floressence	5
Solution Aldehyde Lauric 10%	5
Jasmin Floressence	10
Musk Ketone	10
Musk Ambrette	5
Coumarin	5

Formula No. 2

Phenyl Ethyl Alcohol	10
Violet Ketone	10
Jasmin Flower Oil, Artificial	20
Solution Paracresol Acetate 1%	5
Amylol (Norda)	15
Sweet Orange Oil	1
Solution Duodecyl Aldehyde 10%	5
Cinnamic Alcohol	10
Hyacylene	5
Vanillin	5
Jasmin Floressence	5
Rose	10
Tincture Civet (4/128)	10
Opoponax (Samuelson)	5
Amyl Salicylate	5
Lily Valley (De Laire)	4

Formula No. 3

Phenyl Ethyl Alcohol	15
Methyl Ionone	10
Amylol (Norda)	15
Orange Absolute	1
Solution Lauric Aldehyde 10%	20
Vanillin	5
Opoponax (Guillendome)	15
Bergamot Oil Terpeneless	10
Amyl Salicylate	20
Benzyl Iso Eugenol	4
Rose Absolute	10
Jasminette (Heine)	5
Otto Rose, Genuine	2
Acetophenone	1
Coumarin	4
Hydroxycitronellol	10
Cyclafol (Agfa)	1
Civet Artificial (100%) (Polak Fruital Works)	1
Ylang Ylang Bourbon	10
Dianthine	5
Musk Ketone	5
Benzyl Acetate	5
Muguettol (DuPont)	26

Formula No. 4

Jasmin Floressence	20
Terpineol	20
Persian Ambergris (Norda)	4
Amyl Cinamic Aldehyde	5
Cyclafol (Agfa)	1
Hydroxycitronellol	20
Cinnamic Alcohol from Styrax	10
Styrax Oil	4

Geraniol	10
Citronellol	18
Amylol (Norda)	5
Ylang Ylang Manila	10
Otto Rose, Genuine	25
Phenyl Ethyl Alcohol	5
Solution Methyl Nonyl Acetaldehyde 10%	3
Solution Lauric Aldehyde (10%)	1
Aubepine	10
Rhodinol No. 1 (SCUR)	4
Oil Bergamot, (Trapenetto)	10
Musk Ketone	10
Heliotropine	5

Formula No. 5

Hydroxycitronellol	48
Persian Ambergris	4
Terpineol	40
Jasmin, Absolute	4
Amyl Acetate, Pure	1
Amylol (Norda)	9
Ylang Ylang Oil	4
Dianthine	2
Oil Cinnamon Ceylon	2
Butyl Cinnamic Aldehyde	2
Orange Floressence	2
Solution Benzyl Aldehyde (50%)	1
Rose Otto Genuine	8
Hyacinthol (Norda)	4
Musk Ketone	4
Heliotropine	5
Perrol (Van Ameringen)	10

Lavender

Formula No. 1

French Lavender Oil	500
Spike Lavender Oil	100
Bergamot Oil	200
Geraniol	100
Sandalwood Oil	60
Rosemary Oil	80
Thyme Oil	20
Coumarin	30
Dimethyl-Hydroquinone	10
Artificial Musk	3
Tincture of Civet	10
Mousse de Chêne	3
Labdanum Resin	3
Styrax Resin	3

Formula No. 2

Lavender Oil	75 g.
Lavender Spike Oil	75 g.
Geranium Oil	75 g.
Coumarin	2 g.
Sandal Wood Oil	2 g.
Bergamot Oil	100 g.
Lemon Oil	25 g.

Sandalwood

Formula No. 1

Sandalwood Oil	200
Cedarwood Oil	150
Patchouli Oil	15
Bergamot Oil	30
Eugenol	10
Vetiver Oil	20
Artificial Musk	5
Geranium Oil	30
Cassia Oil	5
Cananga Oil	5
Extract of Mousse de Chêne	10
Styrax Resin	5
Coumarin	5
Dimethyl-Hydroquinone	3
Tincture of Civet	20

Formula No. 2

Sandalwood Oil	100
Cedarwood Oil	120
Geraniol	20
Terpineol	50
Hydroxy-Citronellol	10
Artificial Musk	3
Styrax Resin	3

Medicated Perfume

Lavender Oil (42% Ester)	30
Camphor	10
Menthol	5
Thymol	5
Rosemary Oil	25
Methyl Salicylate	15
Benzaldehyde	5
Bay Oil, Terpeneless	5

Lilac

Formula No. 1

Terpineol	30
Hydroxycitronellal	15
Cinnamyl Alcohol	10
Rhodinol	10
Heliotropin	7
Rose, Absolute	2
Jasmin, Absolute	5
Phenyl Ethyl Alcohol	5
Anisic Aldehyde	7
Phenyl Acetaldehyde (50%)	5
Musk Xylene	3
Sandalwood Oil	1

Formula No. 2

Anisic Aldehyde	10 cc.
Jasmin, Synthetic	10 cc.
Heliotropin	5 cc.
Phenyl Ethyl Alcohol	5 cc.
Phenyl Acetaldehyde	5 cc.
Bergamot Oil	3 cc.
Musk Ketone	3 cc.
Styrax Resin	2 cc.
Ylang Ylang Oil	2 cc.
Terpineol	55 cc.

Individual touches may be imparted to the above by the sparing use of any or all of the following: amyl salicylate, acetophenone, methyl anthranilate, benzyl acetate, cinnamic alcohol, benzyl benzoate, hydroxycitronellol, and oil nutmeg.

Formula No. 3

Ylang Ylang Oil, Manila	1 g.
Jasmine Flower Oil, Artificial	12 g.
Rhodinol	6 g.
Acacia Flower Oil, Artificial	2 g.
Hydroxycitronellal Diethylacetal	30 g.
Terpineol, Extra	20 g.
Phenylacetaldehyde Dimethylacetal	4 g.
Aubépine (from Anethol)	2 g.
Heliotropin	12 g.
Iso-Eugenol	1.5 g.
Vanillin	0.5 g.
Octyl Acetate (10%) in Benzyl Alcohol	0.5 g.

Formula No. 4

Phenylacetaldehyde, (50%)	10 g.
Hydroxycitronellal, Pure	30 g.
Cinnamic Alcohol	20 g.
Amyl Cinnamic Aldehyde	20 g.
Phenyl Ethyl Alcohol	10 g.
Linalool	9 g.
Aldehyde C_{12}, (10%)	1 g.

This formula can be modified by cutting down such products as hydroxycitronellal and cinnamic alcohol and replacing them by 5 per cent jasmin natural, 1 to 2 per cent of rose de mai, one gram of musk ketone. Other variants are heliotropin crystals from 1 to 2 per cent, vanillin 0.5 per cent, methyl ionone 1 per cent, styralyl acetate 1 per cent, terpineol extra (at most) 1 per cent, and benzyl acetate 1 per cent. Any of these products with the exception of vanillin and heliotropin are satisfactory for powders and creams.

Formula No. 5

(For Soaps)

Hydroxycitronellal Residue	25 g.
Phenylacetaldehyde, (50%)	5 g.
Terpineol	40 g.
Amyl Cinnamic Aldehyde	10 g.
Cinnamic Alcohol	10 g.
Bois de Rose, Femelle	9 g.
Styralyl Acetate	1 g.

Patchouli may be added as a fixative but not more than 1 per cent should be added.

Lilac for Disinfectants and Sprays:

Styralyl Acetate	1 g.
Benzyl Acetate	20 g.
Terpineol	60 g.
Hydroxycitronellal	10 g.
Amyl Cinnamic Aldehyde	9 g.

Variants—

20 grams of terpineol, 10 grams of phenylacetaldehyde, 10 grams of benzyl acetate, 5 grams of bromstyrol 100 per cent.

Ylang Ylang Substitute

Coriander	2
Geraniol	2
Benzyl Acetate	4
Cananga Oil	3

Gardenia

Formula No. 1

Opoponax Oil, Natural (Schimmel)	10
Benzyl Iso Eugenol	10
Eugenol	3
Auriantiol	10
Hydroxycitronellal	5
Linalool	50
Amylol (Norda)	10
Musk Ambrette	5
Coumarin	2
Ylang Ylang Manilla	15
Solution Acetophenone (1%)	2
Otto Rose, Genuine	10
Cinnamic Alcohol	20
Amyl Acetate, Pure	1
Solution Aldehyde C_{14}—(1%)	5
Amyl Salicylate	28
Aldehyde C_{18}	10
Solution Lauric Aldehyde (10%)	4

Formula No. 2

Linalool	20
Alpha Ionone	20
Dianthine Naef	15
Ylang Ylang, Bourbon	55
Acetophenone	3
Orange Floressence	20
Jasmin Chassis	20
Amylol (Norda)	25
Hydroxycitronellol	30
Rhodinol No. 1 SCUR (DuPont)	10
Phenyl Ethyl Alcohol	20
Amyl Salicylate	4
Buxine (Givaudan)	8
Musk Ketone	10
Yara Yara	1
Jasmin Floressence	20
Amyl Acetate	5
Solution Oil Dill (10%)	1
Otto Rose, Genuine	5
Hyperessence Orange	8
Aldehyde C 16	5
Opoponax Natural Oil (Schimmel)	5
Cinnamic Alcohol	25
Solution Peach Aldehyde (1%)	5
Benzyl Alcohol	60

Formula No. 3

Phenylacetaldehyde	10 g.
Tincture of Castoreum (4/128)	25 g.
Musk Ketone	10 g.
Lauric Aldehyde (10%)	1 g.
Phenyl Ethyl Alcohol	26 g.
Hydroxycitronellol	18 g.
Gladiol (Lueders)	198 g.
Oil Mandarin	2 g.
Methyl Heptin Carbonate (10%)	1 g.
Orris Liquid, Bruno Court	10 g.
Lavender Oil (38/40% Ester)	3 g.
Heliotropine	3 g.
Iso Eugenol	3 g.
Rhodinol No. 1 SCUR (DuPont)	5 g.
Methyl Ionone	5 g.
Musk Ambrette	5 g.
Solution Methyl Nonyl Acetaldehyde	2 g.
Ylang Ylang Oil	2 g.
Tincture Civette (4/128)	28 g.

Formula No. 4

Lily of the Valley, (DeLaire)	30
Neroli Petale Oil	16
Orange Floressence (Ungerer)	16
Ylang Ylang Oil	25
Phenyl Ethyl Alcohol	15
Aldehyde C 18	120
Indol Crystals (Agfa)	1
Oil Opoponax (Schimmel)	20
Tuberose Aldehyde (Dodge & Olcott)	5
Styralyl Acetate	2
Jasmin Floressence	15
Amylol (Norda)	10
Cinnamic Alcohol	5
Citronellol	5
Iso Eugenol	2
Solution Lauric Aldehyde (10%)	2
Bergamot Oil	6
Violet Ketone	12
Solution Methyl Para Cresol (10%)	1
Musk Ambrette	10

Formula No. 5

Lilac, Synthetic	20
Rose, Synthetic	10
Lily, Synthetic	30
Jasmin, Synthetic	25
Phenyl Acetaldehyde (50%)	2
Methyl Naphthyl Ketone	6
Isoeugenol	2
Vanillin	2
Styralyl Acetate	3

Jasmine

Formula No. 1

Benzyl Acetate	50
Hydroxycitronellal	15
Cinnamyl Alcohol	10
Linalool	7
Ylang Ylang Manila	7
Para Cresyl Caprylate	2
Methyl Ionone	3
Benzyl Formate	1
Benzyl Propionate	3
Amyl Cinnamic Aldehyde	2

Formula No. 2

Benzyl Acetate	10.0 g.
Tolyl Acetate	5.0 g.
Benzyl Propionate	3.0 g.
Phenyl Ethyl Alcohol	8.0 g.
Rhodinol	2.0 g.
Nerol	1.0 g.
Geraniol	2.0 g.
Alpha-amyl Cinnamic Aldehyde (pure)	2.5 g.
Para Methyl Quinoline	0.3 g.

Musk Ketone	0.5 g.
Aldehyde C_{13} (1–10)	0.3 g.
Linalyl Acetate	1.0 g.
Linalol	1.0 g.
Hydroxycitronellol	3.0 g.
Methyl Ionone, Alpha	5.0 g.
Methyl Anthranilate	2.0 g.
Phenyl Acetic Acid	0.1 g.

Formula No. 3

Jasmin Pomade Washings	100 g.
Heliotropin	5 g.
Ylang Ylang Oil	5 g.
Phenylacetaldehyde	5 g.
Terpineol Extra	5 g.
Bromstyrol, (10%)	1 g.
Musk Ketone	1 g.
Civet, Tincture	5 g.

Formula No. 4

Benzyl Acetate	10 g.
Amyl Cinnamic Aldehyde	30 g.
Styrax, Distilled	20 g.
Indol Solution, (1%)	10 g.
Ionone, Alpha	10 g.
Cinnamic Alcohol	10 g.
Phenyl Ethyl Alcohol	9 g.
Musk Ketone	1 g.

(Instead of using 10 grams of indol 1 per cent, one can replace half of it by that amount of civet tincture, 4 oz. to the gallon.)

Formula No. 5

(For Soap)

Cinnamic Alcohol	100 g.
Styrax	100 g.
Amyl Cinnamic Aldehyde	300 g.
Orris, Powdered	50 g.

Linalool can be used in jasmin to the extent of 5 per cent, in which case it can replace some of the styrax. Also, about 10 per cent of hydroxycitronellal can be added.

Formula No. 6

Benzyl Acetate	400
Hydroxycitronellal	100
Linalool	50
Heliotropin	50
Amyl Cinnamic Aldehyde	50
Para Cresyl Caprylate	50
Ylang Ylang Oil	50
Jasmin Absolute	250

Formula No. 7

"J Vegetal"

Jasmin Pomade Washings	10 g.
Tuberose Pomade Washings	5 g.
Hydroxycitronellal	5 g.
Ylang Ylang, Manilla	2 g.
Heliotropin	1 g.
Ionone, Alpha	1 g.
Phenylacetaldehyde	1 g.
Linalool	1 g.
Musk Ketone	1 g.
Tincture of Civet (4 oz. to gallon)	1 g.

Lily

Hydroxycitronellal	30
Terpineol	20
Methyl Ionone	5
Ylang Ylang Oil	5
Rose, Absolute	3
Jasmin, Absolute	2
Heliotropine	5
Cyclamen Aldehyde	3
Phenyl Ethyl Alcohol	10
Vanillin	0.5
Methyl Phenyl Acetate	0.5
Nerol	6
Rhodinol	5
Linalool	5

Violet

Constituents.	*Parma*		*Boise de Nice.*			*Classic.*	*Ordinary.*
Formula	No. 1	No. 2	No. 3	No. 4	No. 5	No. 6	No. 7
Ionone, Alpha	260	400	500	350	350	300	150
Ionone, Beta	140	—	—	—	—	—	250
Methylionone	200	—	—	250	250	—	—
Orris Concrete	—	50	—	25	—	—	—
Orris Resinoid	—	150	—	65	—	100	—
Cassie, Natural	—	20	—	—	10	—	—
Jasmin, Natural	—	15	—	25	—	20	—
Rose, Natural	—	10	—	—	—	10	—
Benzyl Acetate	50	25	100	40	100	30	100

Constituents.	*Parma*		*Boise de Nice.*			*Classic.*	*Ordinary.*
Formula	No. 1	No. 2	No. 3	No. 4	No. 5	No. 6	No. 7
Geraniol	—	—	100	25	—	—	—
Vetiverol	20	35	—	—	—	—	—
Musk Xylol	—	—	—	—	—	—	40
Musk Ketone	—	40	35	50	—	—	—
Methyl Heptin Carbonate	—	—	5	—	10	7.5	10
Methyl Octin Carbonate	5	5	—	—	—	—	—
Coumarin	—	35	—	—	30	—	—
Heliotropin	70	—	100	45	100	100	100
Vanillin	30	10	—	—	—	—	—
Phenylethyl Alcohol	100	60	—	75	—	140	150
Bergamot	—	50	—	—	—	125	50
Hydroxycitronellal	—	50	—	—	—	—	—
Violet Leaf Absolute	—	—	—	10	—	—	—
Methylnonyl Aldehyde	—	—	—	0.5	—	—	—
Linalol	75	—	—	25	—	—	150
Terpineol	—	—	—	—	85	—	—
Linalyl Acetate	50	—	40	—	50	—	—
Geranyl Acetate	—	—	—	—	20	—	—
Aldehyde C_{12}	—	—	—	—	5	—	—
Anisic Aldehyde from Anethol	—	—	60	—	—	—	—

Formula No. 8

Alpha Ionone	200
Beta Ionone	50
Methyl Ionone	150
Orris Resin	100
Cassie Synthetic	50
Jasmin Synthetic	50
Vetiverol Acetate	50
Coumarin	25
Vanillin	25
Bergamot Oil	50
Hydroxycitronellal	50
Isobutyl Phenyl Acetate	50
Musk Ketone	50
Violet Natural	100

Neroli

Formula No. 1

Neroli, Petale	25
French Pettigrain	35
Nerol	10
Rhodinol	5
Linalool	5
Linalyl Acetate	3
Orange Flower, Absolute	5
Methyl Anthranilate	5
Aldehyde (10%)	2
Phenyl Ethyl Alcohol	5

Formula No. 2

Neroli, Petale	250
French Pettigrain	300
Phenyl Ethyl Alcohol	100
Linalyl Anthranilate	100
Linalool	50
Nerol	100
Rhodinol	50
Phenyl Acetic Acid	5
Sweet Italian Orange Oil	45

Formula No. 3

Ionone (100%)	4.0
Ionone, Alpha	2.0
Ionone, Beta	2.0
Methyl Ionone, Alpha	2.0
Orris, Liquid	1.5
Rose, Artificial	1.0
Jasmine, Artificial	1.0
Heliotropin	1.0
Citronella Hydrate	2.0
Musk Ambrette	0.2
Methyl Heptine Carbonate	0.1
Bergamot	3.0
Aldehyde C_{13} (1–10)	1.5
Cassia Absolute	1.5

Manufacturers have a wide divergence of opinion as to what constitutes ionone. Samples vary so much that the first experiments should be made with the smallest possible quantities. Many experiments can be made by the alterations of the ionones, but alpha-methyl-ionone should never be exceeded beyond the given amount, and the total to be about 50 per cent of the formula. Aldehyde C_{13} and methyl heptine carbonate can be slightly increased or decreased, at will of the compounder.

Formula No. 4

Ionone	400
Concrete Orris Oil	20
Cananga Oil	40
Methyl Heptin Carbonate	8
Sandalwood Oil	15
Benzyl Acetate	40
Artificial Otto of Rose	20
Bergamot Oil	20
Phenyl-ethyl Alcohol	10
Heliotropin	35
Cassie Extract	20
Styrax Resin	15
Artificial Musk	2
Extract of Mousse de Chêne	5

Formula No. 5

Bergamot Oil	100 g.
Iris Resinoid	30 g.
Neroli	25 g.
Benzoin Infusion	75 g.
Terpineol	50 g.
Violet (5187, Heine)	125 g.
Jasmine Flower Oil	40 g.
Fixol—Violet	50 g.

Formula No. 6

Violet Oil, Artificial	2
Cananga Oil	3
Jasmine, Artificial	1
Neroli	½
Vanillin	1
Heliotropin	2
Lemongrass	¼
Sandalwood	¼
Jacinth	1

Lily of the Valley

Formula No. 1

Bois de Rose (French distilled), or Linalool, same quantity	20 g.
Mimosa, Concrete	5 g.
Isoeugenol Acetate	1 g.
Rose de Mai	1 g.
Jasmin Concrete	5 g.
Muguet Concrete	10 g.
Orris Concrete	5 g.
Cinnamic Alcohol	10 g.
Phenyl Ethyl Alcohol	5 g.
Tincture Civet (4 oz. to gallon)	5 g.
Musk Ketone	2 g.

If this is too expensive, the natural materials can be cut down and additional linalool, isoeugenol acetate, amyl cinnamic aldehyde, and terpineol can be added. But this means nearly half the materials can be omitted.

For toilet waters, the quantity of bois de rose or linalool should be doubled.

Formula No. 2

Linalool, or Cayenne Linaloe Oil	40 g.
Ylang-Ylang, Manilla	7 g.
Dimethyl Benzyl Carbinyl Acetate	2 g.
Terpineol	7 g.
Hydroxycitronellal	10 g.
Ionone	2 g.

Formula No. 3

Cyclamen Aldehyde	1 g.
Phenylethyl Alcohol	7 g.
Estragon Oil	0.1 g.
Ysminia (Naef)	5 g.
Cassie Absolute	1 g.
Rhodinol	10 g.
Linalyl Isobutyrate	2 g.
Floranal (Flora)	2 g.

Formula No. 4

Hydroxycitronellal	40 g.
Phenylethyl Alcohol	10 g.
Dimethyl Benzyl Carbinol	2 g.
Alpha Ionone	3 g.
Geranium Oil, Terpeneless	3 g.
Cinnamic Alcohol	6 g.
Ylang-Ylang Oil	3 g.
Ysminia	5 g.
Heliotropin	1 g.

Formula No. 5

For Creams

Linaloe Oil, Cayenne	50 g.
Ylang-Ylang, Bourbon	20 g.
Bergamot Oil, Terpeneless	5 g.
Dimethyl Benzyl Carbinol	2 g.
Rose de Mai Absolute	2 g.
Jasmin Absolute	1 g.
Orange Flower Absolute	1 g.
Rosacetol (Givaudan) or Floranal (Flora)	2 g.
Citronellol	5 g.

Formula No. 6

Linalool	40 g.
Hydroxycitronellal	20 g.
Linalyl Acetate	5 g.
Terpinyl Acetate	5 g.
Phenyl Ethyl Alcohol	5 g.
Phenyl Acetic Acid	5 g.

Terpineol	10	g.
Styrax, Distilled	8	g.
Musk Ambrette	2	g.

Formula No. 7

Geraniol, from Palmarosa Oil	25	g.
Linalool, from Rosewood Oil	12.5	g.
Phenylethyl Alcohol	15	g.
Phenylacetaldehyde Dimethylacetal	5	g.
α-Ionone	1.5	g.
Benzaldehyde	0.1	g.
Jasmine Flower Oil, Artificial	10	g.
Rose Oil, Artificial, Extra Fine	8	g.
Lilac Flower Oil, Artificial	25	g.
Ylang Ylang Oil, Manila	4	g.
Rhodinol	10	g.
Coriander Oil, Terpene-Free	0.5	g.
Hydroxycitronellal Dimethylacetal	20	g.
Hydroxycitronellal Diethylacetal	40	g.

Type "Tosca"

Formula No. 1

Orange Oil, Sweet, Calabrian	8.5	cc.
Bergamot Oil, Extra Fine, Reggio	17	cc.
Lemon Oil	19	cc.
Ylang Ylang, Genuine	6	cc.
Rose Oil, Genuine, Bulgarian	2.5	cc.
Jasmine, Pure	1.3	cc.
Coumarin	6.5	g.
Musk, Artificial, Ambrette	1	g.
Musk, Artificial, Ketone	1	g.
Cedar Wood Oil, Rectified	5.5	cc.
Neroli Oil, Genuine	2.5	cc.
Geraniol, C.P.	4	cc.
Phenylethyl Alcohol	1.5	cc.
Benzoin Extract, Filtered	5	cc.
Petitgrain Oil	1.5	cc.
Linaloë Oil, Cayenne	6	cc.
Sandal Wood Oil, East Indian	5.5	cc.
Indol (100%)	0.07	cc.
Iris Oil, Genuine, Concrete	1.5	cc.
Castoreum (100%)	0.05	g.
Basilicum Oil	0.03	cc.
Undecyl Aldehyde (100%)	0.05	cc.
Mousse de Chêne, Liquid	0.5	cc.
Vanillin	3	g.
Menthol	0.5	g.

Formula No. 2

Bergamot Oil, Extra Fine	11	cc.
Lemon Oil	26.5	cc.
Orange Flower Water Oil, Genuine	1	cc.
Ylang Ylang Oil, Genuine	9	cc.
Sandal Wood Oil, East Indian	8	cc.
Amyl Salicylate	3.5	cc.
Iris Oil, Genuine, Concrete	1	cc.
Civet, Genuine (100%)	0.22	cc.
Patchouli Oil	1.5	cc.
Coumarin	4	g.
Vanillin	5	g.
Rose Oil, Bulgarian	3.5	cc.
Petitgrain Oil	1.5	cc.
Musk, Artificial, Ketone	6	g.
Geraniol, C.P.	6.5	cc.
Benzoin Extract, Filtered	5	cc.
Undecyl Aldehyde (100%)	0.2	g.
Birch Tar Oil, Twice Rectified	0.03	cc.
Cedar Wood Oil, Rectified	2	cc.
Neroli Oil, Genuine	0.5	cc.
Linaloë Oil, Cayenne	2	cc.
Opoponax Extract	0.05	cc.
Jasmine Oil, Pure	2	cc.

The above-mentioned perfume compositions should be made up 1–2% in a 90% pure alcohol and kept in the dark, shaking from time to time, and filtering after a few weeks.

Type "Quelques Fleurs"

Tart ("Herb") Type

Formula No. 1

Olibanum Oil	3	cc.
Geraniol, C.P.	7.5	cc.
Alpha Amyl Cinnamic Aldehyde	2.36	cc.
Citral	5	cc.
Geranium Oil, Réunion	3.5	cc.
Benzyl Alcohol	10	cc.
Linalyl Acetate	7	cc.
Hydroxycitronellal, C.P. (100%)	14	cc.
Heliotropin, Crystallized	10	g.
Cananga Oil, Java	13	cc.
Ionone for Soaps	4	cc.
Methylnonyl Acetaldehyde (100%)	0.14	cc.
Benzyl Acetate, Free of Chlorine	6	cc.
Linaloë Oil, Cayenne	3	cc.

Terpineol, C.P.	11	cc.
Musk, Ambrette, Artificial	0.5	g.

Formula No. 2

Benzoin, Extract	3	cc.
Olibanum Oil	1.36	cc.
Citronella Oil, Colombo	3	cc.
Cananga Oil, Java	10	cc.
Heliotropin, Crystallized	6	g.
Linaloë Oil, Cayenne	7	cc.
Hydroxycitronellal, C.P. (100%)	7	cc.
Benzyl Acetate, Chlorine-Free	3	cc.
Terpineol, C.P.	26.5	cc.
Citral	3	cc.
Methylnonyl Acetaldehyde (100%)	0.14	cc.
Geranium Oil, Réunion	5.5	cc.
Ionone for Soaps	5.5	cc.
Phenylethyl Alcohol	5	cc.
Linalyl Acetate	4.5	cc.
Anise Aldehyde	6.5	cc.
Alpha Amylcinnamic Aldehyde	3	cc.

Perfume Oil, Type "Quelques Fleurs"

For Fine Soaps (Soft Type)

Cananga Oil, Java	9	cc.
Benzyl Acetate, Free of Chlorine	5	cc.
Ionone for Soaps	5	cc.
Linalyl Acetate	6	cc.
Linaloë Oil, Cayenne	2.3	cc.
Heliotropin, Crystallized	8	g.
Geraniol, C.P.	8	cc.
Musk, Ambrette, Artificial	3.5	g.
Bergamot Oil	2	cc.
Phenylethyl Alcohol	3.5	cc.
Benzyl Alcohol	9	cc.
Alpha Amylcinnamic Aldehyde	0.5	cc.
Terpineol, C.P.	21	cc.
Indol, Crystallized	0.06	g.
Lemon Oil, Genuine	4	cc.
Anise Aldehyde	4	cc.
Hydroxycitronellal, C.P.	9	cc.
Methylnonyl Acetaldehyde (100%)	0.14	cc.

Type "Chypre Extract"

Formula No. 1

Bergamot Oil	33	cc.
Geranium Oil, Réunion	2	cc.
Rose Oil, Genuine, Bulgarian	3.5	cc.
Ylang Ylang Oil, Genuine	2.5	cc.
Rosemary Oil	4	cc.
Coumarin	8	g.
Lavender Oil, Genuine	6	cc.
Jasmine, C.P.	2.4	cc.
Vanillin	3	g.
Anise Aldehyde	5.5	cc.
Cedar Wood Oil, Rectified	1.5	cc.
Patchouli Oil, Genuine	0.5	cc.
Mousse de Chêne, Decolorized	3	cc.
Opoponax Extract	2	cc.
Linaloë Oil, Cayenne	18	cc.
Civet, Genuine (100%)	0.6	g.
Musk, "Ambrette," Artificial	4.5	g.

Formula No. 2

Lemon Oil	12	cc.
Bergamot Oil	9	cc.
Benzyl Acetate, Free from Chlorine	8	cc.
Cedar Wood Oil, Rectified	9.5	cc.
Benzyl Benzoate	6	cc.
Hydroxycitronellal, Pure (100%)	5	cc.
Geraniol, C.P.	7	cc.
Vanillin	4	g.
Benzoin Extract, Filtered	5.5	cc.
Sandal Wood Oil, East Indian	5	cc.
Geranium Oil, Réunion	3	cc.
Coumarin	2	g.
Rose Oil, Genuine, Bulgarian	1	cc.
Linaloë Oil, Cayenne	2.5	cc.
Musk, "Ambrette," Artificial	1.5	g.
Patchouli Oil, Genuine	1.5	cc.
Labdanum Extract	3	cc.
Civet, Genuine	0.3	g.
Olibanum Extract	0.7	cc.
Iris Oil, Genuine, Concrete	1	cc.
Mousse de Chêne, Decolorized	2	cc.
Ylang Ylang Oil, Genuine	5	cc.
Phenylethyl Alcohol	5.5	cc.

Narcisse

Ylang Bourbon Oil	150
Benzyl Acetate	100
Hydroxycitronellal	200
Terpineol	100
Cinnamyl Alcohol	100
Rose Synthetic	75
Coumarin	50
Jasmin Synthetic	50
Para Cresyl Phenyl Acetate	25
Para Cresyl Acetate	10
Methyl Para Cresol	10

Tuberose

Tuberose, Natural	100
Cinnamyl Alcohol	50
Phenyl Propyl Alcohol	100
Ylang Manilla Oil	300
Benzyl Salicylate	100
Benzoin Resin	50
Tolu Resin	50
Styrax Resin	50
Methyl Ionone	50
Heliotropin	50
Methyl Salicylate	25
Aldehyde C_{12} (10%)	50
Alcohol C_{12} (25%)	25

Jacinthe

Phenyl Acetic Aldehyde (50%)	200
Phenyl Acetic Aldehyde Dimethyl Acetal	50
Hydrotropic Aldehyde	50
Brom Styrol	10
Methyl Octrine Carbonate 10%	15
Clary Sage Oil	20
Ylang Manila Oil	50
Methyl Ionone	50
Phenyl Ethyl Alcohol	100
Cinnamyl Alcohol	200
Rose, Synthetic	50
Phenyl Ethyl Propinate	50
Phenyl Propyl Acetate	50
Terpineol	55
Vanillin	20
Musk Ketone	30

Mimosa

Mimosa, Absolute	100
Dimethyl Acetophenone	100
Isobutyl Salicylate	100
Phenyl Acetic Acid	25
Phenyl Acetic Aldehyde (50%)	25
Linalool	75
Benzyl Acetate	50
Coumarin	50
Cinnamyl Alcohol	200
Cinnamyl Acetate	75
Hydroxycitronellal	150

Hyacinth

Formula No. 1

Phenylacetaldehyde (100%)	500 g.
Jasmin Oil, Synthetic	150 g.
Neroli Oil, Synthetic	150 g.
Terpineol Extra	50 g.
Orris Oil Concrete	50 g.
Phenylethyl Alcohol	50 g.
Phenylethyl Phenylacetate	25 g.
Heliotropin	10 g.
Octyl Alcohol (50%)	10 g.
Octyl Aldehyde (50%)	5 g.

Formula No. 2

Cinnamic Alcohol	200 g.
Geranium Oil, Bourbon	200 g.
Citronellol	100 g.
Benzyl Acetate	100 g.
Ionone, Beta	100 g.
Coumarin	100 g.
Benzyl Benzoate	60 g.
Phenylacetaldehyde	60 g.
Citronellol	50 g.
Clove Oil, Zanzibar	20 g.
Musk Xylol	10 g.

Eau de Quinine

Neroli	5
Patchouli Oil	10
Bay Oil	20
Geraniol	20
Geranium Oil	30
Bergamot Oil	30
Lemon Oil	80
Rosemary Oil	40
Balsam Peru Infusion	50

Ambre (Fixative)

Musk Ketone	30
Musk Ambrette	30
Labdanum Bleached	100
Orris, Absolute	10
Methyl Ionone	50
Vanillin	50
Vetiverol Acetate	50
Coumarin	50
Clary Sage Oil	25
Bergamot Oil	125
Heliotropin	100
Benzyl Cinnamate	100
Resin, Peru	50
Resin, Tolu	50
Santalool Acetate	80
Resin, Benzoin	50
Ambreine or Ambrethene	100

Treflé

Isobutyl Salicylate	250
Benzyl Salicylate	150
Ylang Bourbon Oil	150
Methyl Ionone	100
Isoeugenol	30
Eugenol	30
Bergamot Oil	100
Linalyl Acetate	50
Citronellol Acetate	65
Coumarin	50
Para Cresyl Phenyl Acetate	25

Oregon

Carnation, Synthetic	250
Methyl Ionone	200
Peru Balsam	10
Tolu Balsam	10
Benzoin	50
Ylang Manilla Oil	60
Jasmin, Synthetic	50
Cinnamyl Alcohol	150
Rose Synthetic	50
Oppoponax Resin	5
Castoreum Absolute	5
Ambreine or Ambrethene	150

PERFUMES FOR SOAPS

Perfumes for soaps must be judiciously selected. They must not contain ingredients which will discolor a light soap. They must be stable to alkali and lasting in character. A soap may seem to be well perfumed when made. The final criterion is, how well will it age.

Muguet for Soaps

Linalool	40 g.
Ionone, Alpha	10 g.
Isoeugenol	5 g.
Sandalwood	5 g.
Geranium, Algerian	5 g.
Amyl Cinnamic Aldehyde	10 g.
Aldehyde C_{14}	1 g.
Musk Xylol (dissolved in Diethyl Phthalate or Benzyl Benzoate)	5 g.

Perfume for Soap, Type "Palmolive"

Citral	40 g.
Geranium Oil, Bourbon	40 g.
Citronellal	25 g.
Spike Oil, Lavandér	14 g.
Rosemary Oil	10 g.
Peppermint Oil	8 g.
Lavender Oil	8 g.
Sandal Wood Oil	8 g.
Methyl Acetate	5 g.
Vetivert Oil Bourbon	4.5 g.
Tonkarol	4 g.

Perfume Base for Luxury Soap Fruit

Amyl Acetate	750 g.
Benzaldehyde	50 g.
Aldehyde C_{14}	200 g.

Use 100–200 g. per 100 kg. to the coconut oil soap-base.

Perfume for Wax Coatings of Soap Fruits

Orange

(6 g. Perfume for 1 kg. Coating)

Orange Oil, Sweet, African	800 g.
Citral, C.P.	50 g.
Amyl Acetate	50 g.
Aldehyde C_{10}	10 g.
Heliotropin	90 g.

Apple

(10 g. Perfume for 1 kg. Coating)

Amyl Acetate	300 g.
Amyl Isovalerianate	400 g.
Benzaldehyde	25 g.
Linalyl Acetate (Bois de Rose)	100 g.
Geranyl Acetate, C.P.	50 g.
Heliotropin	30 g.
Coumarin	20 g.
Petit Grain Oil, Paraguay	25 g.
Oenanthic Ether	25 g.
Amyl Formate	25 g.

Apricot

(6 g. Perfume for 1 kg. Coating)

Apricot Composition	700 g.
Amyl Cinnamate	50 g.
Heliotropin	50 g.
Benzyl Isobutyrrate	100 g.
Benzyl Alcohol, Free from Chlorine	100 g.

Pear

(10 g. Perfume for 1 kg. Coating)

Amyl Acetate	775 g.
Eugenol	50 g.
Benzyl Acetate	50 g.
Amyl Formate	25 g.
Lemon Oil, Messina, Extra	25 g.
Benzaldehyde	25 g.
Heliotropin	50 g.

Lemon

Lemon Oil, Messina, Extra	825 g.
Citral, C.P.	50 g.
Amyl Acetate	50 g.
Benzaldehyde	25 g.
Heliotropin	50 g.

Fruit Perfume for Cheap "Soap Fruits"

Amyl Acetate	475 g.
Heliotropin	100 g.
Benzaldehyde	50 g.

Aldehyde C_{14}	100 g.
Aldehyde C_{16}	50 g.
Linalyl Acetate, (from Bois de Rose)	100 g.
Methyl Phenyl Acetate	50 g.
Rose Oil, Artificial	50 g.
Amyl Formate	25 g.

Use 500–750 g. per 100 kg. soap.

Soap Perfume, Tuberose

Cananga Oil	200 g.
Phenylpropyl Alcohol	200 g.
Benzyl Acetate	100 g.
Amyl Salicylate	100 g.
Phenyl Ethyl Alcohol	100 g.
Petitgrain Oil, (Paraguay)	60 g.
Linalol	40 g.
Ionine Beta	50 g.
Heliotropine	50 g.
Musk Xylol	40 g.
Benzoin Resin	60 g.
	1,000

Perfume for Almond Soap

Low Priced Perfume

Soap Chips	100 kg.
Bergamot Oil	150 g.
Palmarosa Oil	75 g.
Bitter Almond Oil	100 g.
Mirbane Oil	75 g.

Pompas Bouquet (for Soap)

Low Priced Perfume

Soap Chips	100 kg.
Cassia Oil	200 g.
Clove Oil	100 g.
Thyme Oil	100 g.
Balsam Peru Tincture	100 g.

Lavender Perfume (for Soaps)

Lavender Oil	45 g.
Geranium Oil, African	25 g.
Bergamot Oil	25 g.
Lemon Oil	10 g.
Coumarin	5 g.
Musk Solution	3 g.

For Shaving-soaps. Use 1–1.5%.

Perfume for Windsor Soap

(Yellow)

Soap Chips	100 kg.
Caraway Oil	250 g.
Cassia Oil	200 g.
Clove Oil	50 g.

Perfume for Windsor Soap

(White)

Soap Chips	100 kg.
Caraway Oil	250 g.
Anise Oil	100 g.
Bergamot Oil	150 g.

Jones' Perfume for Liquid Soap

Syringeol, Synthetic	5 cc.
Artificial Oil of Rose	.5 cc.
Artificial Oil of Jasmine	.5 cc.
Rose Geranium Oil	.5 cc.
Clove Oil	.5 cc.
Terpineol	7.5 cc.
Artificial Musk	.5 g.
Alcohol, to make	20 cc.

Shaving Soap Perfume

Lavender (French) Oil	20 cc.
Lavender Spike Oil	15 cc.
Thyme Oil	2 cc.
Rosemary Oil	3 cc.
Terpinyl Acetate	4 cc.
Bois de Rose	3 cc.
Linalyl Acetate	3 cc.

SHAVING CREAM PERFUMES

Lavender

Lavender Oil	75 oz.
Geranium Oil	75 oz.
Spike Oil	75 oz.
Coumarin	2 oz.
Sandalwood Oil	2 oz.
Bergamot Oil	100 oz.
Lemon Oil	25 oz.

Rose

Pelargol	100 oz.
Diphenyl Oxide 1:1	25 oz.
Vanillin	10 oz.
Geraniol	75 oz.
Terpineol	20 oz.

Phantasy

Lavender Oil	150 oz.
Orange-Peel Oil	450 oz.
Bergamot Oil	750 oz.
Lemon Oil	150 oz.
Benzaldehyde	30 oz.

Eau de Cologne Perfume

Bergamot Oil	100 g.
Lemon Oil	50 g.
Portugal Oil	35 g.
Rosemary Oil	25 g.
Lavender Oil	30 g.
Petitgrain Oil	30 g.
Neroli, Synthetic	20 g.

Bitter Almond Perfume

Bitter Almond Oil	60 cc.
Bergamot Oil	10 cc.
Lavender Oil	5 cc.

Fancy Perfume

Lavender Oil	150 cc.
Portugal Oil	450 cc.
Bergamot Oil, Synthetic	750 cc.
Lemon Oil	150 cc.
Benzaldehyde	30 cc.

Almond Perfume

Peru, Balsam	100 g.
Heliotropin	125 g.
Musk, Tincture	50 g.
Vanillin	15 g.
Almond Oil	10 g.
Neroli, Synthetic	5 g.

PERFUME COMPOSITIONS FOR SHAMPOOS

Rose

Geraniol	60 g.
Rose Oil, Artificial	25 g.
Sandal Wood Oil, East India	15 g.

Violet

Bergamot Oil	50 g.
Cananga Oil	45 g.
Ionone	5 g.

Heliotrope

Heliotropin	90 g.
Vanillin	10 g.

Lavender

Lavender Oil	60 g.
Bergamot Oil	20 g.
Lemon Oil	15 g.
Clove Oil	5 g.

Eau de Cologne

Bergamot Oil	50 g.
Lavender Oil	50 g.
Lemon Oil	50 g.
Citronella Oil	25 g.
Clove Oil	20 g.
Rosemary Oil	10 g.
Orange Peel Oil, Bitter	5 g.

Birch

Birch Bud Oil	6 g.
Lemon Oil	2 g.
Rose Oil, Artificial	2 g.
Vanillin	0.5 g.
Ionone	0.5 g.

Pine Needle

Formula No. 1

Pine Needle Oil, Siberian	125 g.
Palmarosa Oil	25 g.
Lavender Oil	25 g.
Cumin Oil	10 g.

Formula No. 2

Pine Needle Oil, Siberian	108 g.
Juniper Berries Oil	16 g.
Lavender Oil	10 g.
Thyme Oil	14 g.

PERFUME FOR NON-GREASY CREAMS

Formula No. 1

Rose

Phenyl Ethyl Alcohol, Extra	7.0 g.
Geranium Oil, Terpeneless	1.8 g.
Citronellol	10.5 g.
Geraniol	7.0 g.
Rhodinol, Genuine	3.7 g.
Rose Oil, Artificial	70.0 g.

Tea Rose

Formula No. 2

Citronellol	12.5 g.
Geraniol	2.5 g.
Nerol	5.0 g.
Rhodinol, Genuine	5.0 g.
Guaiac Wood Oil, Terpeneless	1.0 g.
Rose Oil, Artificial	74.0 g.

Formula No. 3

Lilas

Ylang-Ylang Oil, Bourbon	2.8 g.
Dihydroxy Citronellal	5.6 g.
Dimethyl Benzyl Carbinol	5.5 g.
Lilac Oil	83.3 g.
Terpineol	2.8 g.

Formula No. 4

Lime Blossom

Citral	5 g.
Benzyl Salicylate	5 g.
Petitgrain Oil, French	4 g.
Bergamot Oil	5 g.
Ketone Musk	1 g.
Nerol	0.5 g.
Citryl (Heine)	79.5 g.

Tabac Blanc

Formula No. 5

Jasmine, Absolute, Free of Indol	2 g.
Benzyl Alcohol	3.5 g.
Naphthyl Methyl Ketone	1 g.
Ylang-Ylang Oil, Bourbon	0.5 g.
Benzyl Acetate	1 g.
Citronellol	1 g.
Cyclamen Aldehyde	2 g.
Dimethyl Benzyl Carbinol	2 g.
Ionone, Alpha	2 g.
l-Linalool	85 g.

Perfume for Cholesterin Creams

1. Orange Flower Water instead of water:

Neroli Oil, Artificial	9 g.
Aubépine	1 g.

2. Rose Water instead of distilled water:

Rose Oil	1 g.
Geranium Oil, African	1 g.
Bergamot Oil	5 g.

3. Rose Water instead of distilled water:

Geranium Oil	5 g.
Anisaldehyde	5 g.
Linalylacetate	2 g.
Eugenol	1 g.

The three mixtures are added to creams made with Rose Water or Orange Flower Water instead of distilled water. (Usual percentage of perfume.)

Peach Blossom

(for toilet creams)

Pure Peach Lactone	840 g.
Amyl Acetate	25 g.
Benzoic Aldehyde	10 g.
Vanillin	90 g.
Ethyl Valerianate	20 g.
Ethyl Butyrate	25 g.

Face Powder Perfume

Jasmin Oil, Artificial	20.0 g.
Neroli, Artificial	2.0 g.
Ylang Ylang	5.0 g.
Anisic Aldehyde	2.0 g.
Phenylacetaldehyde	0.5 g.
Vanillin	0.5 g.
Ionone	0.5 g.
Sandalwood Oil, E.I.	2.0 g.
Orris Oil	0.5 g.
Otto of Rose, Artificial	2.0 g.
Isoeugenol	2.0 g.
Civet, Artificial	0.005 g.

Chypre Perfume Base for Face Powder

Coumarin	10
Santylyl Acetate	5
Musk Ketone	5
Musk Ambrette	2
Vetivertol Acetate	5
Patchouli	2
Isoeugenol	5
Methyl Ionone	5
Bergamot	25
Ylang Ylang Manila	10
Tolu Resin	5
Vanillin	2
Linalool	3
Mousse de Chêne	7.5
Cinnamyl Alcohol	5.0
Labdanum Resin	3.5

Cucumber Juice

Grind clean whole cucumbers from which the juice is then expressed. Boil the juice for a few minutes, strain, add about 25 to 30% of alcohol or preservative or both, allow to stand a day or two and filter into storage bottles. This is an old tried recipe and works well.

Gardenia for Hair Oil

Terpineol	20
Amylol (Norda)	25
Hydroxycitronellol	2
Methyl Anthranilate	1
Phenyl Ethyl Alcohol	12
Bitter Orange Oil	1
Benzyl Acetate	4
Orange Flower Oil, Artificial	15
Benzyl Alcohol	20

Use ½ oz. to 1 gal. Mineral Oil. Color to suit.

Perfume for Sweeping Compound

Use ½% of following

Pine Needle Oil, Siberian	500 g.
Bornyl Acetate	300 g.
Camphorated Oil	150 g.
Juniper Wood Oil	90 g.

Covering Odor for Chlorine Preparations

Use 1–2 drams of tincture of orris per pint of product. Vanillin is less satisfactory but useful in some cases.

Cyclamen Extract

Cyclamen Aldehyde	5 g.
Hydroxycitronellal, (very pure)	25 g.
Benzyl Ethyl Carbinol	10 g.
Terpineol, (very pure, middle distillate)	5 g.
Methyl Ionone	5 g.
Citronellol, purified	10 g.
Benzyl Acetate	2 g.
Citral, (Water-white, very pure)	0.50 g.
Alpha Ionone, (Water-white, extra fine)	10 g.
Phenyl Ethyl Alcohol	10 g.
Rhodinol Ex Geranium	10 g.
Bergamot Oil	5 g.
Cinnamic Alcohol	5 g.
Jasmin Liquid Absolute	2 g.
Grasse Rose Oil	0.50 g.
Heliotropin, Crystallized	2 g.
Infusion of Florentine Orris, (20%)	100 g.

Alcohol (90%) to produce 1 liter.

Rose Extract

Red Rose Flower Oil	40 cc.
Nerol	30 cc.
Phenyl Ethyl Alcohol	20 cc.
Jasmin Aldehyde	16 cc.
Neroli Oil	12 cc.
Ambrette, Musk	10 cc.
Rose Absolute, Synthetic	9 cc.
Iris, Concrete	5 cc.
Tuberose, Artificial	3 cc.
Bergamot Oil	2 cc.
Narcisse, Artificial	2 cc.
Vetivert Oil, Java	1 cc.
Sandal Wood Oil, East India	1 cc.
Alcohol (96%)	1500 cc.
Water	150 cc.

Water "Soluble" Perfumes

All perfume oils can not be solubilized, but the following bases used with 1–3 parts of many oils does render them water "soluble."

Formula No. 1

Isopropyl Alcohol	50 g.
White Oleic Acid	20 g.
Triethanolamine	10 g.

Formula No. 2

White Oleic Acid	140 g.
"Carbitol"	140 g.
Monoethanolamine	30 g.

The formula given below is useful for making non-alcoholic perfumes, toilet waters and hair tonics as well as theatre sprays. In most cases clear solutions result. Where a slight haze forms, it can be removed by filtering through talc. The following mixture is added to 5 gallons (more or less) of water:

Formula No. 3

Perfume Oil	1 oz.
Mulsene	4 oz.

Toilet Waters

Toilet waters are made in a similar fashion to the perfume extracts, excepting that a 60–70% alcoholic concentration is used, and from 3–6 ounces of oil are used per gallon of 60–70% alcohol.

Glycerin Toilette Water

a.	Alcohol	50 g.
	Rose Essence	0.4 g.
b.	Glycerin	50 g.
c.	Borax dissolved in	20 g.
	Water, Warm	880 g.

Add *c* cold to *a* and *b*.

Florida Water

Formula No. 1

Neroli Oil, "Bigarade"	5 cc.
Lavender Oil, English	5 cc.
Bergamot Oil	30 cc.
Limette Oil	2 cc.
Clove Oil	2 cc.
Cassia Oil	3 cc.
Cinnamon Oil	1 cc.
Rose Oil	5 cc.
Ambra, Liquid, Artificial	2 cc.
Orange Flower Water, Triple	100 cc.
Alcohol (90%)	900 cc.

Formula No. 2

Lavender Oil	15 g.
Portugal Oil	5 g.
Bergamot Oil	25 g.
Petitgrain Oil, Paraguay	10 g.
Eugenol	1 g.
Cinnamic Aldehyde	1 g.
Rose Geranium Oil	5 g.
Oleo-resin Orris	2 g.
Musk Ambrette	1 g.
Orange Flower Water, (Triple)	200 g.
Alcohol, (90%)	800 g.

Lavender Water

Lavender Oil	20 g.
Bergamot Oil	10 g.
Lemon Oil	5 g.
Oleo-resin Orris	5 g.
Alcohol (90%)	1,000 g.

Mature for at least 6 months and filter if necessary.

Hungary Water

Rosemary Oil	20 cc.
Verveine Oil	7 cc.
Portugal Oil	1.5 cc.
Limette Oil	1 cc.
Peppermint Oil	0.5 cc.
Rose Water, Triple	100 cc.
Alcohol (90%)	800 cc.

Let stand up to 6 months before marketing.

Birch Water

Birch Bud Oil	10 g.
Glycerin	40 g.
Soap Spirit	250 g.
Alcohol or Isopropyl Alcohol	650 g.
Bergamot Oil	5 g.
Geranium Oil	1 g.
Orange Flower Oil	0.5 g.
Water	50 g.

Eau De Botot (English Type)

(Botot Water)

Tincture of Red Cedar Wood	8 pt.
Tincture of Myrrh	2 pt.
Tincture of Rhatany	2 pt.
Lavender Oil	.75 oz.
Peppermint Oil	1 oz.
Rose Oil	150 gr.

Eau De Botot (French Type)

(Botot Water)

Anise	10 oz.
Cochineal	.75 oz.
Mace	150 gr.
Cloves	150 gr.
Cinnamon	2.75 oz.
Alcohol	6 pt.
Peppermint Oil	.75 oz.

Eau de Quinine

Tincture of Cantharidin	1 dr.
Quinine Hydrochloride	10 gr.
Tincture of Capsicum	20 min.
Glycerin	30 min.
Bay Rum, Prepared with Industrial Spirit	to 20 oz.
Tincture of Cudbear	sufficient to color

For Eau de Cologne and Toilet Water

Base A

Italian Lemon Oil	20 g.
Bergamot Oil	20 g.
Neroli or Neroli Synthetic	35 g.
Italian Sweet Orange Oil	10 g.
Lavender (40–42% Ester)	10 g.
Orris Root, Tincture	2 g.
Ambreine or Ambrethene	3 g.

Use 100 grams to 1 gallon 70% alcohol. Allow to stand for one week. Chill and filter while cold.

Eau de Cologne

Formula No. 1

Lemon Oil	18 g.
Bergamot Oil	16 g.
Orange Oil, Sweet	5 g.
Lavender Oil, Extra	4 g.
Mandarin Oil	3.2 g.
Petitgrain Oil, Grasse	3.2 g.
Benzoin Resinoid	3.2 g.
Neroli Oil, Original	2.8 g.

Orange Oil, Bitter	2.8	g.
Lime Oil	2.7	g.
Rosemary Oil	1	g.
Eugenol	0.6	g.
Cumin Aldehyde (10%)	0.5	g.
Muscatel Sage Oil	0.3	g.
Hysop Oil	0.1	g.
Cardamom Oil	0.1	g.
Iris, Concrete (10%)	0.1	g.
Alcohol (96%)	1800	cc.
Water, Distilled	200	cc.

Formula No. 2

Bergamot Oil	20	g.
Lemon Oil	14	g.
Lavender Oil	5	g.
Benzoin Resinoid	5	g.
Nerosol	5	g.
Orange Oil, Sweet	4	g.
Mandarin Oil	4	g.
Petitgrain Oil, Paraguay	2.6	g.
Rosemary Oil	2.3	g.
Neroli Oil	2	g.
Muscatel Sage Oil	2	g.
Jasmine Aldehyde	0.7	g.
Resinoid Iris	0.5	g.
Alcohol (96%)	1800	cc.
Water, Distilled	200	cc.

Formula No. 3

Lemon Oil	20	g.
Heliotropin	7	g.
Bergamot Oil, Natural	5	g.
Bergamot Oil, Artificial	6	g.
Terpinyl Acetate	4	g.
Neroli Oil, Artificial	4	g.
Orange Oil, Sweet	4	g.
Coumarin	2.5	g.
Benzyl Acetate	1.5	g.
Ketone Musk	0.7	g.
Citral	0.6	g.
Alcohol (96%)	1600	cc.
Water, Distilled	400	cc.

Floral Eau De Colognes (Acacia Type)

Base A	100
Methyl Naphthyl Ketone	2
Anisic Aldehyde	1
Benzyl Acetate	1

Eau de Cologne (50%)

Bergamot Oil	10	cc.
Lemon Oil	14	cc.
Citral	1.4	cc.
Thyme Oil, White	2.6	cc.
Rosemary Oil	3.4	cc.
Lavender Oil	10	cc.
Ixolene, Extra	3.4	cc.
Alcohol	500	cc.
Water	500	cc.

Eau de Cologne for the Bath

Bergamot Oil, Free of Terpenes	17	cc.
Petitgrain Oil, Free of Terpenes	14	cc.
Rosemary Oil	1.75	cc.
Citral	1.75	cc.
Tincture of Benzoin	56	cc.
Orange Flower Water	340	cc.
Alcohol (96%)	1800	cc.
Water, Distilled	3600	cc.

Ambre Eau de Cologne

Bergamot Oil	20	g.
Lemon Oil	20	g.
Heliotropin	7	g.
Ambrette Musk	2.6	g.
Lavender Oil	2.6	g.
Petitgrain Oil, Paraguay	2.6	g.
Methyl Ionone	2.6	g.
Vanillin	2	g.
Rose Oil, Artificial	2	g.
Rosemary Oil	0.7	g.
Neroli Oil	0.7	g.
Coumarin	0.7	g.
Ambre, Artificial	0.6	g.
Rose Absolute, Synthetic	0.1	g.
Alcohol (96%)	1800	cc.
Water, Distilled	200	cc.

Chypre, Eau de Cologne

Lemon Oil	18	g.
Bergamot Oil	16	g.
Rose Oil, Artificial	6	g.
Lavender Oil	4	g.
Coumarin	4	g.
Sandal Wood Oil, East India	2.6	g.
Ketone Musk	2.6	g.
Vetivert Oil, Java	2	g.
Rosemary Oil	2	g.
Muscatel Sage Oil, Artificial	2	g.
Iso-Eugenol	0.7	g.
Patchouli Oil	0.7	g.
Vanillin	0.5	g.
Neroli Oil	0.5	g.
Thyme Oil	0.5	g.
Mousse de Chêne, Absolute	0.5	g.
Alcohol (96%)	1800	cc.
Water, Distilled	200	cc.

Eau de Cologne "Russe"

Lemon Oil	9	g.
Bergamot Oil	9	g.

Methyl Ionone	6	g.
Heliotropin	4	g.
Lavender Oil	4	g.
Iso-Eugenol	3	g.
Vanillin	2.6	g.
Ketone Musk	2	g.
Rosemary Oil	2	g.
Linalyl Acetate	2	g.
Ambrette, Musk	0.7	g.
Neroli Oil	0.7	g.
Coumarin	0.6	g.
Ambre, Artificial	0.6	g.
Alcohol (96%)	1800	cc.
Water, Distilled	200	cc.

Solid Eau de Cologne

1.3 parts of sodium hydroxide are dissolved in 40 parts water; and 8.5 parts of stearic acid are dissolved in 50 parts of 90% alcohol. Then the two solutions are thoroughly mixed and heated slowly until the liquid turns clear. The essence of Eau de Cologne is then added and the liquid cooled to avoid evaporation of the oils, but not enough to allow it to congeal. After the oil has become thoroughly mixed with the base, the solution is then poured into moulds and allowed to cool.

Solidified Perfume (Oils)

Trihydroxyethylamine Linoleate	1
Orange or other Oil	1
Water	1

Add in above order stirring well.

Eau de Lavende

Lavender Oil, Barrême (France)	40	cc.
Musk Infusion	12	cc.
Ambre Infusion	12	cc.
Bergamot Oil	12	cc.
Lemon Oil	6	cc.
Jasmine Aldehyde	2	cc.
Phenyl Ethyl Alcohol	0.6	cc.
Alcohol (96%)	1100	cc.
Water, Distilled	300	cc.

Eau de Lavende, Ambrée

Lavender Oil, French	50	cc.
Bergamot Oil	12	cc.
Musk Infusion	12	cc.
Ambreine	8	cc.
Lemon Oil	6	cc.
Benzoin Infusion	6	cc.
Idola	2	cc.
Alcohol (96%)	2500	cc.
Water, Distilled	500	cc.

Eau de Lubin

Alcohol	650	cc.
Portugal Oil	1.2	cc.
Neroli Oil	0.6	cc.
Jasmine, Absolute	0.6	cc.
Myrtle Oil	3	cc.
Geranium Oil, French	1.2	cc.
Lemon Oil	3	cc.
Bergamot Oil	9	cc.
Civet Tincture	3	cc.
Castoreum Tincture	3	cc.
Peruvian Balm	3	cc.
Musk Tincture	3	cc.
Tolu Balm Tincture	6	cc.
Benzoin Tincture	24	cc.
Myrrh Tincture	6	cc.
Clove Tincture	60	cc.

Aqua Mellis

Honey	5	g.
Bergamot Oil	8	cc.
Lavender Oil, French	1	cc.
Clove Oil	1	cc.
Mace Oil	0.5	cc.
Coriander Oil	1	cc.
Sandal Wood Oil	3.5	cc.
Benzoin Resinoid	5	cc.
Musk Tincture (2%)	2	cc.
Rose Water, Triple	100	cc.
Orange Flower Water, Triple	100	cc.
Alcohol	800	cc.

Acqui Di Lubin (Lubin Water)

Alcohol	2000	cc.
Tincture of Orange Peel	350	g.
Tincture of Musk Seed	300	g.
Tincture of Tonka Bean	100	g.
Tincture of Tuberose	50	g.
Tincture of Styrax	50	g.
Tincture of Benzoin	50	g.
Tincture of Vanilla	30	g.
Lemon Oil	40	g.
Bergamot Oil	4	g.
Neroli Oil	1	g.
Tincture of Musk	4	g.
Tincture of Civet	3	g.
Orange Flower Water	250	g.

Ice—Bay Rum

Bay Oil	8	g.
Menthol	16	g.
Glycerin, C.P.	16	g.
Glycerin (Soap Lye)	20	g.
Rum Essence	80	g.
Alcohol (96%)	2000	cc.
Water, Distilled	800	cc.

Fancy Cologne

Terpeneless Lemon Oil	3
Terpeneless Bergamot Oil	20
Neroli, Petale	25
Nerol	15
Phenyl Ethyl Alcohol	10
Hydroxycitronellal	15
Cinnamyl Acetate	5
Ambreine or Ambrethene	5

Chypre Cologne

Base A	100
Oak Moss, Absolute	3
Vetiverol Acetate	5
Patchouli	3
Coumarin	5
Santalol Acetate	4

Lilac Cologne

Base A	100
Benzyl Acetate	5
Terpineol	5
Anisic Aldehyde	1
Phenyl Acetic Aldehyde	1
Hydroxycitronellal	5

Orchidee or Treflé Cologne

Base A	100
Isobutyl Salicylate	10
Musk Ambrette 20% in Benzyl Benzoate	5

Gardenia Cologne

Base A	100
Styralyl Acetate	2
Hydrotropic Aldehyde	0.5

Carnation Cologne

Base A	100
Isoeugenol	5
Eugenol	5
Vanillin	2
Methyl Ionone	3
Phenyl Ethyl Alcohol	5

Rose Cologne

Base A	100
Rose Geranium	2.5
Rhodinol	5
Phenyl Ethyl Alcohol	7.5
Citronellal Acetate	2.5

Jasmin Cologne

Base A	100
Benzyl Acetate	5
Amyl Cinnamic Aldehyde	2
Hydroxycitronellal	3

Toilet Vinegar

(a) Glacial Acetic Acid	33 g.
Citric Acid	9 g.
Water, Distilled	600 g.
(b) Toilet Vinegar Essence	18 g.
Alcohol	340 g.

Perfume Diluent and Solvent ("Tescol")

A new perfume diluent which is soluble in alcohol and water and which permits the oil to be dissolved in diluted alcohol.

Mix one part of the perfume compound with one or two parts of Tescol. Dissolve this in alcohol and then add water slowly with stirring.

Pot-Pourri

Formula No. 1

Rose Leaves	16 oz.
Lavender Flowers	16 oz.
Orris Root (Coarse Powder)	8 oz.
Cloves (Coarse Powder)	2 oz.
Cinnamon (Coarse Powder)	2 oz.
Allspice (Coarse Powder)	2 oz.
Table Salt	16 oz.

Formula No. 2

Sandal Wood	16 oz.
Gum Benzoin	2 oz.
Orris Root	12 oz.
Cloves	2 oz.
Mace	1 oz.
Tonka Beans	2 gr.
Musk	40 gr.
Rose Oil	40 drops
Lavender Oil	1 dr.
Bergamot Oil	2 dr.
Lemon Oil	2 dr.

Formula No. 3

Powdered Cloves	2 oz.
Powdered Pimento	2 oz.
Powdered Benzoin	2 oz.
Essence of Musk	1 oz.
Essence of Bergamot	4 dr.
Lavender Oil	4 dr.
Cloves Oil	2.5 dr.
Cassia Oil	2.5 dr.
Rose Oil	80 drops
Rose Leaves	4 oz.
Powdered Jamaica Pepper, to make	48 oz.

Perfume Sticks

The most suitable base for these perfumed crayons is acetanilide. It is used in proportion of 87.5 parts by weight. It is melted on water bath or over flame, provided it is carefully stirred while being heated. Temperature must not rise above 80° C. When it is molten, 10.5 parts of pulverized magnesium carbonate are mixed in until it dissolves entirely. Then there are added 35 parts of xylene musk, 17.5 parts of heliotropin, and 3.5 parts of Japan wax. When all ingredients have been melted, 8.4 parts of perfume dissolved in 4.2 parts of benzyl alcohol are added.

The mass will solidify rapidly and can be formed into shape while still warm. Amount of heliotropine added is maximum allowable limit, for more of this substance will make mass soft. Perfume must not be added in excess of that prescribed above, for the excess will simply ooze out of mass. When these perfumed crayons are properly packed in air-tight containers, they will last for years. When acetanilide and magnesium carbonate are used alone, then about 15% menthol or menthol and camphor should be added.

Concentrated Fixative for Perfumes

Alcohol	2	cc.
Benzyl Benzoate	8	cc.
Auramia 100%	0.4	g.
Heliotropine	1	g.
Musk, Xylol	1	g.
Civet, Tincture	2	cc.

To be used in place of a single fixative in about the same proportion.

Solubility of Perfume and Cosmetic Products in Alcohol

The following table of the solubility of various perfume and cosmetic ingredients in alcohol, intended to serve as a guide, gives only practical indications and not exact physical constants. Column 1 gives the parts of alcohol required to dissolve one part of the product by weight. Column 2 shows the strength solution of alcohol required.

PRODUCT	COLUMN 1	COLUMN 2
Acetate, Benzyl	1.5	70%
Acetate, Bornyl	2.5–3.5	70%
Acetate, Geranyl	7 –8.5	70%
Acetate, Linalyl	3 –5	70%
Acetate, Terpinyl	4.5	70%
Alcohol, Benzyl	1	50%
Alcohol, Cinnamic	3.5–4.5	50%
Alcohol, Phenyl Ethyl	2	50%
Alcohol, Phenyl Propyl	3	50%
Aldehyde, Cinnamic	1.5–2.5	70%
Anthranilate, Methyl	2.5–3.5	70%
Aubepine	6 –6.5	50%
Benzoate, Benzyl	7.5	80%
Benzoate, Ethyl	6 –7	60%
Benzoate, Methyl	3.5	60%
Cinnamate, Ethyl	4 –6	70%
Cinnamate, Methyl	1.5	70%
Citral	7	60%
Citronellal	5	70%
Citronellol	4	60%
Coumarin	8 –9	70%
Dimethylhydroquinone	8 –9	95%
Eugenol	4.5–5	50%
Geraniol Pure	2.5–3.5	60%
Heliotropine	10	70%
Irisone Pure	2.5–3	70%
Isoeugenol	4.5–5	50%
Laurine	6.5–7	30%
Linalool	4 –5.5	60%
Methyleugenol	3.5	60%
Musk Ambrette	60	95%
Musk Ketone	80 –100	95%
Musk Xylol	200	95%
Phenyl Acetaldehyde	2.5	70%
Rosacetol	20 –22	95%
Salicylate, Amyl	2.5	90%
Salicylate, Ethyl	3	80%
Salicylate, Methyl	4.5–6	70%
Terpineol	3 –5	60%
Toncarin	25	70%
Vanillin	5 –6	70%

Perfumery Raw Materials Comparative Volatilities

VERY VOLATILE		B.P. of Esters, etc. in degrees Centigrade
p-Cresyl Methyl Ether d-Limonene	Phellandrene	174–196
Acetophenone Benzaldehyde	Methyl Benzoate Phenylacetaldehyde	196–207

		B. P. of Esters, etc. in degrees Centigrade
Benzyl Acetate	Methyl Heptin Carbonate	
Citronellal	Octyl Acetate	
m-Cresol	Octyl Methyl Ketone	
p-Cresyl Acetate	Pine Needle Oil	
Dimethyl Hydroquinone	Propiophenone	
Ethyl Benzoate	Salicyl Aldehyde	
Menthone	Styralyl Acetate	
Methyl Chavicol	Tolylaldehyde	207–217

VOLATILE

Benzyl Propionate	Methyl Acetophenone	
Bergamot Oil	Methyl Heptenone	
Bois de Rose Oil	Methyl Phenylacetate	
Bornyl Acetate	Methyl Salicylate	
Bromstyrol	n-Octyl Alcohol	
Lavender Oil	Spike Lavender Oil	
Linalyl Acetate	Terpenyl Acetate	
I-Menthyl Acetate		217–228
Aldehyde C_{10}	Ethyl Salicylate	
Benzyl Alcohol	Isobutyl Benzoate	
Carvone	Linalool	
Cuminic Aldehyde	Methyl Nonyl Ketone	
Dill Oil	Phenylethyl Acetate	
Dimethyl Acetophenone	Safrol	
Ethyl Pelargonate	Thymol	
Ethyl Phenylacetate		228–238
Anethol	Geranyl Formate	
Benzyl Butyrate	Isobutyl Phenylacetate	
Borneol	Isopulegol	
Carvacrol	Menthol	
Citral	Nonyl Alcohol	
Citronellyl Acetate	Phenylethyl Propionate	
Fenchyl Alcohol	Piperonal	
Geranyl Acetate	Star Anise Oil	238–248

MEDIUM LASTING

Aldehyde C_{11}	Indol	
Anisic Aldehyde	Isosafrol	
Cedarwood Oil	Jasmone	
Cedrene	p-Methoxy Acetophenone	
Citronellol	Methyl Anisate	
Copaiba Oil	Myrtenol	
Decyl Alcohol	Phenylethyl Alcohol	
Diphenyl Ether	Rhodinol	
Eugenol	Terpineol	
Eugenol Methyl Ether		248–259
Benzylidine Acetone	Lauric Aldehyde	
Cinnamyl Acetate	Methyl Anthranilate	
Cinnamic Aldehyde	Methyl Cinnamate	
Diphenyl Methane	Methyl Ionone	
Duodecyl Aldehyde	Methyl Nonyl Carbinol	
Geraniol	Nerol	
Geranium Oils	Orris Concrete	

		B. P. of Esters, etc. in degrees Centigrade
Geranyl butyrate	Phenylacetic Acid	
Geranyl Propionate	Phenylpropyl Alcohol	
Ionone	Resedal	
Isoamyl Benzoate	Rhodanyl Propionate	
Isobutyl Salicylate	Skatole	
Isoeugenol		259–269

LONG-LASTING

Alcohol C_{10}	Hydroxycitronellal	
Cuminic Alcohol	Isoamyl Salicylate	
Ethyl Anisate	Myristic Aldehyde	
Ethyl Cinnamate	b-Naphthyl Methyl Ether	269–280
Aceteugenol	Coumarin	
Anisic Alcohol	Isoeugenol Methyl Ether	
Benzyl Ether	Beta Naphthol	
n-Butyl Salicylate	Beta Naphthyl Ethyl Ether	
Cinnamyl Alcohol	Phenylpropyl Aldehyde	
Cinnamic Aldehyde		280–290
Amyl Cinnamic Aldehyde	Nerolidol	
Celery Seed Oil	Oak-Moss Resin	
Clary Sage Oil	Parsley Oil	
Ethyl Citrate	Patchouli Oil	
Ethyl Myristinate	Vanillin	
Naphthyl Methyl Ketone		290–300
Benzophenone	Ethyl Vanillin	
Cinnamic Acid	Labdanum	
Ethyl Sebacate	Styrax Balsam	300–311
Benzyl Phenylacetate	Muscone (from Animal Musk)	
Benzyl Salicylate	Phenylethyl Phenylacetate	
Costus Oil	Salol	
p-Cresyl Phenylacetate	Sandalwood Oil	
Dibutyl Phthalate	Santalyl Phenylacetate	
Elemol	Tolu Balsam	
Farnesol	Vetiver Oil	
Linalyl Phenylacetate		311–321
Benzyl Cinnamate	Moskene	
Benzyl Isoeugenol	Musk Ambrette	
Benzyl Ketone	Musk Ketone	
Civettone	Musk Xylol	over 321

CHAPTER XIV

SHAVING PREPARATIONS

SHAVING CREAMS

Shaving creams are special types of soaps.

A shaving cream must

1. Lather freely and rapidly.
2. Lather in hot or cold water.
3. Be dense and firm.
4. Be capable of being worked into a dense and voluminous lather.
5. Must not form too soluble a lather which would wash off with excess water.
6. Lather must not dry rapidly but should remain moist for some time.
7. Must be a powerful emulsifying agent, cut surface tension and have good degreasing properties.
8. Must be stable in tube or jar and not dry out or turn hard and gummy and maintain the same consistency for all reasonable temperatures.

The problem of the shaving soap is a problem of balance, so as to obtain a combination which most nearly gives the desired result.

The addition of a sufficient amount of glycerin will help keep the lather moist. The amount generally used is about 10% of the finished cream.

Analysis of the average shaving cream will generally show as follows:

Actual soap content	40%
Water	50%
Glycerin	10%

For the rapid lather a very "soluble" soap is required. If the cream consists entirely of rapid lathering soap, it will be too soluble and will wash away in hot water or on vigorous rubbing, therefore, a large quantity of the "less-soluble" soap is required. The more soluble soaps are made from the more soluble oils. These are represented by coconut oil and palm kernel oil. Because of their solubility, they will give a rapid lather, will lather up in cold water or in hard water, but will wash away in hot water or on vigorous rubbing. Because both coconut and palm kernel contain lower molecular weight acids, they will irritate the face if used in too high concentrations. They are generally limited to about 15% or less of the total fat content. While both are satisfactory, coconut is the more widely used, since the odor of palm kernel is more likely to occur in the finished soap. However, a type of deodorized palm kernel has recently been made available.

The soap required to give a more lasting lather, which will retain its body in hot water, must contain a soap such as tallow, stearic acid or palm oil. If a very dense, persistent lather is required, fats containing large amounts of behenic acid may be used.

The consistency desired is obtained not only by a balancing of soap according to the fatty acids contained, but also by the proper balancing of sodium and potassium soaps. Too much sodium soap cannot be used because of its hardness.

The proper blends of soaps, glycerin and water, is all that a shaving cream consists of. Some contain borax and other fillers. A typical shaving cream formula would be as follows:

Coconut Oil	9 oz.
Tallow	3 oz.
Stearic Acid	28 oz.
Sodium Hydroxide	1.0 oz.
Potassium Hydroxide	7.0 oz.
Glycerin	10 oz.
Water	45 oz.

Sodium hydroxide is prepared as a 20° Bé. solution, using part of the water, in the formula.

Potassium hydroxide is prepared as a 35° Bé. solution.

Glycerin, coconut oil and tallow are melted in the tank. The sodium hydroxide is run in slowly making sure that saponification is complete.

The excess fat is now saponified with potash; ½ the potash is added to the tank and the mass agitated until saponification appears to be complete. The stearic acid is melted and added and finally the remainder of the potash solution. The mass is stirred until neutralization is complete, and then adjusted to the amount of free stearic acid desired. Three per cent excess stearic acid is commonly used.

This soap when made will be very thick while hot, but will soften on cooling. It is possible to keep the soap thin while hot as by finishing with a large excess of stearic acid which may be later neutralized by adding the appropriate amount of potash solution to the cold soap with suitable agitation.

Shaving Cream

Formula No. 1

15 parts by weight of stearin, 5 parts arachis oil, 7 parts coconut oil, 16 parts 38° Bé. caustic potash and 16 parts water.

Formula No. 2

25 parts stearic acid, 8 parts lauric acid, 16 parts 50° Bé. potash solution, 50 parts water, and 1 part perfume. The potash is dissolved in hot water and the fatty acid mixture poured in, with stirring. A creamy product is formed which, after a short time, exhibits the silvery sheen of stearin crystals.

Formula No. 3

Lard	100 g.
Olive-oil or Sesame-oil	80 g.
Coconut-oil (Cochin)	70 g.
Glycosterin	5 g.
Caustic Potash 40° Bé.	125 g.
Solution of Potash 20° Bé.	15 g.

Melt fats and Glycosterin, saponify with caustic potash lye; add the potash solution, perfume and pass through a 3-roll-mill. By addition of a little alcohol during the rolling the cream will get a silky shine.

Formula No. 4

Stearin	25 oz.
Coconut Oil Fatty Acids	8 oz.
Caustic Potash, (50° Bé.)	15 oz.
Water	50 oz.
Glycerin	4 oz.
Stearin	2 oz.

Melt the fats together, except for the 2 parts of stearin, by heating to 70–80° C. Mix the caustic potash, water and glycerin and heat to about the same temperature. Add the warm fat mixture in a slow stream with stirring, to the alkali. Let the cream cool slowly, after saponification is complete, still stirring continuously. Heat up the 2 parts of stearin and stir into the cooled mass. If lumps should form, warm the cream in a drying oven with constant stirring. After the stearin has been taken up, and well worked through the mass cover and let stand over night in a cool room. The next morning mix the cream again and add perfume. The perfume should consist of essential oils that will be non irritating to the skin. Perfume is added dissolved in a small amount of alcohol. The alcohol aids in dispersing the perfume and also gives the cream more sheen. Let stand a day after adding the alcohol and perfume. Transfer to glazed stoneware and keep in this for 8–10 days, mixing at least once every day. The cream becomes softer with this treatment. After several days in a cool room, transfer to tubes or jars. If after 10 days, the cream is still too hard, warm it slightly and stir in a dilute solution of potash. Such addition must be made with great care, as it is easy to make the cream too soft. Other formulas which may be used in the same way, are as follows:

Formula No. 5

Stearin	30 oz.
Peanut Oil	10 oz.
Coconut Oil	14 oz.
Caustic Potash (38° Bé.)	28 oz.
Water	20 oz.
Glycerin	12 oz.
Stearin	5 oz.

Formula No. 6

Stearin	60 oz.
Coconut Oil	11 oz.
Caustic Potash (50° Bé.)	17 oz.
Water	30 oz.
Glycerin	10 oz.
Turkey Red Oil (100 per cent)	2 oz.

The stearin and vaseline are melted together at 70° C. and stirred into the mixture of triethanolamine, water and borax which has been warmed to 60° C. The temperature of the liquid must be kept down in order to avoid decomposition of the triethanolamine. The mass is mixed and just before it becomes cold, the alcohol and perfume are stirred in. When cold, it can be transferred immediately to tubes. This cream is especially suitable for persons with dry, non-oily skins.

Shaving Creams

The following formulas illustrate creams of various consistency employing different ingredients. Consistency can be adjusted to suit requirements by increasing or decreasing the percentage of water.

Formula No. 7

Stearic Acid	33.6 lb.
Coconut Oil (Cochin)	6.4 lb.
Glycerin	4. lb.
Sodium Lauryl Sulphate	3. lb.
Boric Acid	1.4 lb.
Potassium Hydroxide (42° Bé.)	18.4 lb.
Sodium Hydroxide (42° Bé.)	2.8 lb.
Water	29.9 lb.
Perfume	.5 lb.

Melt one-half of the stearic acid and the coconut oil in a kettle. Put the water, boric acid and sulphate glycerin into another kettle and heat until the boric acid dissolves. Add to this solution the potassium hydroxide and sodium hydroxide and mix. Run the melted stearic acid into a steam jacketed mixer, and then add the hot alkali solution with the agitator in motion. Keep the steam on for a half hour while mixing. Meanwhile, in a separate kettle, have the remainder of the stearic acid melted and now run it slowly into the soap. Continue the stirring, not too rapidly, until the soap is smooth and homogeneous. Then add the perfume and mix it in well. Dump the batch and age it for three days.

If the cream appears spongy this is due to the incorporation of air owing to excessive rapid mixing or the use of improperly shaped paddles. Flat paddle mixers, whether of the epicylic; the pony or interacting type, are best. If air has been incorporated it can be removed by running the cream through an ointment mill. In large production the cream is sometimes run over chilling drums.

Formula No. 8

Stearic Acid	28.0 lb.
Cetyl Alcohol	2. lb.
Coconut Oil	6. lb.
Potassium Hydroxide (50° Bé.)	18.8 lb.
Sodium Hydroxide (20° Tw.)	1.6 lb.
Glycerin	3. lb.
Water	38.5 lb.
Boric Acid	1.6 lb.
Perfume	.5 lb.

Melt one-half of the stearic acid and coconut oil in one kettle. In another kettle melt the remainder of the stearic acid and the cetyl alcohol. In a third kettle heat the water; dissolve the boric acid in it, and add the glycerin. Then to this solution add the potassium and sodium hydroxides. Strain the melted stearic acid and coconut oil into a steam packeted mixer. Start the agitator and run in the alkali solution. Mix for a half hour with the heat on and then add the stearic acid, cetyl alcohol mixture very slowly. Continue the mixing until the soap is smooth; add the perfume and mix it in well. Dump the batch in portable tanks and allow to age for three days.

Formula No. 9

Palm-Kernel Oil	5.72 lb.
Stearic Acid	25.50 lb.
Coconut Oil	6.36 lb.
Potassium Hydroxide (85%)	8.57 lb.
Sodium Hydroxide (85%)	.63 lb.
Glycerin	6.54 lb.
Boric Acid	1.59 lb.
Water	44.00 lb.
Bay Oil	.87 lb.
Menthol Crystals	.22 lb.

Put one-half of the stearic acid, all of the coconut and palm-kernel oils into one kettle. Melt the remainder of the stearic acid in another. Put the water, boric acid and glycerin into another kettle and heat until the boric acid dissolves. Then add the alkalies and stir with a wooden paddle until completely dissolved. Run the mixture of stearic acid, palm-kernel and coconut oils into a hot steam jacketed mixer. Start the agitator and add the hot alkali solution. Mix for a half hour with the steam on. Shut the steam off and slowly add the remainder of the melted stearic acid from the other kettle. Mix until a smooth, homogeneous cream is obtained. Then add the menthol dissolved in the bay oil. Allow the cream to stand for three days and mill if desired.

Formula No. 10

Olive Oil	2.0 lb.
Stearic Acid	25.0 lb.
Coconut Oil (Cochin)	8.0 lb.
Potassium Hydroxide (42° Bé.)	18.0 lb.
Sodium Hydroxide (42° Bé.)	2.5 lb.
Water	39.0 lb.
Boric Acid	1.5 lb.
Glycerin	3.5 lb.
Perfume	.5 lb.

Melt one-half of the stearic acid and coconut oil in one kettle. Melt the remainder of the stearic acid and olive oil in another. Heat the water; add the boric acid and glycerin and when dissolved add the potassium and sodium hydroxides. Strain the stearic acid, coconut oil mixture into a mixing kettle; start the agitator and run in the alkali solution. Keep the heat on for one-half hour and then add the stearic acid, olive oil mixture. Mix in the perfume; age for three days.

Formula No. 11

Stearic Acid	25.00 lb.
Coconut Oil (Cochin)	5.13 lb.
Sodium Cholate	.12 lb.
Lecithin	1.00 lb.
Potassium Hydroxide (50° Bé.)	21.15 lb.
Water	42.50 lb.
Glycerin	4.60 lb.
Perfume	.50 lb.

Melt one-half of the stearic acid and coconut oil in one kettle and the remainder of the stearic acid and lecithin in another. Dissolve the sodium cholate in the water and glycerin; then proceed with the mixing of the soap as before.

Formula No. 12

Stearic Acid	28.50 lb.
Cetyl Alcohol	4.00 lb.
Sodium Cholate	.20 lb.
Coconut Oil (Cochin)	12.80 lb.
Potassium Hydroxide (85%)	9.57 lb.
Sodium Hydroxide (85%)	.63 lb.
Boric Acid	1.50 lb.
Glycerin	5.00 lb.
Water	37.30 lb.
Perfume	.50 lb.

Melt one-half of the stearic acid and the coconut oil in one kettle, and the remainder of the stearic acid and cetyl alcohol in another. Heat the water; dissolve in it the boric acid; and add the glycerin and sodium cholate. Then add the alkalies and proceed as before.

Formula No. 13

a.	Stearin	25 g.
	Coconut Oil Fatty Acid	8 g.
b.	Caustic Potash (50° Bé.)	15 g.
	Water	50 cc.
	Glycerin	4 g.
c.	Stearin	3 g.

Melt up *a,* then introduce the solution *b* with stirring. Stir until cooled, then introduce *c.* When homogeneous, cover container and let stand over night. Perfume is added the next morning, optionally together with alcohol. Keep 8–14 days in earthenware jars, stir with a wooden rod on each day. In this time, the cream should become softer. If not, treat with a little caustic potash solution (20° Bé).

Perfume: Lavender, Rose, Violet, Benzaldehyde, or with Eau de Cologne or Chypre.

Formula No. 14

Palm Oil Fatty Acid, Bleached	25 g.
Olive Oil Fatty Acid	25 g.
Coconut Oil Fatty Acid	10 g.
Water	35 cc.
Caustic Potash (50° Bé.)	25 g.

Method as above.

Formula No. 15

Stearin	30 g.
Coconut Oil, or Fatty Acid	15 g.
Olive Oil, or Fatty Acid	10 g.
Caustic Potash (28° Bé.)	27 g.
Water	32 cc.
Glycerin	6 g.
Stearin	3 g.

Method as above.

Formula No. 16

Stearin	30 g.
Coconut Oil	11 g.
Caustic Potash (50° Bé.)	17 g.
Water	30 cc.
Glycerin	10 g.
Turkey Red Oil (100%)	2 g.

to neutralize alkali

Formula No. 17

a.	Stearin	30 g.
	Peanut Oil, or Fatty Acid	10 g.
	Coconut Oil, or Fatty Acid	14 g.
b.	Caustic Potash (38° Bé.)	28 g.
	Water	20 g.
	Glycerin (28° Bé.)	12 g.
c.	Stearin	5 g.

Mix *a* in the order of their melting points (lowest first), melt up to 60–70° C., then stir in *b*, warm to 65° C. Stir until cool, add *c* (melted), stir thoroughly, let stand over night. Next morning stir up thoroughly, adding perfume. Cover, let stand, and fill into earthenware jars on next day.

Formula No. 18

Bleached Palm Oil Fatty Acid	50 g.
Olive Oil Fatty Acid	50 g.
Coconut Oil Fatty Acid	20 g.
Water	70 g.
Caustic Potash (50° Bé.)	50 g.

Method as in No. 1.

Formula No. 19

a.	Stearin	90 g.
	Coconut Oil	10 g.
b.	Caustic Potash (50° Bé.)	42 g.
	Glycerin	20 g.
	Water	100 g.
c.	Stearin	10 g.

As in No. 13.

Formula No. 20

a.	Pig Fat	80 g.
	Olive Oil	100 g.
	Tallow	75 g.
	Coconut Oil	60 g.
b.	Caustic Potash (38° Bé.)	160 g.
	Glycerin	25 g.
	Water	15 g.
c.	Stearin	10 g.

As in No. 1.

Formula No. 21

1.	Mineral Oil	2 oz.
	Tallow, Edible	4½ oz.
	Stearic Acid	10 oz.
	Cochin Cocoanut Oil	5 oz.
	Glyco Wax A	½ oz.
2.	Caustic Potash Lye (36° Be.)	17 oz.
	Caustic Soda Lye (36° Be.)	1½ oz.
3.	Water	23 oz.
	Boric Acid	1¼ oz.
	Triethylene Glycol	2 oz.
4.	Stearic Acid	10 oz.
5.	Perfume	⅓ oz.

The above formula gives a profuse lathering cream equal to the best creams on the market. It gives a thick, rich, non-drying lather of the small bubble type, which softens the beard quickly and contains no uncombined alkali, making it non-irritating to the skin. This cream is pearly and the pearliness increases with age.

Heat (1) until melted and keep melted. Heat (3) until dissolved; then cool. Now add (2) to (3) and stir; then add this to (1) slowly with good stirring, keeping batch hot on a steam-bath; continue stirring until homogeneous. Keep hot and allow to stand covered for 30 minutes. Stir for 5 minutes. Melt (4) in a separate pot and run it into the above batch with good stirring; allow to stand covered for 30 minutes; take off steam-bath and stir until thick; add (5) when almost cold; stir thoroughly. Allow to stand covered for week or ten days, stirring each day for five minutes.

Formula No. 22

1. Stearic Acid	30.0 oz.
2. Cocoanut Oil	3.3 oz.
3. Caustic Potash, (50° Bé.)	18.8 oz.
4. Caustic Soda, (20° Tw.)	1.6 oz.
5. Glycerin	5.0 oz.
6. Water	41.3 oz.
Perfume	to suit

Formula No. 23

Melted mutton tallow (250 g.) and 50 g. ox tallow are saponified with 178 cc. 50° Bé. potassium hydroxide solution and boiled to sticky mass. Cool and mix with boiled solution of 150 g. stearin, 40 g. anhydrous lanolin, 50 g. potassium carbonate and 1200 g. water. Make up to 3000 g. with water.

Formula No. 24

Cocoanut Oil	18 lb.
Stearic Acid	73 lb.

Caustic Potash Lye (39° Bé.)	54 lb.
Glycerin	33 lb.
Water	27 lb.

Put oil and glycerin in kettle and heat to 120° F. and stir thoroughly. Add slowly 35 lb. lye and continue to stir until it thickens. Add balance of lye mixed with the water slowly with constant stirring until smooth. Allow to stand in kettle 24 hours, then add perfume. Fill into tubes.

Formula No. 25

Stearic Acid	28 kg.
Coconut Oil	10 kg.
Caustic Potash (50° Bé)	15.5 kg.
Glycerin	10.5 kg.
Water	34 kg.
Sulphonated Castor Oil, 100%	2 kg.

Formula No. 26

Stearic Acid	10 kg.
Coconut Oil	3 kg.
Peanut Oil	5 kg.
Caustic Potash (50° Bé)	6.33 kg.
Caustic Soda (50° Bé)	1.93 kg.
Glycerin	1 kg.
Water	14 kg.

Formula No. 27

Stearic Acid	2 kg.
Coconut Oil	0.5 kg.
Oleic Acid	0.45 kg.
Caustic Potash (36° Bé)	1.7 kg.
Caustic Soda (36° Bé)	0.15 kg.
Glycerin	0.5 kg.
Water	2.5 kg.
Boric Acid	0.125 kg.

Formula No. 28

Coconut Oil	40 kg.
Palm Oil, Bleached	100 kg.
Olive Oil	100 kg.
Caustic Potash (50° Bé)	100 kg.
Water	140 kg.

Formula No. 29

Stearic Acid	29 kg.
Coconut Oil	10 kg.
Caustic Potash (50° Bé)	18 kg.
Glycerin	12 kg.
Water	30 kg.

Formula No. 30

Stearic Acid	15 kg.
Coconut Oil	7 kg.
Peanut Oil	5 kg.
Caustic Potash, 38° Bé	14 kg.
Water	16 kg.

Formula No. 31

Stearin, White	15 g.
Olive or Peanut Oil	5 g.
Coconut Oil	7 g.
Caustic Potash (38° Bé)	15 g.
Water	16 g.
Triethanolamine Oleate	5 g.

Saponify at 75–80° C, adding half the stearin (which should be retained) at the end. Keep standing for several days, stirring up occasionally. Add perfume (in alcohol).

Formula No. 32

Stearic Acid	15
Peanut Oil	5
Coconut-oil (Cochin)	7
Caustic Potash Lye 40° Bé.	14
Water	16
Glycosterin	2

Stir as usual, add to the melted fats at 70° Celsius the mixed potash lye and water till sufficiently thick, leave till fully saponified and cooled. The melted Glycosterin and perfume is then stirred into the soft mass.

Shaving Soaps (Solid)

Formula No. 1

1.	Stearin, White	80 g.
	Coconut Oil	20 g.
2.	Caustic Potash (38° Bé)	50 g.
	Caustic Soda (38° Bé)	12 g.
	Glycerin	10 g.

Saponify at 75–80° C, running the hot mixture (2.) into the melted fats (1.), and stirring until homogeneous.

Keep at elevated temperature, stirring up intermittently, and testing each time the alkalinity and the degree of saponification.

Formula No. 2

French Patent 794,877

Magnesium Peroxide	1500 g.
Gum Arabic	300 g.
Magnesium Carbonate	3500 g.

Carbamide-Hydrogen Peroxide 60 g.
Lactose 200 g.

Mix dry and pack in air-tight container.

Brushless (Latherless) Shaving Creams

These are essentially soft vanishing creams which are applied by the fingers, without a brush, and do not lather or foam.

Brushless Shaving Cream

Formula No. 1

Stearic Acid	21.00 lb.
Lanolin, Anhydrous	3.50 lb.
White Mineral Oil	.80 lb.
Alcohol	1.50 lb.
Triethanolamine	1.60 lb.
Borax	1.51 lb.
Distilled Water	70.00 lb.

Melt the stearic acid together with the oil, add the lanolin and heat to 70° C. Dissolve borax and triethanolamine in water and heat to boiling point. Add the fat solution while agitating rapidly. When smooth add perfume dissolved in alcohol. Stir at slow speed until cold. Consistency of cream can be regulated by changing quantity of water.

Formula No. 2

Stearic Acid	15.00 oz.
Spermaceti	2.00 oz.
Sulphonated Castor Oil	4.00 oz.
Ammonia (26°)	6.75 oz.
Sodium Hydroxide (Sticks)	.25 oz.
"Carbitol"	7.00 oz.
Water	64.50 oz.
Perfume	.50 oz.

Mix the ammonia with the water; add the sodium hydroxide and "carbitol" and when it dissolves bring the temperature of the solution to about 70° C. Melt the spermaceti and stearic acid and add the sulphonated castor oil. Run the melted fats into the alkali solution and mix rapidly until emulsified. When the temperature drops to 40° C. add the perfume.

Formula No. 3

Stearic Acid	19.00 oz.
Cocoa Butter	2.00 oz.
Potassium Hydroxide (Sticks)	1.25 oz.
Glycerin	7.00 oz.
Alcohol	5.00 oz.
Gum Tragacanth Powder	1.50 oz.
Water	63.75 oz.
Perfume	.50 oz.

Mix the gum tragacanth with the alcohol, add a part of the water. Dissolve the potassium hydroxide in the remainder of the water, add the glycerin. Melt the stearic acid and cocoa butter. Heat the alkali solution to the temperature of the melted fats acid and add them very rapidly. When emulsified add the gum tragacanth. Mix thoroughly and when the temperature drops to about 40° C. add the perfume.

Formula No. 4

Glyceryl Monostearate	6.5 oz.
Stearic Acid	6.5 oz.
Mineral Oil	2.0 oz.
Sulphonated Olive Oil	6.0 oz.
Glycerin	10.0 oz.
Potassium Hydroxide (Sticks)	.2 oz.
Water	68.3 oz.
Perfume	.5 oz.

Dissolve the potassium hydroxide in water, then add all the ingredients with the exception of the perfume, and with continuous mixing heat until the mass becomes homogeneous. Continue the mixing until the temperature drops to 40° C., then add the perfume. Adjust consistency with water.

Formula No. 5

Stearic Acid	20.00 oz.
Lanolin	1.50 oz.
Mineral Oil	2.00 oz.
Ethylene Glycol	1.50 oz.
Triethanolamine	1.65 oz.
Borax	1.85 oz.
Water	71.00 oz.
Perfume	.50 oz.

Melt the stearic acid; add the lanolin and mineral oil, bringing the temperature to about 70° C. Put the borax and triethanolamine into the water and bring it to a boil; then add the melted fats with rapid agitation. When the temperature drops to about 40° C. add the perfume, mixing with the ethylene glycol.

Formula No. 6

Stearic Acid	20.0 oz.
Anhydrous Lanolin	1.8 oz.

Peanut Oil	3.2 oz.
Triethanolamine	1.7 oz.
Borax	1.9 oz.
Water	70.9 oz.
Perfume	.5 oz.

Melt the stearic acid; add the lanolin and the peanut oil, bringing the temperature to 70° C. Put the triethanolamine and borax into the water; bring to the boiling point and add the melted fats. Mix rapidly until smooth, white cream results. Add the perfume at 40° C.

Formula No. 7

Stearic Acid	20.0 oz.
Hydrogenated Cotton Seed Oil	4.5 oz.
Ethylene Glycol	1.5 oz.
Triethanolamine	1.5 oz.
Alcohol	1.0 oz.
Water	71.0 oz.
Perfume	.5 oz.

Melt the stearic acid; add the hydrogenated cotton seed oil and the ethylene glycol. Put the borax and triethanolamine into the water; bring to the boiling point and add the melted fats with vigorous stirring. Continue stirring until the temperature drops to 40° C. and add the perfume.

Formula No. 8

Stearic Acid	10.00 g.
Sulphonated Olive Oil	15.00 g.
Sodium Lauryl Sulfonate	1.00 g.
Lecithin	2.00 g.
Triethanolamine	1.25 g.
Water	65.25 cc.
Glycerin	5.00 g.
Perfume	.50 g.

Melt the stearic acid, add the sodium lauryl sulfonate and the lecithin and then the sulphonated oil. Dissolve the triethanolamine in the water. Add the glycerin and bring to a temperature of 60 or 70° C. Add the hot oil and stir rapidly until cool. Perfume.

Formula No. 9

Stearic Acid	1000 g.
Glycerin	600 g.
Ammonia (sp.g. 0.97)	400 g.
Water, Distilled	8000 g.

Formula No. 10

Stearic Acid	2000 g.
Mineral Oil, White	200 g.
Ammonia (sp.g. 0.97)	800 g.
Water, Distilled	16500 g.

Formula No. 11

Stearic Acid	1440 g.
Ammonia (sp.g. 0.97)	580 g.
Borax	50 g.
Water	9000 g.
Soap, (Freshly Powdered)	250 g.
Water, Hot	1000 g.

The soap solution is added to the molten stearin before saponification. Caustic potash (35° Bé) can be used with advantage in the place of the ammonia. Use 25 g. for each 100 g. of stearic acid.

Formula No. 12

Any soft or medium vanishing cream is very effective as a brushless cream. The addition of 2% Parachol (melted into the stearic acid) improves it greatly. If a cooling effect is desired, 0.1% of menthol is used with the perfume.

Formula No. 13

Stearic Acid	50 g.
Cocoa Butter	9 g.
Sodium Carbonate, Monohydrated	10 g.
Borax	20 g.
Glycerin	40 cc.
Alcohol	32 cc.
Water	400 cc.
Perfume	to suit

Dissolve the sodium carbonate, borax, and glycerin in hot water. Melt the fats and waxes and add the alkali solution. Stir briskly until effervescence ceases and a smooth white soap is formed. Stir slowly until cold; then add the perfume mixed with alcohol.

Formula No. 14

Stearic Acid	75 lb.
Sesame Oil	70 lb.
Spermaceti	10 lb.
Strong Ammonia Solution	10 lb.
Hot Water	315 lb.
Glycerin	30 lb.
Perfume	to suit

Melt waxes and fats. Boil water, add ammonia, and pour into melted fats with constant agitation. When completely saponified stir slowly until quite cold. Add perfume.

Formula No. 15

Deramin	4 lb.
Water	5 gal.

Heat to 180° F. and pour into

Stearic Acid	15 lb.
Lanolin	1 lb.

previously heated to 180° F. while mixing moderately.

Add perfume 4 oz. when thick and mix until cold. If a cooling effect on the skin is desired 1 oz. Menthol may be added with the perfume.

This gives a non-irritating, soothing cream, which washes off readily.

Formula No. 16

Glycosterin	25 oz.
Mineral Oil	10 oz.
Peanut Oil	5 oz.
Water	60 oz.
Moldex or Other Good Preservative	0.2 oz.

Formula No. 17

Stearic Acid	20 oz.
Olive Oil	6 oz.
Lanolin	2 oz.
Glycerin	6 oz.
Triethanolamine	2 oz.
Sodium Carbonate	1 oz.
Water	63 oz.
Perfume	to suit

Formula No. 18.

Stearic Acid	12 oz.
White Mineral Oil	12 oz.
Paraffin Wax	5 oz.
Soap Flakes	3 oz.
Water	72 oz.

Formula No. 19

Stearic Acid	1 lb. 12 oz.
Mineral Oil	5¼ oz.
Potassium Hydroxide	1¾ oz.
Glycerin	8¾ oz.
Water	7 lb. 5 oz.
Perfume	sufficient

Melt stearic acid in mineral oil. Dissolve potassium hydroxide in the water, warm, add glycerin and stir in briskly, the melted fats. Mix until a smooth cream results. When temperature drops to about 40° C., add perfume and mix thoroughly. Put in tubes or jars. Menthol may be added, if desired. Makes about 10 lb. cream.

Formula No. 20

Liquid Creams

Stearic Acid	200 g.
Triethanolamine	10 g.
Water	800 g.

Formula No. 21

Thicker Creams

Stearic Acid	200 g.
Triethanolamine	10 g.
Anhydrous Sodium Carbonate	10 g.
Water	800 g.

Formula No. 22

Soapless Type

Glyceryl Monostearate	6.5 oz.
Stearic Acid	6.5 oz.
Mineral Oil	4.0 oz.
Peanut Oil	4.0 oz.
Glycerin	10.0 oz.
Water	69.0 oz.

German Patent 604,774

Formula No. 23

Glycol Stearate	100 g.
Water	400 g.

Formula No. 24

Absorption Base (Parachol)	100 g.
White Beeswax	25 g.
Water	100 g.

Formula No. 25

Glycol Palmitate	100 g.
Petrolatum	100 g.
Water	200 g.

Formula No. 26

Diglycol Laurate	100 g.
Lanolin	100 g.
Petrolatum	50 g.
Water	100 g.

Formula No. 27

Stearic Anilide	100 g.
Glycol Stearate	300 g.

Absorption Base	100 g.
Water	1500 g.

Formula No. 28

Glycol Stearate	30 g.
Absorption Base (Parachol)	100 g.
White Beeswax	30 g.
Sesame Oil	800 g.
Water	600 g.
Saponin	16 g.

Formula No. 29

Water	1280 cc.
Potassium Hydroxide	8 g.
Stearic Acid	160 g.
White Petrolatum	96 g.

Water is heated to boiling and stearic acid and petrolatum is added. When acid is melted the potassium hydroxide in the form of 20% solution is added. The whole is mixed well until it is almost cold, when perfume is added to suit.

Formula No. 30

Stearic Acid	50 lb.
Lanolin (Anhydrous)	9 lb.
"Carbitol"	3 lb.
Triethanolamine	1.5 lb.
Borax	1.7 lb.
Water	135 lb.

Formula No. 31

Stearic Acid	40 lb.
Lanolin (anhydrous)	7 lb.
Mineral Oil (white)	18 lb.
"Carbitol"	3 lb.
Triethanolamine	3.3 lb.
Borax	3.7 lb.
Water	125 lb.

Preparation

Melt the stearic acid, which should be the purest grade obtainable, either alone or with the mineral oil depending upon which formula is followed. Add the lanolin and bring the temperature to about 70° C. Heat the water, Triethanolamine and borax in a separate container and when at the boiling point, add the acid solution. Stir vigorously until a smooth emulsion is obtained and then add the perfume dissolved in the Carbitol. During the further cooling of the cream, stir gently but continuously taking care to avoid rapid stirring, as this tends to aerate the cream.

Properties

Cream No. 30 is a white, pearly product somewhat like a vanishing cream and is preferable for oily skins. Cream No. 31 is a smooth white cream of greater body than the other, and is preferred for use on dry skins. Both creams are readily applied to give a smooth coating on the face, have a soothing after-effect and are readily washable. The consistency of these creams can be varied by altering the proportion of water, and other changes can be made along the lines indicated by the difference in the two formulae. A cream of good consistency can be made by combining the two formulae given above.

Formula No. 32

Glycosterin	10 lb.
Ethylene Glycol	10 lb.
Mineral Oil White	8 lb.
Lanoline	2 lb.
Stearic Acid	34 lb.
Glycerin	2 lb.
Water	134 lb.
Menthol	0.2 lb.

Formula No. 33

Creams of this type are made without heat. Merely beat together.

Ammonium Stearate (Paste)	250 oz.
Mineral Oil, White	25 oz.
Perfume to suit.	

Stir until most of the ammonia has evaporated.

This cream is particularly soothing to the skin and combines the properties of a vanishing and cold cream.

Formula No. 34

U. S. Patent 1,979,385

Stearic Acid	350 g.
Lanolin (Anhydrous)	67.5 g.
White Mineral Oil	169 g.
Triethanolamine	34 g.
Sodium Tetraborate	34 g.
"Carbitol"	22.5 g.
Water	1170 g.

Formula No. 35

Stearin	75 oz.
Vaseline	13 oz.
Triethanolamine	2 oz.
Borax	2 oz.
Water	195 oz.
Alcohol	6 oz.

Formula No. 36

U. S. Patent 1,991,501

Stearic acid 11 g., lanolin 10 g., coconut oil 0.3 g., concentrated ammonium hydroxide 1.35 g., paraffin wax 6 g., spermaceti wax 2 g., boric acid 1.5 g., water 75 g., and having a trace each of menthol, camphor and perfume.

Stearic acid and hydrous lanolin containing 20% water, together with coconut oil are melted together, and to this mixture is added the concentrated ammonium hydroxide, which contains approximately 25% of ammonia.

The waxes are then added and heating is continued until the entire mixture is liquefied. The resulting mixture is subsequently removed from the heat and a warm solution of the boric acid in approximately 75 g. of water is added while continuously stirring.

At this point, or at any point previously, the menthol, camphor and selected perfumes are added in amounts which give the most pleasing effect.

The mixture is then violently stirred until cold, and the final resulting product is a white cream.

Formula No. 37

a.	Stearin	75 g.
	Vaseline	13 g.
b.	Triethanolamine	2 g.
	Borax	2 g.
	Water	195 g.
c.	Alcohol	6 g.

Melt up *a* to 70° C., mix *b* and heat up to 60° C., then pour *a* into *b* with stirring. Shortly before the cooling (solidification) add perfume in the alcohol *c*, stir until cold. Fill into collapsible tubes.

Formula No. 38

Stearin	36 g.
Aminostearin	10 g.
Vaseline	5 g.
Glycerin	5 g.
Water	130 g.

Formula No. 39

Stearin	30 g.
Triethanolamine	10 g.
Witch Hazel	100 g.
Water	45 g.
Glycerin	10 g.

Formula No. 40

a.	Stearin	50 g.
	Vaseline	10 g.
b.	Triethanolamine	1.5 g.
	Borax	1.5 g.
	Water	130 cc.
c.	Alcohol (Perfume)	3 g.

Pour *a*, 70° C., into *b*, 60° C. Cool stirring; add *c* before solidification. Pack in collapsible tubes.

Formula No. 41

Stearin	45 g.
Triethanolamine	2.5 g.
Glycerin	15 g.
Water	67.5 cc.
Witch Hazel	50 cc.

Method as above.

Formula No. 42

1	Stearin	20 g.
2	Olive Oil	4.5 g.
3	Spermaceti	1 g.
4	Glycerin	3 g.
5	Water	10 g.
6	Potash (30° Tw.)	1.5 g.
7	Water	120 cc.

Items 1, 2, 3, 4 and 5 are placed in the pan and brought to a temperature of 40° C. The potash and remaining water are mixed in a separate vessel and heated to the same temperature. When both mixtures are at 40° C. the caustic and water are plunged rapidly into the fatty materials and strongly agitated. The mass is, at first, a thin emulsion which soon changes to a transparent gel which, with continued stirring, again changes to an opaque, thin cream. This soon begins to thicken. When it can stand alone, stirring must immediately cease and the pan left at rest until quite cold; or the contents may be run off into smaller vessels to cool. When quite cold, the cream is fairly firm, but upon kneading or further stirring in the pan, it assumes the consistency at which it may be placed into tubes or pots.

The perfume is added during the cold mixing.

Formula No. 43

Stearic Acid	20.00 oz.
Cetyl Alcohol	1.50 oz.
Mineral Oil	2.00 oz.
Ethylene Glycol	1.50 oz.
Triethanolamine	1.65 oz.
Borax	1.85 oz.
Water	71.00 oz.
Perfume	0.50 oz.

Melt the stearic acid, add the cetyl alcohol and mineral oil, bringing the temperature to about 70° C. Put the borax and triethanolamine into the water and bring to a boil. Then add the melted fats with rapid agitation. When the temperature drops to about 40° C., add the perfume mixed with the ethylene glycol.

Formula No. 44

Stearic Acid	14.0 oz.
Cetyl Alcohol	2.0 oz.
Potassium Hydroxide	1.0 oz.
Glycerin	5.0 oz.
Water	77.5 oz.
Perfume	0.5 oz.

Melt the stearic acid, cetyl alcohol and mineral oil. Dissolve the potassium hydroxide in the water; add the glycerin and stir in the melted fats. Mix until a smooth white cream is formed and when the temperature drops to about 40° C., add the perfume. It will not evaporate at that heat.

Formula No. 45

A.	Coconut Oil	20.0 g.
	Suet	15.0 g.
B.	Caustic Potash (90%)	31.0 g.
	Caustic Soda (90%)	4.0 g.
	Borax	2.5 g.
	Water	142.5 cc.
C.	Water	140.0 cc.
D.	Stearic Acid	145.0 g.
E.	Glyceryl Monostearate	40.0 g.
	Stearic Acid	80.0 g.
	Water	380.0 cc.

"A" must be saponified with "B." To this add "C" and then "D," which has already been melted. The whole mass should be stirred for a few minutes at a temperature of about 80° C., so as to be sure that no lumps will form. It should then be allowed to cool without stirring. After one to two days, the mass will take on a pearly appearance. Then an emulsion made with "E" should be added while both are cold. In order to make the emulsion "E" smooth, it is advisable to take ten parts of the combined mass resulting from "A," "B," "C" and "D," and add this to "E" while the latter is still hot. The pearly appearance will temporarily vanish but after two days will again appear.

Formula No. 46

(Non Alkaline)

1. Diglycol Stearate	24 oz.
2. Diglycol Laurate	8 oz.
3. Albacer	6 oz.
4. Ceraflux	6 oz.
5. "Carbitol"	6 oz.
6. Diethylene Glycol	6 oz.
7. Sulfatate	.5 oz.
8. Water	141.5 oz.
9. Perfume	2. oz.

Heat 1, 2, 3, 4, 5, 6, till liquid. Heat 7 and 8 to boiling, and add slowly to the melted wax mixture, stirring rapidly. When cooled to 120° F. add perfume and stir till cold. This gives a very white smooth cream, which spreads well, and washes off easily.

Formula No. 47

Borated Brushless Shaving Cream

1. Acimul	11 oz.
2. Stearic Acid	13 oz.
3. Diglycol Laurate	9 oz.
4. "Carbitol"	4 oz.
5. Diethylene Glycol	2 oz.
6. Boracic Acid	1.5 oz.
7. Water	57.5 oz.
8. Perfume	1 oz.

Heat 1, 2, 3, 4, and 5 together till melted. Heat 6 and 7 to boiling and add slowly to the melted waxes, stirring rapidly. When cooled to 120° F. add perfume and stir till cool. This gives a cream of good consistency, which spreads well and washes off readily.

	No. 48	No. 49	No. 50	No. 51	No. 52
Lanolin	4.3	3.3%	—	1.0%	— g.
Stearic Acid	23.8	19.5%	10.0%	16.0	14.5 g.
Mineral Oil, Light	—	7.5%	—	4.0	— g.
Cocoa Butter	—	—	5.0	—	— g.
Sesame Oil	—	—	—	—	— g.
Spermaceti	—	—	—	—	13.5 g.
Glycerin	—	—	—	2.0	1.9 g.
Sodium Carbonate, Monohydrated	—	—	10.0	5.0	6.0 g.
Triethanolamine Oleate	0.7	1.5	—	—	— g.
Water	69.1	65.7	70.0	67.0	62.0 g.
Alcohol	1.4	1.0	—	—	— g.
Borax	0.7	1.5	—	—	— g.
Triethanolamine Stearate	—	—	5.0	5.0	— g.
Perfume			to suit		
Ammonia Water, Stronger	—	—	—	—	1.9 g.

Shaving Soap Powder

Formula No. 1

Soap

Stearic Acid	60 kg.
Coconut Oil	5 kg.
Caustic Potash, (40° Bé)	21 kg.
Caustic Soda, (40° Bé)	14 kg.

Finish up with an excess of stearic acid (1–2%) to make free of caustic alkali. Cut the soap-plates and let stand for several weeks; dry, grind and sift.

This soap is used for a

Shaving Powder

Soap Powder, as above	45 kg.
Rice Flour	5 kg.
Mineral Oil, White	0.2 kg.
Boric Acid	0.25 kg.
Perfume	to suit

½ g. is enough for 1 application.

Formula No. 2

Coconut Oil	113 lb.
Soda Lye (35° Bé.)	140 lb.
Potash Lye (50° Bé.)	170 lb.
Stearic Acid	550 lb.

This soap is made in a crutcher. It may be dried in a dryer by keeping the temperature low. It is advisable, however, during the pulverizing operation to add from 25 to 50 per cent dry tallow soap chips, and about 5 per cent talc.

Shaving Sticks

Formula No. 1

High-Titer Tallow	54 kg.
Coconut Oil	10 kg.
Caustic Potash (40° Bé)	21 kg.
Caustic Soda (40° Bé)	13 kg.
Potassium Carbonate	0.36 kg.
Water	1.64 kg.

Formula No. 2

Tallow	34 kg.
Coconut Oil	6 kg.
Castor Oil	1.5 kg.
Caustic Potash (40° Bé)	14.5 kg.
Caustic Soda (40° Bé)	7.5 kg.
Potassium Carbonate	0.2 kg.
Water	0.4 kg.

Formula No. 3

Stearic Acid	40 oz.
Coconut-oil	10 oz.
Caustic Potash (38° Bé.)	23 oz.
Caustic Soda (38° Bé.)	6 oz.
Glycosterin	4 oz.

Fats must be saponified at 70° C. The reaction is rather strong, therefore the lye must be added more quickly than usual; to the saponified mass add Glycosterin and leave to the self-induced heating process for three hours, but stir through hourly. Put into forms or pass through a drying machine. A soap put into forms takes very long to harden. Good drying is necessary. The freshly machined sticks are too soft for cutting and must be left to harden several hours. After cutting wrap in tinfoil for preserving their soft and pliant quality.

Shaving Soap, Liquid

Formula No. 1

Olein, Light	9 g.
Coconut Oil, Cochin	3 g.
Caustic Potash (50° Bé.)	5.3 g.

Alcohol	1 g.
Glycerin	8 g.
Water	73 g.
Rose Water	1 g.

Formula No. 2

Shaving Soap, "Rasibloc" Type

a.	Stearin	100 g.
	Glycerin	5 g.
b.	Caustic Potash (39° Bé.)	40.2 g.
	Caustic Soda (37° Bé.)	11.4 g.
c.	Coconut Soap	30 g.

Warm each portion and mix together in above order.

Formula No. 3

Coconut Oil	30 g.
Tallow	90 g.
Stearic Acid	90 g.
Caustic Potash (50%)	90 g.
Potassium Carbonate	1 g.
Distilled or Softened Water	370 g.
Glycerin	120 g.
Alcohol	210 g.
Perfume	2.5–10 g.

Formula No. 4

Tallow	30 kg.
Coconut Oil	12 kg.
Caustic Potash (50° Bé.)	18.5 kg.
Potash Carbonate	4 kg.
Water	30 kg.
Alcohol	30 kg.

To keep clear in the cold use oleic acid instead of tallow.

Formula No. 5

Coconut Oil	420 g.
Stearic Acid	420 g.
Glycerin, Double Distilled	420 g.
Caustic Potash, 35%	405 g.
Alcohol	120 g.
Water	2400 g.

A small amount of stearic acid in excess will change the consistency from thin to heavy.

Transparent Liquid Shaving Soap

Olein, Clear, Pale	13.5 g.
Coconut Oil	1.575 g.
Caustic Potash (50%)	about 6.33 g.
Distilled Water (or Softened Water)	79 g.

Shaving Milks

Formula No. 1

Mix in warmed mortar:

Wool Fat	10 g.
Borax	2 g.
Glycerin	15 g.
Orange Flower Water	40 g.
Rose Water	40 g.
Tincture of Benzoin	10 g.

Formula No. 2

Make up emulsion of:

Almond Oil	20 g.
Glycerin	20 g.
Gum Arabic	20 g.
Rose Water	440 g.

And add:

Glycerin	50 g.
Tincture of Benzoin	40 g.
Perfume	10 g.

Formula No. 3

Grind:

Lanolin, Pure, Pale	50 g.
Coconut Oil	25 g.
Borax	8 g.
Neutral Soap Powder	25 g.
Water	80 g.
Rose Water	400 cc.
Orange Flower Water (Tepid)	400 cc.
Peppermint Oil	2 cc.

Formula No. 4

Stearic Acid	10 kg.
Coconut Oil	10 kg.
Caustic Potash, 38° Bé.	10 kg.
Water	80 kg.
Lanolin	0.5 kg.
Glycerin	0.5 kg.

Astringent After Shaving Milk

Formula No. 1

Glyceryl Monostearate	10 g.
Vegetable Oils	8 g.
White Paraffin Oil, Odorless	2 g.
Distilled Water	73 g.
Acetic Acid (50%)	5 g.
Glycerin (28° Bé.)	2 g.

Add perfume resistant to acids.

Formula No. 2

Camphor	2 g.
Eau de Cologne Oil	4 g.
Alcohol	300 g.
Glycerin (28° Bé.)	80 g.
Rose Water	614 g.

Camphor Shaving Milk

Camphor, Spirits of	50 g.
Glycerin	50 g.
Lavender Oil	2 g.
Alcohol	600 g.
Add:	
Borax, Powdered	25 g.
Distilled Water	1200 g.
Fresh Lemon Juice	200 g.

Stir; allow to stand over night; filter.

After-Shave Lotions

Formula No. 1

Alcohol	25.00 g.
Glycerin	5.00 g.
Menthol	0.50 g.
Boric Acid	0.50 g.
Water	69.00 g.
Perfume } Color }	to suit

Formula No. 2

Acetic Acid, (80%)	20 g.
Glycerin	20 g.
Perfume Composition	20 g.
Alcohol	440 g.
Water, Distilled	500 g.

Formula No. 3

Glycerin	50 cc.
Alcohol	650 cc.
Water	300 cc.
Menthol	5 g.
Salicylic Acid	1 g.
Ferric Chloride (Dilute Solution)	1 drop

Formula No. 4

Glycerin	100 cc.
Alcohol	500 cc.
Water	400 cc.
Menthol	2 g.
Salicylic Acid	1 g.
Ferric Chloride (Dilute Solution)	1 drop

Formula No. 5

Glycerin	200 cc.
Alcohol	400 cc.
Water	400 cc.
Menthol	1 g.
Salicylic Acid	1 g.
Ferric Chloride (Dilute Solution)	1 drop

For most skins, Formula No. 1 is desirable; it dries quickly and has a pleasant after glow. Formula No. 3 gives an oily product which should be wiped off with a towel. The intensity of the color can be varied by the amount of ferric chloride used.

Formula No. 6

Glycerin	2 g.
Lactic, Citric, or Phosphoric Acid	0.2 g.
Menthol	0.5 g.
Alum	0.3 g.
Perfume	0.5 g.
Alcohol (45%)	96.5 g.

Formula No. 7

Glycerin	5 g.
Alum	1 g.
Zinc Sulphophenolate	0.5 g.
Propyl Alcohol	10 g.
Rose Water	10 g.
Perfume	0.5 g.
Alcohol (45%)	72.5 g.

Formula No. 8

Alcohol (40%)	1000 cc.
Glycerin, C.P.	40 g.
Aluminum Lactate	3 g.
Citric Acid	2 g.

Formula No. 9

Zinc Sulphophenolate	0.5 g.
Alcohol (96%)	15 cc.
Witch Hazel	10 g.
Peruvian Balm	0.25 g.
Glycerin	1 g.

Formula No. 10

Distilled Water	20 cc.
Isopropyl Alcohol	4 cc.
Alcohol	4 cc.
Alum	1 g.
Glycerin	0.5 cc.
Zinc Sulphophenolate	0.25 g.

Formula No. 11 (Cloudy)

Emulsone B	50 g.
Boric Acid	50 g.
Isopropyl Alcohol	100 g.
Diethylene Glycol	200 g.

Titanium Dioxide	60 g.
Distilled Water	4 l.
Menthol	2 g.
Moldex or Other Preservative	2 g.

Formula No. 12

Alcohol (95%)	680 g.
Perfume Oil	6 g.
Glycerin	15 g.
Tannic Acid	5 g.
Distilled Water	294 g.

To the alcohol perfume-solution add glycerin, then the water-tannic acid solution.

Formula No. 13

Menthol	1 dr.
Boric Acid	2½ oz.
Glycerin	5 oz.
Alcohol	5 qt.
Water, to make	5 gal.
Perfume	

Dissolve menthol in alcohol. Add boric acid, perfume, and glycerin. Stir thoroughly until everything is dissolved. Add water. Filter. This preparation may be colored by adding enough color to give shade desired.

Formula No. 14

Tragacanth	8 oz.
Formalin	2 dr.
Menthol	2 oz.
Cologne Oil	2½ oz.
Red Coloring	a sufficiency
Industrial Spirit	3 pt.
Water	5 gal.

Anesthetic Shaving Lotion

Boric Acid	160 gr.
Menthol	8 gr.
Benzocaine	6 gr.
Alcohol	6 oz.
Water	to 1 pt.

Dissolve the menthol and benzocaine in the alcohol and add gradually to the water in which the acid has been dissolved.

"Bestol" After Shaving Lotion

Alcohol (95%)	98 cc.
Distilled Water	92 cc.
Glycerin	10 cc.
Menthol	0.2 g.
Bay Oil	3 drops

Color with 2 drops of a 0.5% alcoholic solution of Dimethyl amidoazobenzol (Butter Color). Dissolve menthol and oil in the alcohol. Mix with the water and glycerin, and make brilliant by filtering through diatomaceous earth.

Vinegar After Shave Lotion

Acetic Acid (80%)	20 g.
Glycerin (28° Bé.)	20 g.
Perfume Composition	20 g.
Alcohol	440 g.
Water, Distilled	500 g.

Antiseptic After-Shave Lotion

1. Gum Tragacol	50 g.
2. Boric Acid	50 g.
3. Isohol	100 g.
4. Phenol	1 dr.
5. Menthol	1 dr.
6. Oil of Rose	1 dr.
7. Polycol	400 g.
8. Water	7 pt.
9. Titanium Dioxide	2 oz.

Rub No. 1 and No. 2 together with No. 3, add and mix in thoroughly Nos. 4, 5, 6 and 7. Mix Nos. 8 and 9 and stir into previous mixture rapidly for 4 minutes only. Strain through cheese-cloth and bottle. This gives a thick soothing cream which is very popular.

Smooth-Skin Balm

The lotion formula given above is used with the exception that the phenol is replaced by 1 dram bismuth oxychloride.

Swedish Face Tonic

1. Zinc Phenolsulfonate	½ oz.
2. Witch Hazel	15 oz.
3. Isohol	10 oz.
4. Glycerin	1 oz.
5. Balsam Peru	¼ oz.
6. Lavender Oil	10 g.

Dissolve Nos. 1 and 2 and then dissolve Nos. 4, 5 and 6 in No. 3. Mix both solutions and stir thoroughly. Allow to stand overnight and filter.

Aromatic Bay Rum

Jamaica Rum	12 fl. oz.
Alcohol	45 fl. oz.
Glycerin	5 fl. oz.
Bay Oil	2 fl. oz.
Water	36 fl. oz.

Mix the perfume with the alcohol, add the glycerin, Jamaica rum and water. Mix and filter.

Almond Cream for After Shaving

Formula No. 1

Gum Tragacanth	175 gr.
Glycerin	10 oz.
Borax	1 oz.
Distilled Water	64 oz.
Perfume, Almond	as required

In 20 oz. hot water dissolve Borax then add Gum Tragacanth and Glycerin. Allow to stand 12 hours, stirring frequently. When gum has formed mucilage add the remaining 44 oz. of water while stirring and strain through muslin.

Formula No. 2

Stearic Acid (triple pressed)	5 oz. 260 gr.
Sweet Almond Oil	3 oz.
Ethyl Amino Benzoate	½ oz.

Melt acid and oil together and add Ethyl Amino Benzoate. Stir until dissolved and adjust temperature to 70° C.

After Shaving Cream

Formula No. 1

Stearic Acid	13 g.
Triethanolamine	.8 g.
"Carbitol"	.8 g.
Menthol Crystals	.3 g.
Alcohol	.5 g.
Water	85 cc.

Formula No. 2

U. S. Patent 1,979,385

Stearic Acid	15 g.
Triethanolamine	0.75 g.
"Carbitol"	8 g.
Menthol	0.75 g.
Ethyl Alcohol (Anhydrous)	0.5 g.
Water	75 g.

Styptic Powder

An excellent styptic powder results from the mixture of 50% powdered talc and 50% phthalyl peroxide. The latter often contains up to 40% of its weight as phthalic acid; this is beneficial and acts as a stabilizer. The mixture is antiseptic.

Styptic Pencils

The following are the methods adopted for the manufacture of alum pencils:

Formula No. 1

White: Liquefy 100 g. of potassium alum crystals by the aid of heat. Remove any scum and avoid overheating, particularly of the sides of the vessel in which liquefaction is being carried out. The molten liquid should be perfectly clear. Triturate a mixture of French chalk in fine powder, 5 g., glycerin 5 g. to a paste, incorporate with the liquefied alum and pour into suitable molds. A white appearance can be imparted to the resulting pencils by the addition of more French chalk.

Formula No. 2

Clear: Carefully liquefy potassium alum crystals so as to avoid loss of water of crystallization, adding a small amount of glycerin and water (about 5 per cent) until a clear liquid is obtained. This is poured, whilst hot, into suitable moulds, previously smeared with fat. The solidified pencils are rendered smooth by rubbing them with a moistened piece of cloth.

CHAPTER XV

DENTIFRICES

Tooth Paste

TOOTH PASTES consist essentially of an abrasive, a cleaner, a non-drying liquid, a binder and a flavor. Because of the complexity of the average tooth-paste formula it is next to impossible to predict how it will stand up under varying conditions except by rigorous testing and the experience of past mistakes. Poor formulation will produce products which separate, harden or liquefy.

Ingredients of Tooth Pastes

Abrasives	*Soaps and Cleaners*	*Carriers and Softeners*	*Binders*	*Other Ingredients*
Bentonite	Diglycol Laurate	Alcohol	Acacia, Gum	Alum
Calcium Phosphates	(Diglycol Stearate)	Calcium Chloride	Agar	Aromatics (Flavors)
Calcium Sulfate	Glycosterin	Glucarin	Colloidal Clays	Benzoic Acid
Chalk	Hard Soaps	Glucose	Free fatty acid (set free from soap)	Bicarbonate of Soda
China Clay (Kaolin)	Soft Soaps	Glycerin	Glycerite of Starch	Boric Acid
Cuttle Fish Bone Ground	Sulfonated Alcohols	Glycols	India Gum	Camphor
Hydrated Magnesia	Sulfonated Oils	Honey	Irish Moss	Citric Acid
Magnesia		Invert Sugars	Karaya, Gum	Dyestuffs
Magnesium Carbonate		Mineral Oil	Locust Bean Gum	Iodine
Pumice (very fine)		Simple Syrup	Pectin	Malic Acid
Silica (very fine)		Water	Petrolatum	Moldex
Sodium Metaphosphate			Silica Gel	Phenols
Talc			Starch	Potassium Chlorate
Tin Oxide			Tragacanth	Saccharine
Whiting				Salt
				Sugars
				Sodium Benzoate
				Sodium Perborate
				Thymol
				Ultramarine

An ideal abrasive is one which will not scratch the tooth enamel and yet exert a sufficiently fine scouring effect to clean and polish the teeth. It should not react with the other ingredients or spoil the taste or appearance of the finished product. In addition it must not segregate or lump together on aging.

Because soaps have good detergent properties they appear in most of the older tooth-pastes. The recent trend has been away from soaps because of their undesired action on the saliva. Soaps are being replaced by glycol and glyceryl fatty acid esters (glycosterin and glyceryl mono-stearate). The latter possess high emulsifying and cleaning powers. The former is neutral and the latter much less alkaline than the purest soaps.

Carriers and softeners are used to suspend the abrasive and to prevent drying out. Binders are incorporated as carriers and colloiding agents. When the latter are vegetable products they must be preserved properly to avoid decomposition. Medicinal and antiseptic ingredients of little practical value are often incorporated.

Tooth Paste

Formula No. 1

Glycerin	448	lb.
Starch	64	lb.
Cold Water	12	gal.
Magnesium Carbonate	15	lb.
Powdered Castile Soap	15	lb.
Precipitated Chalk—Light	350	lb.
Water	2	lb.
Saccharin (dissolve Saccharin in the water)	6½	oz.
1 oz. National Fast Pink "B" Dry Color; 16 oz. Water	Dissolve color in the water	
Glycerin	9	gal.

Flavoring for above

Methyl Salicylate	48	oz.
Peppermint Oil	40	oz.
Cloves Oil	4	oz.
Cassia Oil	12	oz.
Menthol	1 oz. 343	gr.

Directions: Heat glycerin in steam jacketed kettle with an agitator. Bring the mix up to 212° F. Mix starch in cold water and add slowly to hot glycerin with constant agitation. Allow to cook until it forms a clear jelly. Now add powders by sifting in small amount at a time and mix thoroughly after each addition. When all powder is added, mix paste for about five hours and add perfume oils during the last half hour of mixing. If pony mixer is to be used, make glycerite of starch in jacketed kettle first, then transfer to pony mixer and add balance of ingredients.

Formula No. 2

Sodium Bicarbonate	11.0	g.
Borax	4.0	g.
Powdered Soap	14.0	g.
Precipitated Chalk	4.0	g.
Magnesium Carbonate	10.0	g.
Powdered Cuttlefish Bone	10.0	g.
Glycerin	50.0	g.
Menthol	0.4	g.
Anise Oil	2.0	g.
Peppermint Oil	3.0	g.
Cinnamon Oil	2.0	g.
Carmine	0.4	g.

Formula No. 3

Glycerin	25.5	g.
Calcium Carbonate, Precipitated	30.1	g.
Neutral Soap Powdered	1.2	g.
Magnesium Hydroxide	4.9	g.
Gum Tragacanth, Powdered	0.9	g.
Flavoring	1.7	g.
Saccharine	0.07	g.
Water, to make	100	cc.

Formula No. 4

Calcium Carbonate, Precipitated	32.00	g.
Magnesium Carbonate Precipitated	3.50	g.
Soap, Powdered	5.60	g.
Glycerin	30.00	g.
Water	26.60	cc.
Saccharin	0.06	g.
Flavoring	1.80	g.
Gum Karaya	0.30	g.
Irish Moss	0.30	g.
Color	sufficient	

Formula No. 5

Calcium Carbonate, Precipitated	55.00	g.
Soap, Powdered	6.00	g.
Glycerin	34.00	g.
Petrolatum	1.25	g.
Saccharin	0.25	g.

Peppermint Oil	0.10 g.
Water	2.26 cc.
Potassium Iodide	0.24 g.

Formula No. 6

Soap, Powdered	2500 g.
Calcium Carbonate	500 g.
Lactose	150 g.
Glycerin	2000 g.
Water	400 cc.
Peppermint Oil	100 g.
Alcohol	100 g.
Carmine	10–20 g.

Formula No. 7

Calcium Carbonate, Precipitated	50 g.
White Bolus	10 g.
Glycerin	20 g.
Water	18 cc.
Tragacanth	1 g.
Perfume (as below)	
Peppermint Oil	50 cc.
Menthol	5 cc.
Anise Oil	25 cc.
Clove Oil	5 cc.
Fennel Oil	5 cc.
Ceylon Cinnamon Oil	1 cc.
Lemon Oil	1 cc.

Formula No. 8

Soap	33.00 g.
Precipitated Chalk	25.00 g.
Absolute Alcohol	20.00 g.
Glycerin	15.00 g.
Benzoic Acid	3.00 g.
Eucalyptus Oil	2.00 g.
Peppermint Oil	2.00 g.
Saccharin	0.50 g.
Thymol	0.25 g.

Formula No. 9

Calcium Carbonate	22.0 g.
Castile Soap, Neutral	24.0 g.
Thymol	.20 g.
Benzoic Acid	.35 g.
Saccharin Soluble	.50 g.
Eucalyptus Oil	1.80 g.
Peppermint Oil	2.00 g.
Glycerin	28.00 g.
Alcohol	21.15 g.

Formula No. 10

Soap Powdered	2000 g.
Chalk Precipitated	800 g.
Glycerin	sufficient
Peppermint Oil	10 g.
Alcohol	100 cc.

The soap and chalk are mixed with a sufficient quantity of glycerin to make a paste of the desired consistency and then the oil of peppermint, dissolved in the alcohol, is added.

Formula No. 11

Magnesium Hydroxide	3.700 g.
Glycerin	31.300 g.
Corn Starch	4.700 g.
Saccharin, Soluble	0.015 g.
Calcium Carbonate, Precipitated	46.900 g.
Soap	2.300 g.
Flavoring	0.700 g.
Water	10.44 cc.

Formula No. 12

Precipitated Chalk	100 g.
Sugar	10 g.
Magnesium Carbonate	50 g.
Glycerin	10 g.
White Soap, Powdered	50 g.
Peppermint Oil	5 g.
Carmine	0.3 g.

Formula No. 13

Sodium Carbonate	3.7 g.
Sodium Bicarbonate	45.8 g.
Glycerin	32.1 g.
Soap	4.3 g.
Water	12.7 cc.
Flavoring	1.4 g.

Formula No. 14

Chalk, Precipitated	35 oz.
White Neutral Soap	20 oz.
Sugar, Powdered	10 oz.
Purified Talc	10 oz.
Glycerin	25 oz.
Peppermint Oil	to suit

Mix the powders thoroughly together and then work into a paste with the glycerin. Add oil peppermint.

Formula No. 15

Glycerin	28.0 g.
Soap, Powdered	5.0 g.
Calcium Carbonate, Powdered	35.7 g.
Precipitated Chalk	7.6 g.
Sodium Benzoate	2.1 g.

Flavoring Oils	0.9 g.
Corn Starch	6.5 g.
Water	14.2 cc.

Soapless Tooth Paste

Formula No. 1

Calcium Carbonate, Precipitated	50	g.
Sodium Bicarbonate	10	g.
Pancreatin	3	g.
Peppermint Oil	1.5	g.
Menthol	0.3	g.
Tragacanth—Glycerin *	100–130	g.

* Tragacanth Gum	0.75	g.
Alcohol	5	g.
Glycerin	95	g.

Wet the gum with the alcohol and add the glycerin. Stir until smooth.

Formula No. 2

(a)	Whiting, Finest	90.0	g.
	Magnesium Carbonate	7.5	g.
	Soap Wort Powder	2.5	g.
(b)	Clove Oil	0.06	g.
	Cassia Oil	0.06	g.
(c)	Orange Oil	0.06	g.
	Lavender Flower Oil	0.06	g.
	Geranium Oil	2.0	g.
(d)	Glycerin	30.0	g.
	Water	22.5	g.

Mix (a), add (b), mix, add (c), mix thoroughly again, add (d). Stir up well.

Formula No. 3

Chalk, Precipitated	120	g.
Violet Root Powder	60	g.
Carmine	3.75	g.
Geranium Oil	1.0	g.
Sandal Wood Oil	0.33	g.
Glycerin	to paste	

Grind the chalk with the carmine, add the violet root powder, add the perfume oils and the glycerin.

Formula No. 4

Calcium Carbonate, Precipitated	500	g.
Magnesium Carbonate	70	g.
Peppermint Oil	4	g.
Eucalyptus Oil	1.5	g.
Calamus Oil	0.5	g.
Glycerin	200	g.
Gum Arabic Mucilage	sufficient	

Tooth Paste with Low Soap Content

Glycerite of Starch	60	lb.
Irish Moss Infusion (2% Moss in Water)	48	lb.
Neutral White Soap	9¼	lb.
Benzoic Acid	2 lb. 6	oz.
Saccharin	5	oz.
Calcium Phosphate	6	lb.
Light Precipitated Chalk	77	lb.
Flavor	2½	lb.

The solids are mixed into the liquids and the benzoic acid is added to the glycerite of starch and moss infusion and the powdered soap first added and mixed about 15 minutes so that the benzoic acid has sufficient time to set free and thoroughly distribute the free fatty acids derived from the soap. Then the chalk is mixed in.

(Acid) Tooth Paste

Glycerin	200.0 g.
† Flavor	9.6 g.
* Acid Solution	64.0 g.
Benzoic Acid	0.8 g.
Calcium Chloride	2.4 g.
Corn Sugar	40.0 g.
Powdered Gum Tragacanth	6.4 g.
Powdered Gum Karaya	7.2 g.
Calcium Sulphate	304.0 g.
Tricalcium Phosphate	90.4 g.
	724.8

* The acid solution is made as follows: 5 g. each of citric, boric, and tartaric acids dissolved in 100 g. cold water.

Procedure:

(a) Mix the glycerin, flavor, acid solution benzoic acid, calcium chloride, and cerelose. Mix for 15 minutes.

(b) Mix the powdered gums, calcium sulfate and the tricalcium phosphate.

(c) Add (b) to (a) and mix at least two hours.

Mill through a paint or ointment mill before filling tubes.

† Flavor is composed of 8.0 parts peppermint oil, 1/.1 parts spearmint oil, 0.3 parts menthol and 0.4 parts cassia oil.

Tooth Paste, Waterless

Formula No. 1

German Patent 630,344

Mineral Oil	200 g.
Tragacanth	20 g.

added to form a thin paste, bearing in mind that the paste becomes firmer on keeping. The paste should be packed in tubes as soon as possible after manufacture.

Soap Tooth-Paste Base

Formula No. 1

Precipitated Calcium Carbonate	50.00 g.
Soft Soap U. S. P.	12.59 g.
Glycerin	18.88 cc.

Make into a paste.

Add the glycerin gradually to the soft soap in a mortar and triturate until soap is dissolved. Then add the resulting liquid in small amounts to the carbonate, triturating well after each addition until a smooth, creamy paste results. The glycerin and soft soap will first cause considerable foam which will cease and a clear liquid remain. It may be used while foaming, if desired.

An easy and very satisfactory method to make this paste is as follows:

Flavor: The following formula per 100 g. of paste gives a pleasing taste:

Benzoic Acid	0.25 g.
Thymol	0.25 g.
Saccharin, Soluble	0.25 g.
Eucalyptus Oil	1.50 cc.
Peppermint Oil	1.50 cc.

If the paste is to be flavored, the above ingredients, after first being mixed, are added to the excipient. Dissolve the thymol and benzoic acid in the volatile oils and the saccharin in the water used in the excipient. Deduct the quantity of flavor used from the general excipient so that the paste will not become too soft.

This paste produces a rich, soapy foam when brushed on the teeth and leaves a cool, clean sensation in the mouth if above flavor is used. The flavor may be changed, if desired, by using other volatile oils. It will have a yellow tint due to the soft soap.

Formula No. 2

Precipitated Calcium Carbonate	55.25 g.
Powdered Castile Soap	6.00 g.
Glycerin	34.00 cc.
Liquid Petrolatum	1.50 cc.
Saccharin, Soluble	0.05 g.
Water	2.50 cc.

Make a paste and dispense in a tube with large opening at cap end. A suitable flavor may be obtained by adding 1 cc. of peppermint oil.

Mix the calcium carbonate and soap together by sieving through a No. 60-mesh sieve. Dissolve saccharin in water and add to the mixture of glycerin, the volatile oil, if used, and the liquid petrolatum. This makes a smooth, creamy white paste which may be colored pink if desired by using 0.154 g. of Cherry Red No. 2.

This is not a soap paste; the soap is used as a binder and will not cause a lather.

The oil of peppermint may be replaced by any other volatile oil or combination of volatile oils used as a flavor. The taste may be increased or decreased as desired by adding to or limiting the amount of flavor.

Tooth Powders

In mixing tooth powder the flavor is first mixed with part of the abrasive. The other ingredients are then mixed in thoroughly and the whole is mixed in a ball mill or good powder mixer. Care must be taken that there is no great increase in temperature or the flavoring materials will dissipate or alter in character.

Dentifrice powders consist of an abrasive, a soap and an odor. Abrasives may be chalk (either precipitated or prepared); activated carbon; calcium triphosphate; calcium di-phosphate; calcium oxide; magnesium carbonate; magnesium oxide; sodium bicarbonate; borax; sodium perborate. Some makers have used calcium sulphate but this material delivers such a coarse gritty product that its use is not advisable. All powders should be of the finest possible grain.

Formula No. 1

Calcium Tri-Phosphate	90	lb.
Magnesium Carbonate	3 to 5	lb.

Soap, Powdered	2 to 4 lb.
Saponin	1 lb.
Odor-Flavor	1 to 1½ lb.

Formula No. 2

Calcium Carbonate, Precipitated	60.0 g.
Magnesium Carbonate	1.0 g.
Magnesium Oxide	2.0 g.
Sodium Bicarbonate	30.0 g.
Castile Soap Powdered	6.0 g.
Sodium Chloride, Powdered	5.0 g.
Saccharin	0.2 g.
Wintergreen Oil	1.0 g.
Peppermint Oil	0.4 g.

Formula No. 3

Salt	59.5 oz.
Sodium Bicarbonate	19.8 oz.
Magnesium Carbonate	4.9 oz.
Sodium Perborate	14.9 oz.
Clove Oil	0.3 oz.
Methyl Salicylate	0.6 oz.

Formula No. 4

450 grams of saponin, 225 grams of calcium sulfocyanide and 111.3 grams of saccharin dissolved in one liter of water. The solution is agitated in a mixing machine. Then 12.9 kilograms of anhydrous gypsum are added gradually in small proportions and the mixing is continued until powder is obtained, which is only slightly moist and non-dusting. The mixture is then dried at a temperature of 70 to 80° C. Calcium sulfocyanide is perfectly protected in the powder by the gypsum and the saponine from coming in contact with moisture.

Formula No. 5

525 parts of tartaric acid intimately mixed with 900 parts of gum tragacanth. About 100 to 200 parts of ethyl alcohol are added and worked into the mixture until a crumbly, slightly moist mass is obtained, which is then dried at a moderate temperature. The two powders are then mixed together to give the finished dentifrice.

Formula No. 6

Glycerin	24.50 g.
Dicalcium Phosphate (400 mesh)	54.00 g.
Galactonic Acid Lactone	3.00 g.
Water	10.00 g.
Alcohol	4.00 g.
Petrolatum	1.00 g.
Gum Tragacanth	0.75 g.
Gum Karaya	0.75 g.
Malic Acid	0.25 g.
Salt	0.60 g.
Saccharin	0.07 g.
Menthol	0.05 g.
Peppermint Oil	0.75 g.

Alkaline Tooth Powder

Sodium Bicarbonate	150.00 g.
Carmine No. 40, Powder	0.01 g.
Methyl Salicylate	1.00 cc.
Clove Oil	1.00 cc.

Make into tooth powder and dispense in glass bottles.

Add the carmine to a small amount of sodium bicarbonate in a mortar and triturate until color is thoroughly distributed, then add to it the balance of the bicarbonate of soda and mix until uniform color results. Finally incorporate the volatile oils and place in a bottle. This makes a harmless, pleasant tooth powder.

Foaming Tooth Powder

Chalk, Dense	180 lb.
Soap, Powdered	20 lb.
Saccharin	5 oz.
Flavor	5 lb.

In this type formula the chalk may be replaced entirely or in part by any desired abrasive and the powdered soap may also be varied as desired.

Charcoal Tooth Powder

Willow Charcoal, Ground	100 lb.
Chalk, Dense	90 lb.
Powdered Soap	30 lb.
Saccharin	6 oz.
Flavor	5 lb.

Camphorated Tooth Powder

Chalk or Other Abrasive	200 lb.
Camphor, Finely Ground	2 lb.
Powdered Sugar	10 lb.
Flavor	4 lb.

Peroxide Tooth Powder

Chalk or Other Abrasive	200 lb.
Sodium Perborate or Magnesium or Calcium Peroxide	25 lb.
Flavor	4 lb.

Tooth Powder Containing Wax

U. S. Patent 2,024,146

To produce a 75-pound batch of the new dentifrice powder, the following ingredients are suggested: Sodium perborate, 16 lb., 6½ oz.; magnesium oxide powder heavy, 16 lb., 6½ oz.; sodium bicarbonate, 10 lb., 2½ oz.; sodium chloride powder, 10 lb., 2½ oz.; calcium carbonate, 4 lb., 4¾ oz.; powdered borax, 5 lb., 1¼ oz.; powdered castile soap, 8 lb., 3¼ oz.; ceresin, 25 oz.; saccharin soluble, 4 oz., 125½ g.; menthol, 6 oz., 375 g.; thymol, 2 oz., 250 g.; clove oil, 3⅛ oz.; cassia oil, 3⅛ oz.; peppermint oil, 4 oz., 205 min.; spearmint oil, 10 oz., 325 min.; ether, 64 oz.

All the solid materials are thoroughly dried and are then sifted through a very fine sieve, about No. 60, before mixing. These dry materials are then thoroughly mixed. The ceresin is now melted. The oils, the menthol and the thymol, are then mixed and this mixture is added to the melted ceresine. The ceresin is now removed from the fire and the ether is added thereto. The mixture of ceresin, oils, and ether is now incorporated with a quarter of the entire amount of mixed powders by constantly stirring this quantity of powder in a closed electrically heated mixing machine, the powder, of course, being stirred continuously during the spraying of the liquid thereon and the machine remaining closed during this mixing process.

''When the powders and the liquids are thoroughly mixed, the remaining three-quarters of the powder is added thereto, the powder being stirred continuously during this mixing process. When all the ingredients are now thoroughly mixed the cover is removed and the mixer is allowed to continue running for one hour while the powder is maintained at a temperature which will drive away all the ether which was used to facilitate impregnating the powder with the ceresine.

''Following the compounding of the dentifrice as above noted, the entire mixture is then passed through a No. 40 sieve and placed in air-tight containers.''

Salt Dentifrice

Salt	25 g.
Calcium Carbonate	33 g.
Orris Powder	6 g.
Soap	3 g.
Glycerin	33 g.

Dentifrice Massing Fluid

Formula No. 1

Water	4 oz.
Gelatin	1 to 2 oz.
Glycerin	7 oz.

Dissolve gelatin in water by heat and add glycerin.

Formula No. 2

Glycerin	1 oz.
Mucilage of Acacia	1 oz.

Dental Paste

Tooth Powder	600 parts
Massing Fluid	300 to 400 parts

"Vince" Type Powder

Propyl *para* hydroxy-benzoate ⅝ grain, magnesium carbonate 1½ grains, calcium phosphate 2½ grains, rubin 1/50 grain, soluble saccharin 4 grains, aromatics 3 grains, sodium perborate to 1 ounce.

Action and Uses: For oral disinfection and as a dentifrice. In treatment of Vincent's disease.

Directions: To be used on a wet tooth-brush or made into a paste with water.

Tooth "Bleach"

(For removing Nicotine Stains)

Formula No. 1

Sodium Bicarbonate	50 oz.
Precipitated Chalk	50 oz.

Flavor as desired.

Formula No. 2

Lactic Acid	3 oz.
Talc	30 oz.

Flavor as desired.

Artificial Denture Cleaner

Formula No. 1

Chalk, Precipitated	4 oz.
Heavy Magnesium Carbonate	1 oz.
Light Magnesium Carbonate	½ oz.
Soap, Powdered	2 dr.

The dental plate brush should be slightly damp when using this powder.

Formula No. 2

Cuttlefish Bone	1 oz.
Pumice, Finely Powdered	2 oz.
Borax	2 oz.
Chalk, Precipitated	16 oz.
Thymol	10 gr.
Peppermint Oil	10 drops
Aniseed Oil	10 drops

Formula No. 3

Glycerite of Starch	36 g.
Diglycol Laurate	1 g.
Sugar Syrup	2.25 g.
Magnesium Carbonate	1.13 g.
Gum Tragacanth	.07 g.
Chalk Precipitated	41 g.
Sodium Bicarbonate	6 g.
Water	10.5 g.
Flavor	to suit

Mouth Wash

Formula No. 1

Alcohol, 95%	1200 g.
Water	200 g.
Glycerin	100 g.
Triethanolamine Oleate	15 g.
Tincture of Myrrh	100 g.
Peppermint Oil	60 g.
Menthol	15 g.
Vanillin	3 g.
Cinnamon Oil	3 g.

Formula No. 2

Alcohol	250 g.
Glycerin, C.P.	25 g.
Potash Soap, Neutral, Free of Filler (38%)	10 g.
Water	90 g.
Tincture of Myrrh	20 g.
Tincture of Rhatania	20 g.
Menthol	2 g.
Anise Oil	3 g.
Cinnamon Oil	1 g.
Dyestuff, Red, Alcohol-Soluble	

Formula No. 3

Benzoic Acid	1 lb.
Boric Acid	1 lb.
Borax	1 lb.
Alcohol	1½ gal.
Eucalyptus	3 fl. oz.
Thyme Oil	1 fl. oz.
Wintergreen Oil	2 fl. oz.
Water	15 gal.
Caramel Coloring	1¼ fl. oz.

The boric acid and borax are added to part of the water and dissolved by boiling. The solution is cooled by the addition of the rest of the water and left to become quite cold. The benzoic acid is dissolved in half the alcohol, and the essential oils in the remaining half, and the two mixed and added to the water solution. The caramel color is added while stirring, and thorough mixing is continued for four hours.

Formula No. 4

Benzoic Acid	12 g.
Tincture of Rhatany	60 g.
Alcohol	400 g.
Peppermint Oil	3 g.

A teaspoonful in a small wine-glassful of water is used.

Formula No. 5

Eucalyptus Oil	10 drops
Wintergreen Oil	10 drops
Menthol	10 gr.
Thymol	10 gr.
Boric Acid	½ oz.
Alcohol	4½ oz.
Water	16 oz.

Formula No. 6

Salol	5 g.
Peppermint Oil	1 g.
Clove Oil	0.04 g.
Fennel Oil	0.04 g.
Saccharin	0.004 g.
Alcohol	190 g.

Formula No. 7

Tannic Acid	1 dr.
Spirits Lavender Compound	1 oz.
Water	3 oz.

Formula No. 8

Chlorthymol	.1 oz.
Alcohol	25 oz.
Glycerin	7.5 oz.
Water	67.5 cc.

This preparation is said to have a Phenol Coefficient of about 110.

Formula No. 9

Saccharin, Soluble	0.10 g.
Fuchsin, Basic	0.02 g.
Cinnamon Oil	0.25 cc.

Peppermint Oil	0.25 cc.
Clove Oil	0.50 cc.
Alcohol	300.00 cc.
Talc	10.00 g.
Distilled water to make	1000.00 cc.

Dissolve the saccharin in 10 cc. of water and the fuchsin and volatile oils in 250 cc. of alcohol. Add slowly to the 700 cc. of water and filter through talc. Finally add the remaining 50 cc. of alcohol.

Formula No. 10

Saccharin, Soluble	0.10 g.
Fuchsin, Basic	0.02 g.
Cinnamon Oil	0.25 cc.
Peppermint Oil	0.25 cc.
Clove Oil	0.50 cc.
Alcohol	300.00 cc.
Talc	10.00 g.
Distilled Water, to make	1000.00 cc.

This makes a pleasant sweet spicy mouth rinse when diluted with 2–3 parts of water. No medication is intended in this formula. Especially suitable for the Spray Bottle.

Formula No. 11

Thymol	0.50 g.
Menthol	1.00 g.
Peppermint Oil	3.00 cc.
Alcohol	300.00 cc.
Distilled Water, to make	1000.00 cc.

Color to suit.

A pleasant mint-flavored mouth wash to be used diluted 2–3 times with water. Especially suitable for the Spray Bottle.

Astringent Mouth Wash

Formula No. 1

Zinc Chloride	2.0 g.
Menthol	0.6 g.
Cinnamon Oil	1.4 cc.
Clove Oil	0.3 cc.
Formaldehyde	0.4 cc.
Saccharin	0.4 g.
Alcohol	40 cc.
Water, to make	1000 cc.

Formula No. 2

Zinc Chloride	1 g.
Alcohol	12 cc.
Eucalyptol	20 dr.
Cinnamon Oil	2 dr.
Peppermint Oil	3 dr.
Distilled Water to make	100 cc.

Formula No. 3

Zinc Chloride	2.0 g.
Menthol	0.6 g.
Cinnamon Oil	1.4 cc.
Clove Oil	0.3 cc.
Formaldehyde	0.4 cc.
Saccharin	0.4 g.
Alcohol	40.0 cc.
Water to make	1000.0 cc.

Formula No. 4
("Lavoris" type)

Zinc Chloride	5.0 g.
Saccharin	0.2 g.
Fuchsin	0.005 g.
Cinnamon Oil	0.5 cc.
Peppermint Oil	0.5 cc.
Clove Oil	1.0 cc.
Glycerin	10.0 cc.
Alcohol	75.0 cc.
Distilled Water to make	100.0 cc.

Formula No. 5
(Aromatic)

Zinc Chloride	1.065 g.
Formaldehyde	1.0135 g.
Menthol	.00858 g.
Cassia Oil	.0312 g.
Clove Oil	.0064 g.
Saccharin	.0017 g.
Glycerin	.010 g.
Alcohol	.050 g.

Mouth Wash, Analgesic

Anaesthesin is used in analgesic mouth washes. This substance is easily soluble in alcohol and difficultly soluble in water and hence adheres to mucuous membrane with which it contacts.

Formula No. 1

Two grams of anaesthesin are dissolved in 90 parts alcohol and 20 parts water are added. Peppermint oil, anise oil and clove oil may be added to finish preparation. Another product used in these mouth washes is ethyl paraphenol-sulfo-para-aminobenzoate in 2% solution. Novocaine hydrochloride may be used with addition of taste correctives.

Formula No. 2

800 parts tincture of pyrethrum, 40 parts tincture of Spanish pepper, 40 parts clove oil, 20 parts menthol, 20

parts camphor and 80 parts chloroform.

The following mouth washes may be used for treating pain caused by cariotic teeth.

Formula No. 3

Four parts red saunders are mixed with 2 parts guaiacum wood, 5 parts myrrh, 5 parts cloves and one part cinnamon bark. This mixture is digested with 290 parts 90% alcohol, filtered, and 0.1 part clove oil and 0.1 part cinnamon oil is added.

Formula No. 4

16 parts tincture of myrrh are mixed with 8 parts tincture of catechu, 4 parts tincture of guaiac, 4 parts tincture of rhatany, 3 parts tincture of cloves, 2 parts spirits of cochlearia, a few drops cinnamon oil and 63 parts 50% alcohol.

Formula No. 5

2 parts oil of black mustard and 30 parts spirits of cochlearia.

Formula No. 6

8 parts tannic acid are mixed with 5 parts tincture of iodine, 1 part potassium iodide, 5 parts tincture of myrrh and 200 parts rose water.

Formula No. 7

Five parts tannic acid are also mixed with 5 parts tincture of pyrethrum, 4 parts lavender water, 40 parts 90% alcohol and 20 parts distilled water.

Formula No. 8

6 parts tannic acid are mixed with 3 parts tincture of iodine, 6 parts tincture of myrrh, 70 parts 90% alcohol and 240 parts rose water.

Antiseptic Mouth Wash

Formula No. 1

Menthol	1 oz.
Thymol	1 oz.
Benzoic Acid	4 oz.
Boric Acid	21 oz.
Glycerin	26 oz.
Ethyl Alcohol	250 oz.
Water to make	1000 oz.

This mouth wash when diluted 1 to 3 will still show negative against the organisms Staphylococcus Pyogenes Aureus and Staphylococcus Pyogenes Albus when tested by the Hygienic Laboratory method for one minute.

Formula No. 2

("Listerine" Type)

Boric Acid	50 g.
Benzoic Acid	1 g.
Thymol	1 g.
Eucalyptol	0.125 cc.
Peppermint Oil	0.5 cc.
Wintergreen Oil	0.25 cc.
Thyme	0.1 cc.
Grain Alcohol	250 cc.
Water to make up to	1000 cc.
Caramel	to color

The boric acid is dissolved in the water or about 700 cc. of same. All the other products are dissolved in the alcohol and the two solutions mixed and colored to a very pale straw. The above product must be labeled 25% grain alcohol.

Mouth Wash Tablets

Peppermint Oil	30 cc.
Saponin, Best	100 g.
Sodium Benzoate	500 g.

Mouth Rinse

Salt	30 g.
Sugar	20 g.
Cinnamon Oil	¼ cc.
Clove Oil	½ cc.
Peppermint Oil	¼ cc.

Gingivitis Mouth Wash

Boric Acid	4 g.
Potassium Chlorate	8 g.
Peppermint Water	350 cc.

Breath Deodorant

Dissolve one 4.6 grain tablet chloramine in 1 oz. water. Brush teeth and tongue, and rinse out mouth with this solution, while fresh.

Immediately and permanently rids breath of even such odors as those of garlic and onions.

Sodium Perborate Mouth Wash

Sodium Perborate	100.00 g.
Carmine No. 40	0.03 g.
Cinnamon Oil	2.00 cc.

Dispense in glass bottle.

Add the carmine to a small amount of the powder in a mortar and triturate until the color is distributed. Add this to the remainder of the powder and triturate until a uniform color results. Lastly add the cinnamon oil.

Plain sodium perborate is more or less disagreeable to taste but with the addition of cinnamon oil the taste is largely disguised. The color is also pleasing.

Dissolve one drachm in a glass of warm water and rinse mouth. It may be used as a tooth-powder if desired, on moistened tooth-brush.

Mouth Wash (Salol)

Salol	8 g.
Spearmint Oil	2 g.
Clove Oil	1 g.
Cinnamon Oil	1 g.
Star Anise Oil	1 g.
Alcohol, to make	400 cc.

Mouth Wash (Thymol)

Thymol	0.3 g.
Alcohol	160 g.
Rose Geranium Oil	15 drops
Calamus Oil	10 drops
Glycerin	120 g.
Venetian Soap	16 g.
Sassafras Oil	15 drops
Eucalyptus Oil	6 drops
Pine Needle Oil	40 drops
Distilled Water	700 g.

Mouth Wash (Phenol)

Phenol	4 dr.
Camphor	1 oz.
Chloroform	2 oz.
Cajeput Oil to make	4 oz.

Triturate the phenol with the camphor; add the chloroform and then the oil of cajeput.

Chloro-Phenol Mouth Wash

Benzoic Acid	4 oz.
Cinnamon Oil	8 oz.
Phenol	6 oz.
Chloroform	6 oz.
Alcohol	150 oz.
Peppermint Oil	2 oz.
Glycerin	to make 400 oz.

Dissolve the benzoic acid in the chloroform, add the glycerin and mix. Dissolve the cinnamon, peppermint, and phenol in alcohol and mix the two solutions together. Mix for two hours, chill, and filter.

Alkaline Mouth Wash

Potassium Bicarbonate	21.0 g.
Borax	20.0 g.
Sassafras Oil	1.0 cc.
Thymol	0.5 cc.
Eucalyptol	1.0 cc.
Methyl Salicylate	0.5 cc.
Cudbear	2.0 g.
Alcohol	50.0 cc.
Glycerin	90.0 cc.
Magnesium Carbonate	10.0 g.
Water	to 1,000 cc.

Mix the potassium bicarbonate and sodium borate with 100 c.c. of water. When the effervescence ceases, add this solution to 500 c.c. of water. This is then added to the alcohol in which the essential oils have been previously dissolved. The tincture of cudbear and the rest of the water are next added with the magnesium carbonate. The whole is mixed thoroughly for 2 hours and allowed to stand for 48 hours, chilled, and filtered. Purified talc may be used in place of the magnesium carbonate.

Mouth Wash (Quinosol)

Quinosol	30 g.
Glycerin	100 g.
Rose Water	900 cc.
Carmine	Sufficient

Mouth Wash (Peroxide)

Solution of Hydrogen Dioxide	250 g.
Peppermint Oil	1 drop
Ponceau R R	0.01 g.

Mouth Wash (Lactic Acid)

Lactic Acid	40 g.
Cochineal	1 g.
Peppermint Oil	30 g.
Clove Oil	3 g.
Cinnamon Oil	6 g.
Distilled Water	400 cc.
Alcohol	1600 cc.

Mouth Wash (Peppermint)

Powdered Angelica Root	25 g.
Powdered Anise Seed	30 g.
Powdered Cinnamon	6 g.
Powdered Nutmeg	3 g.
Powdered Cloves	10 g.
Alcohol (90%)	1000 cc.
Vanillin	1 g.
Peppermint Oil	8 g.
Tincture of Cochineal	sufficient

Mix and allow to stand for a few days. Mix again and filter.

Spearmint Mouth Wash

Menthol	38 g.
Gaultheria Oil	.26 g.
Spearmint Oil	1.5 g.
Glycerin	66 g.
Alcohol	100 g.
Water to make	1000 cc.

Resorcin Mouth Wash

Resorcin	50.0 g.
Zinc Chloride	0.3 g.
Menthol	5.0 g.
Thymol	2.0 g.
Eucalyptol	0.3 g.
Camphor	0.3 g.
Peppermint Oil	0.5 g.
Alcohol	250.0 g.
Solution Hydrogen Dioxide	200.0 g.
Water to make	1,000 g.

Dissolve the resorcin and zinc chloride in water, and the thymol, eucalyptol, wintergreen, menthol, and camphor in the alcohol. Mix the two solutions together, add the peroxide; stir for one hour, chill, and filter.

Zinc Chloride Mouth Wash

Tincture of Myrrh	2 fl. oz.
Thymol	5 gr.
Powdered Borax	½ oz.
Red Saunders	enough to color
Clove Oil	5 dr.
Cinnamon Oil	5 dr.
Zinc Chloride	4 gr.
Diluted Alcohol	1 pt.

Macerate three days with occasional shaking. Then filter.

Mouth Wash, Swedish (Amykos)

Boric Acid	50 g.
Tincture of Cloves	25 g.
Borax	5 g.
Water	4000 cc.

Mentholated Throat and Mouth Wash

Alcohol		4¾ gal.
Ethyl Amino Benzoate	12 oz.	350 gr.
Thymol	1 oz.	120 gr.
Eucalyptol		1 oz.
Wintergreen Oil		¾ oz.
Menthol		100 gr.
Boric Acid		3 lb.
Distilled Water		5¼ gal.

Dissolve ethyl amino benzoate, thymol, eucalyptol, wintergreen oil and menthol in alcohol. Dissolve boric Acid in hot distilled water, cool and filter. Add this aqueous solution slowly while stirring to the alcoholic solution and filter.

Perfection Mouth Wash and Antiseptic

Zinc Chloride	4.4 g.
Menthol	0.750 g.
Cinnamon and Clove Oils each	3 or 4 drops
Formalin	1 cc.
Saccharin	0.720 g.

Dissolve oils, menthol and saccharin in 86 cc. alcohol. Dissolve zinc chloride and formalin in water, mix, make up to 2000 cc. with water, filter through diatomaceous earth and color with a few drops of a saturated aqueous solution of Napthol Yellow.

Iodo-Phenol Gargle

Liquefied Phenol	2 oz.
Tincture of Iodine	16 oz.
Glycerite of Tannic Acid	54 oz.
Glycerin	54 oz.
Aromatic Elixir, to make	1 gal.

Mix the ingredients in the order given.

Dilute one part to sixteen parts of water to use.

Coloring Matter for Mouth Washes

A dilute ethyl alcohol extract of red sandal wood or/and cochineal is suitable for coloring mouth washes containing about 60% hydrogen peroxide. Reddish, non-poisonous food colors may also be used, such as raspberry red. Deep color is obtained even when the color is added in small proportions. The mouth wash prepared in this manner does not flocculate. 10 to 12 grams of coloring matter are used per 100 kilograms of the mouth wash.

CHAPTER XVI

MISCELLANEOUS

Air Purifiers

Formula No. 1

Alcohol	2000 cc.
Formalin (40%)	400 cc.
Pine Needle Oil	190 cc.
Thyme Oil	10 cc.

For use dilute with water 1:50.

Formula No. 2

Alcohol	850 cc.
Pine Needle Oil, Siberian	50 cc.
Dwarf-Pine Oil	10 cc.
Juniper Oil	10 cc.
Lemon Oil	10 cc.
Eucalyptus Oil	10 cc.
Lavender Oil	5 cc.
Rosemary Oil	5 cc.
Ethyl Acetate	10 cc.
Formaldehyde Solution (Formalin)	60 cc.

Solid, Volatile Preparations to Perfume and Disinfect the Air

Formula No. 1

Naphthalene, Pure

Formula No. 2

Paradichlorobenzol, Pure

Formula No. 3 *

Naphthalene, Scales	70 g.
Camphor, Sublimed	10 g.
Paradichlorobenzol	20 g.

Formula No. 4

Naphthalene	80 g.
Carbolic Acid (Phenol)	20 g.

Heat the mixtures gently, very little beyond the melting point (color optionally with yellow, red, blue, oil-soluble dyestuffs) and pour into molds. Work in well ventilated rooms.

"Air-Purifier" for Lavatories

Soft Soap without Fillers	25 lb.
Alcohol	35 lb.
Formaldehyde	5 lb.
Perfume Mixture * †	35 lb.

† 0.5% of Citral may be added.

* *Perfume Mixture:*

Pine Needle Oil, Siberian	10 oz.
Eucalyptus Oil	1 oz.
Rosemary Oil	3 oz.
Coumarin	1 oz.
Musk, Tincture	1 oz.
Pinus Montana Oil	2 oz.

The "purifier"-mixture is applied in a dilution in water of 25:1000.

Disinfectant for Telephones

Solution 1

Wintergreen Oil	0.5 g.
Eucalyptus Oil	0.25 g.
Denatured Alcohol	15 g.

Solution 2

Formaldehyde	25 cc.
Water	225 cc.

Add solution 1 to solution 2 and dilute with water to 1000 cc.

"Creolin" Disinfectant

Sulphonated Castor Oil	100 kg.
Caustic Soda (36° Bé.)	51.2 kg.

Heat above at 80–100° C., then add

Rosin	104 kg.

Mix with heating until uniform and add

Tar Oils (200–320° C.)	775 kg.

Mix until dissolved and then add

Water to make	1000 kg.

Water Soluble Bactericide

U. S. Patent 1,930,474

A 1 : 1 mixture (200 g.) of chlorothymol and olive oil is treated with sulphuric acid (60 g.) at 20° for 2 days, and then washed free from acid with saturated aqueous sodium sulphate; the product is readily dispersed in water.

Nail Biting Deterrent

Carnauba Wax, Emulsion (Bright Drying) 100 cc.
Quinine 1 to 3 g.

Ingrown Toe Nail Remedy

Powdered exsiccated alum is inserted between the nail and the fleshy part once a day for two or three days; (b) then applied ointment of phenol during several days.

Frost Bite Pencil

Camphor	25 g.
Iodine	50 g.
Olive Oil	500 g.
Paraffin, solid	450 g.
Alcohol	sufficient

Dissolve the camphor in the oil, and the iodine in the least possible amount of alcohol. Melt the paraffin and add the mixed solutions. When homogeneous, pour out into suitable molds.

Wrap the pencils in paraffin paper or tin foil, and pack in wooden boxes. By using more or less olive oil the pencils may be made of any desired consistency.

Frost Bite Ointment

Formula No. 1

Ichthyol	3 g.
Lanolin	4 g.
Camphor	2 g.
Petrolatum	60 g.

Warm and stir until dissolved. Rub into skin and bandage.

Formula No. 2

Euresol (Acetyl Resorcinol)	2 g.
Eucalyptol	2 g.
Turpentine	2 g.
Collodion	16 g.

Formula No. 3 (Soap)

Euresol (Acetyl Resorcinol)	2 g.
Eucalyptol	2 g.
Turpentine Oil	2 g.
Salve Soap*	

* *Salve Soap:*

Caustic Potash (20° Bé.)	40 g.
Hog Fat	40 g.
Alcohol	4 g.
Glycerin	15 g.

This salve soap can also be combined with other remedies for frost lesions. It dissolves:

10% of Peru Balsam
or 5% of Camphor
or 10% of Carbolic Acid
or 10% of Ichthyol
or 10% of Thymol

to form useful medicinal salves.

Foot Creams

Formula No. 1

Potash Soap	50 g.
Yellow Vaseline	15 g.
Water	29 g.
Zinc Oxide	6 g.
Caustic Soda	11 drops

Formula No. 2

Potash Soap	52 g.
Vaseline	15 g.
Water	27 g.
Zinc Oxide	6 g.

Formula No. 3

Soap	35 g.
Vaseline	15 g.
Water	45 g.
Zinc Oxide	5 g.
Lavender Oil	to suit

Formula No. 4

Lamb Tallow	100 g.
Pig Fat	100 g.
Creosote	1 g.
Juniper Oil	10 g.

Formula No. 5

Wool Fat	20 g.
Vaseline	10 g.
Formalin	10 g.

Formula No. 6

Glyceryl Monostearate	20 g.
Glycerin	5 g.
Paraffin Oil	5 g.
Formaldehyde Solution	15 cc.
Water	55 cc.

Melt up to 60° C. Stir until cold.

Athlete's Foot Ointment

Formula No. 1

Benzoic Acid	5 g.
Salicylic Acid	3 g.
Absorption Base (Parachol)	50 g.
Distilled Water	10 cc.
Petrolatum White to make	100 g.

1% Thymol is sometimes included to increase fungicidal activity.

Formula No. 2

Salicylic Acid	8 oz.
Ammoniated Mercury	4 oz.
Bismuth Subnitrate	12 oz.
Eucalyptus Oil	12 oz.
Hydrous Wool Fat	64 oz.

Mix and make into an ointment.

Athlete's Foot Powder

Sodium Thiosulphate	20 oz.
Boric Acid	50 oz.
Purified Talc (Sterilized)	30 oz.

Triturate thoroughly. This may be used as a prophylactic powder applied to the feet and dusted in the shoes.

Athlete's Foot Treatment

Immerse feet two or three times a day in a warm saturated aqueous solution of furfural. Always have a little free furfural floating around to make sure of an excess. Continue treatment until all signs of the disease disappear. Then treat feet once a day for several weeks to prevent recurrence. Shoes and socks should also be treated with this solution to disinfect them.

Athlete's Foot Remedy

Gentian Violet	1 g.
Alcohol	100 cc.
Water	100 cc.

Stir until dissolved.

Bunion Remover

Salicylic Acid	6 g.
Lanolin	60 g.

Soak foot in hot water; cut off thick skin and apply twice a day.

Callous Skin Remover

Stearoricinol	40 g.
Diglycol Laurate	10 g.
Salicylic Acid	50 g.

Warm together until dissolved. Pour at lowest possible temperature. Apply to callous or hard skin and allow to remain overnight. Do not repeat treatment for seven days. Penetrates better than usual preparations for skin peeling. Do not use on tender skin.

Peeling Paste for Corns or Hard Skin

(Not to be put on normal skin, as it is irritating).

Formula No. 1

Lard	50 g.
Salicylic Acid	50 g.

Formula No. 2

Salicylic Acid	30 g.
Vaseline, White	70 g.

Formula No. 3

Mild-acting paste (stir warm):

a.	Rosin	8 g.	Melt
	Wax, Yellow	30 g.	Melt
	Larch Turpentine	12 g.	
	Vaseline, Yellow	16 g.	
b.	Salicylic Acid	8 g.	
	Anaesthesin	3 g.	
	Peanut Oil	14.5 g.	

Mix warm, stir until clear; cool while stirring; when thickening starts, add

Methyl Salicylate	0.5 g.
Peru Balsam	8 g.

Stir until cold.

Wart Removers

Formula No. 1

Green Soap	50 g.
Acetyl-Salicylic Acid	2.5 g.
Petrolatum, White	5 g.
Cocoa Butter	10 g.
Camphor	1 g.

To each 100 g. of the above add:
1 drop of Butyl Aldehyde.

It may be perfumed with oil of Eucalyptus or any other essential oil.

Formula No. 2

Cellulose Acetate	4 oz.
Acetone	70 oz.
Trichloracetic Acid	10 oz.

Boil Ointment

Ichthyol	15 g.
Lanolin	68 g.

Apply thickly on gauze and hold in place with adhesive.

Carbuncle Ointment

Ichthyol	25 g.
Lanolin	35 g.
Zinc Oxide Ointment	90 g.

Apply thickly daily.

Itching, Scaling, Skin Astringent

Salicylic Acid	12.5 gr.
Ethyl Amino Benzoate	1.0 gr.
Lanolin to make	1 oz.

Warm together and mix until dissolved.

Skin Disinfectant

Mercuric Chloride	.1 g.
Hydrochloric Acid	6.0 cc.
Distilled Water	30.0 cc.
Alcohol to make	100.0 cc.

Apply locally.

Fish Poisoning, Lotion for Skin

Mercurochrome	2 g.
Acetone	10 g.
Alcohol	35 g.
Distilled Water	53 g.

Fishery workers frequently suffer from skin or blood infections. To avoid this trouble workers should wash with water containing 2 per cent of "lysol." This is followed by a good soap washing; drying with clean towels and applying the above solution.

Skin Ointment

Formula No. 1

Amber Petrolatum	270 oz.
Amber Liquid Petrolatum	78 oz.
Paraffin Wax	16 oz.
Lanolin, Anhydrous	10 oz.
Zinc Oxide	12 oz.
Ethylamino Benzoate	8 oz.
Phenol	2 oz.
Thyme Oil	½ oz.
Thymol	¼ oz.
Eucalyptus Oil	½ oz.
Ichthyol	1 oz.

Mix oil, wax and fats together. Mix zinc oxide and ethyl aminobenzoate and sift through No. 100 mesh sieve. Then add to melted oil mixture. Stir until cooled to about 50° C. to prevent powder from settling. Mix phenol and thymol with essential oils and warm to effect solution. Add to ointment at 45°–50° and stir well. Grind Ichthyol with a few pounds of the ointment and mix with bulk of ointment while still warm. Finally pass through ointment mill.

Note: For special treatment of burns add 4 oz. Picric Acid.

For acute eczema and other inflammatory conditions of the skin add 4 oz. Resorcin.

Formula No. 2

Titanium Oxide	20 g.
Titanium Borate	5 g.
Titanium Salicylate	5 g.
Lanolin	70 g.

Danish Ointment

Sublimed Sulphur	125 g.
Potassium Hydroxide	125 g.
Distilled Water	125 cc.

Dissolve the potassium hydroxide in the water. Add the sulphur to this liquid, heating gently until dissolved. Incorporate this yellow liquid in a mixture of the following:

Petrolatum	225 g.
Wool Fat	225 g.

To the mixture so obtained add the following combination:

Zinc Sulphate	28 g.
Sodium Hydroxide	8 g.
Distilled Water	40 cc.
Liquid Petrolatum to make	1000 g.

Add the zinc sulphate to the solution of sodium hydroxide in water, producing zinc hydroxide.

Finally add sufficient liquid petrolatum to make the product weigh 1000 g. Add 5 cc. of benzaldehyde to mask the unpleasant odor.

Soothing Ointment

Menthol	1 g.
Phenyl Salicylate	5 g.
Lanolin	54 g.
White Mineral oil (65–75)	20 g.
Cetyl Alcohol	5 g.
White Beeswax	15 g.

Procedure: Melt the last four ingredients together with constant stirring. Add the menthol and phenyl salicylate and stir until semi-solid. Adjust consistency to suit by means of the beeswax.

Compound Ointment Base

Glycerin	10.0 cc.
Boric Acid	5.0 g.
Lavender Oil	0.5 cc.
Concentrated Carob Mucilage (4%) to make	100.0 g.

Antiseptic Ointment

Chlorthymol	1 g.
Benzoic Acid	1 g.
Salicylic Acid	1 g.
Coconut Oil	12 g.
Petrolatum	16 g.

Zinc Ointment

White Beeswax	60 g.
Spermaceti	60 g.
Sweet Almond Oil	300 g.
Digest 2 hours on water bath.	
Gum Benzoin, Siam	20 g.
Add while cooling.	
Zinc Oxide	100 g.
Boric Acid	2 g.
Carmine	enough to color

Perfume with extract of rose leaves.

Compound Benzoic Acid Ointment

Salicylic Acid	1 g.
Benzoic Acid	2 g.
Ointment of Rose Water	30 g.

Apply locally twice daily. Strength may be doubled, if necessary.

Chrysarobin Ointment

Chrysarobin	1.5 g.
Petrolatum	30 g.

Apply with care against getting it in the eyes.

Dermatologist's White Drying Salve

Make salve of:

Petrolatum, White	2 oz.
Zinc Oxide Ointment	2 oz.
Powdered Gum Camphor	2 oz.
Phenol Crystals	2 oz.
Mix this with a salve of:	
Corn Starch	4 oz.

with amount necessary of white petrolatum.

Dermatitis Ointment

Lanolin	100 parts
Phenyl Mercuric Nitrate (1–1500)	100 parts
Glycerin	10 parts

Dermatitis Lotion

"Lysol"	10.0 cc.
Castor Oil	4.0 cc.
Methyl Salicylate	2.5 cc.
Clove Oil	2.5 cc.
Alcohol to make	100.0 cc.

Acne Ointment

Sulphur, Precipitated	10 g.
Kaolin	10 g.
Ointment, Zinc Oxide to make	100 g.

Resorcin may be substituted for the Sulphur (in like amount)

Glycerin-Sulphur-Kaolin-Acne Paste

Kaolin	10 g.
Sulphur, Colloidal	7.5 g.
Glycerin (24%)	to pasty consistency

Acne Face Lotion

Formula No. 1

Acetic Acid (96%) or Benzoic Acid	5 g.
Alcohol	500 g.
Lavender Oil	4 g.
Water	466 g.
Glycerin	25 g.

Let stand several weeks. Filter.

Formula No. 2

Potassium Soap from Olive Oil (Neutralized)	100 g.
Alcohol (90%)	500 g.
Lavender Oil	5 g.
Rose Oil, Artificial	5 g.
Water	390 g.

Formula No. 3

Triethanolamine	10.0 g.
Stearin	22.0 g.
Petroleum Jelly	3.0 g.

Preparations for Scabies

Ointment

Potassium Sulphide	50 oz.
Water	250 oz.
Petrolatum	250 oz.

Lanolin	250 oz.
Titanium Dioxide	5 oz.
Mineral Oil	200 oz.
Perfume to suit.	

Procedure: Dissolve the potassium in the water. Take part of the petrolatum and mill in the titanium. Melt the rest of the petrolatum, the lanolin and the mineral oil and add the potassium solution. Then add the titanium mass. Mix thoroughly and mill again.

Eczema Preparations

Ointments

Formula No. 1

Lanolin	200 oz.
Petrolatum	200 oz.
Beeswax	50 oz.
Phenol	5 oz.
Camphor	10 oz.
Eucalyptus Oil	50 oz.
Salicylic Acid	10 oz.
Perfume to suit.	—
	525 oz.

Formula No. 2

Ichthyol	10.0 g.
Salicylic Acid	3.0 g.
Petrolatum	to make 100.0 g.

Formula No. 3

Icthyol	10 g.
Starch	25 g.
Zinc Oxide	25 g.
Petrolatum	to make 100 g.

Psoriasis Ointment

Formula No. 1

Cade Oil	10 cc.
Salicylic Acid	3 g.
Petrolatum	to make 100 g.

Formula No. 2

Chrysarobin	3 oz.
Salicylic Acid	1 oz.
Rectified Pine Tar Oil	10 oz.
Soft Soap	15 oz.
Petrolatum	28 oz.
Absorption Base (Parachol)	5 oz.
Perfume	to suit

Procedure: Mill the salicylic and the chrysarobin with a part of the petrolatum. Melt the rest of the petrolatum and the absorption base, add the soap, the pine tar and the chrysarobin-salicylic mass and mix thoroughly.

Formula No. 3

Salicylic Acid	10 g.
Cade Oil	25 cc.
Soft Soap	25 g.
Alcohol	to make 100 cc.

Paint over patches, permit to dry, and wash off excess in bath.

Formula No. 4

Salicylic Acid	10 g.
Chrysarobin	20 cc.
Cade Oil	20 cc.
Soft Soap	25 g.
Petrolatum	25 g.

Label: Apply to patches.

Psoriasis Lotion

Picis Pini	170 g.
Liquor Picis Carbonis	690 g.
Olive Oil	190 g.
Bitumen Sulphonatum	60 g.
Bismuth Subnitrate	175 g.
Water enough to make	3785 g.

Rub the pine tar with the liquor picis carbonis and then slowly work in the olive oil. Rub up the bitumen sulphonatum with some of the water, add the bismuth subnitrate to this mixture and incorporate this aqueous mixture with the first mix above. Triturate well till thoroughly mixed and bring up to required amount with additional water.

Sulphur Ointment

Precipitated Sulphur	1.5 g.
Petrolatum	30 g.

Rub in gently once or twice daily. Strength may gradually be increased up to 20 per cent.

Chapped Skin Ointment

Phenyl Salicylate	8 g.
Menthol	4 g.
Olive Oil	40 cc.
Lanolin	125 g.

Warm together and mix until dissolved.

Jelly-Fish Sting Ointment

Lanolin	1 dr.
Paraffin Ointment	3 dr.
Almond Oil	4 fl. dr.
Lime Water	1 oz.

Strong Solution of Lead Subacetate	½ oz.
Clove oil	5 min.

Burn Ointment

Formula No. 1

Liquid Petrolatum	5 oz.
Snow White Petrolatum	5 oz.
Lanolin	¾ oz.
White Wax	¾ oz.
Spermaceti	¼ oz.
Sodium Borate	1/10 oz.
Ethylamino Benzoate	⅕ oz.
Distilled Water	to make 1 lb.
Perfume	to suit

Formula No. 2

Tannic Acid	2 g.
Ichthyol	33 g.
Lanolin	62 g.

Burn Dressing

Tannic Acid	5.0 g.
Chlorbutanol	0.2 g.
Distilled Water	to make 100.0 cc.

Dose: Use as wet dressing, or as spray.

Modern Burn Treatment

Remove the burned tissue, and apply, first a 5 per cent solution of tannic acid, and then, immediately, a 10 per cent solution of silver nitrate. This forms, almost instantly, a black, leather-like, antiseptic, protective dressing. This is dried quickly and kept dry. No other dressing is applied.

Greaseless Burn Jelly

Five per cent tragacanth jelly preserved by the addition of 1:500 salicylic acid can be medicated with 5 per cent tannic acid. While the salicylic acid would be stainless, the tannic acid might darken the hair temporarily.

Nasal Balm Ointment

Boric Acid	30 gr.
Menthol	1½ gr.
Sodium Chloride	5 gr.
Eucalyptus Oil	1 min.
Ethyl Amino Benzoate	10 gr.
Parachol (Absorption Base)	1 oz.

Cod Liver Oil Healing Salve

Cod Liver Oil	100 cc.
Petrolatum	100 g.
Vitamin Concentrate	1½ g.
Japan Wax	10 g.

Warm together and mix

The above is useful for

Fresh superficial wounds, older wounds which have started to fester, chronic ulcers, burns, frostbite, severe injuries to the extremities, and healing of open stumps of arms and legs after amputations.

Poison Ivy Treatment and Preventative

A very good remedy, not as well known as it deserves to be, is a five per cent. solution of potassium permanganate in water. Puncture all blisters, and swab up their watery contents with absorbent cotton or sterile gauze. Then thoroughly moisten all poisoned skin areas with the solution. It will turn the skin brown, but this can be cleaned up after a time with lemon juice.

A highly successful preventive treatment is a five per cent. solution of ferrous sulphate in a half-and-half mixture of water and alcohol, with a little glycerin added. Wash this solution on all exposed parts of the skin, before going into the woods. Do not rinse or dry the skin; let the solution dry in place. The iron in the compound unites with the poison and renders it insoluble and harmless. This "iron treatment" has been used by thousands of persons, and has given complete protection to all except a very few unlucky extreme-susceptibles.

Analgesic Balm

Menthol	5 oz.
Methyl Salicylate	10 oz.
Hydrous Wool Fat	75 oz.
White Petrolatum	10 oz.

Camphor Ice

Camphor ice contains from 10 to 25 per cent. of camphor, which is added to the melted fats when they have cooled. It is then poured into molds and the blocks wrapped in tinfoil.

Camphor Flowers	150 g.
Ceresin, White	50 g.
Hard Paraffin Wax	250 g.
Soft Paraffin Wax, White	550 g.

Arthritis Ointment

Ichthyol	20 g.
Lanolin	30 g.

Apply freely to joint and cover with bandage.

Witch Hazel Jelly

Boric Acid	1 oz.
Tragacanth	2 oz.
Witch Hazel	1 gal.

Zinc Oxide-Vaseline

Yellow Vaseline	50 g.
Zinc Oxide	5 g.

Methyleugenol Antiseptic Lotion

Methyleugenol	4 fl. oz.
Alcoholic Soap	14 fl. oz.
Distilled Water	20 fl. oz.

Two teaspoonfuls diluted to a pint may be used as a soluble antiseptic lotion.

Stainless Iodine Solution

Resublimed Iodine	4 g.
Potassium Iodide	10 g.
Hyposulphite of Soda	10 g.
Alcohol, Anhydrous	200 cc.

Non-Irritating Iodine Antiseptic

Iodine	2 g.
Potassium Iodide	2.4 g.
Alcohol	55 g.
Water	45 g.

Mercurochrome Antiseptic

"Mercurochrome"	4.0 g.
Acetone	10.0 cc.
Alcohol	50.0 cc.
Distilled Water to make	100.0 cc.

Counter Irritant, Extra Strong

Menthol	2 g.
Volatile Oil of Mustard	2 cc.
Alcohol	50 cc.

Apply a few drops to affected area. (Must not be used in the vicinity of the eyes.)

Smelling Salts

Formula No. 1

If a solid smelling salt is desired, a successful product is obtained by combining 47 g. of potassium carbonate granular, 10 g. of ammonium carbonate granular, 38 g. of ammonium chloride, 4½ g. of camphor powder and perfume to make 100 g.

Formula No. 2

If a liquid smelling salt is required, cubes are made of ammonium carbonate or potassium sulphate and a mixture is added consisting of 4 g. of ammonia water, 90 g. of alcohol, 1 g. of perfume and 5 g. of water.

Formula No. 3

Phenol	1 g.
Menthol	1 g.
Camphor	2 g.
Weak Solution of Iodine (2.5%)	1 g.
Pumilio Pine Oil	1 g.
Eucalyptus Oil	1 g.
Strong Solution of Ammonia	3 g.
Ammonium Carbonate	90 cc.

The ammonium carbonate should be packed into the bottle, the strong solution of ammonia added, then the other ingredients, previously mixed. Sodium sesquicarbonate is sometimes substituted for ammonium carbonate.

Hiccough Remedy

Take one teaspoonful of tincture of castoreum and repeat in a half hour if needed.

Solidified "Hydrogen Peroxide"

Hydrogen Peroxide (30%)	114 g.
Urea	60 g.

Mix together until dissolved and evaporate by stirring at room temperature without heating.

Hydrogen Peroxide Preservative

Formula No. 1

The addition of 20 g. phenacetin to 5 kg. hydrogen peroxide acts as a good preservative.

Formula No. 2

According to French chemists the best preservative for hydrogen peroxide solution is phenetidine lactate in the proportion of 0.5 g. per liter of solution. Less effective are glucose, gelatin (0.2

g. per liter); ethyl alcohol (16 g. per liter); and hippuric acid (0.2%).

Formula No. 3

The addition of 0.1% barbituric acid stabilizes hydrogen peroxide solutions.

Formula No. 4

Canadian Patent 337,601

A hydrogen peroxide solution is stabilized by adjusting the acidity to pH 2–6 and adding an amount of sodium stannite equivalent to 5–100 milligrams of tin per liter of solution and 0.01–0.2 grams of sodium pyrophosphate per liter of solution.

Formula No. 5

Tests run for some time show that amounts as small as 0.15% of methyl para-oxybenzoate will preserve peroxide solutions. Controls showed a loss of almost 15 times more than those so preserved. This is indeed a help in the formulation of peroxide lotions for bleaching, etc.

Removing Tattoo Marks

The following procedure for the removal of tattoo marks has been used with excellent results; however, in view of the possibility of complications, the method should only be applied under the direction of a medical practitioner. The skin surrounding the tattoo marks is covered with a thick layer of zinc paste. A piece of cambric, the size of the tattooed region, spread with the following recently prepared cream.

Formula No. 1

Pyrogallic Acid	7 g.
Salicylic Acid	7 g.
Resorcin	7 g.
Glycerin	5 g.
Alcohol (70%)	5 g.
Tragacanth	1 g.

is applied in such a way that its edge rests on the layer of zinc paste. The whole is covered with a few layers of gauze and held in place by means of an elastoplast bandage. Care must be taken to ensure that the coated piece of Billroth's cambric does not slip. After twenty-four hours the bandage is taken off, whereupon the epidermis may be easily removed. Another application as described above is then made, which is allowed to remain in place for forty-eight hours, at the end of which, in most instances, the whole of the tattooed area will be found to have become necrotic. This is treated by the daily application of Desitin paste dressings until healthy granulation occurs. In view of the painful nature of this treatment it is advisable to confine the application of the caustic cream to small areas at a time.

Formula No. 2

Pepsin and papain have been proposed as applications to remove the epidermis. A glycerol solution of either is tattooed into the skin over the disfigured part; and it is said that the operation has proved successful. Papain, 5; water, 25; glycerol, 75; diluted hydrochloric acid, 1. Rub the papain with the water and hydrochloric acid, allow the mixture to stand for an hour, add the glycerin, let it stand for three hours and filter.

Formula No. 3

Apply a highly concentrated tannin solution to the tattooed places and treat them with a tattooing needle as the tattooer does. Next vigorously rub the places with a lunar caustic stick and allow the silver nitrate to act for some time until the tattooed portions have turned entirely black. Then take off by dabbing. At first a silver tannate forms on the upper layers of the skin, which dyes the tattooing black; with slight symptoms of inflammation a scurf ensues, which comes off after fourteen or sixteen days leaving behind a reddish scar. The latter assumes the natural color of the skin after some time. The process is said to have good results.

Obviously such treatments are heroic and carry along with them the risk of permanent scarring. It is therefore a job for a trained dermatologist rather than for a layman.

Formula No. 4

First the skin is vigorously rubbed until the outer epidermis comes off; then a paste of quicklime, just slacked, to which pulverized phosphorus (two tablespoonfuls to a pint) is added and thoroughly mixed, is applied to the tattooed surface and held by a bandage, which is taken off two days later. The crust is left to dry and then fall off itself; in about fifteen days. A second application should be made; a third is rarely necessary. Thus treated, the tattooing disappears completely without the least scar.

Cacao Butter Substitute

Hydrogenated Oil (m.p. 35.5° C.)	96 g.
Yellow Beeswax	2 g.
Anhydrous Lanolin	2 g.

Warm together and stir until uniform. This product melts at 38–39° C.

COLORING

The coloring of cosmetic and allied products is usually done with aniline dyes. They must be selected judiciously or they will fade or change color because of interaction with certain chemicals present in the formula. Information as to stability should be gotten from the sellers of the dye.

Popular dyes for coloring are given below. Mixtures, of course, can be made to get other tints. Three types of colors are used. The first type is called water-soluble as it dissolves in water; the second, alcohol or spirit soluble as it dissolves in alcohol; the third type, oil soluble as it dissolves in oils and melted fats or waxes.

Water Soluble Dyes

Yellow	Auramine O
Rose	Rhodamine B
Purple	Pylam Purple
Peacock Blue	Patent Blue
Green	Pylam Brilliant Green
Pink	Eosin
Cerise	Rose Bengale

Alcohol Soluble Dyes

Pink	Rhodamine B
Red	Safranine Y
Blue	Methylene Blue ZF
Violet	Methyl Violet
Green	Malachite Green
Yellow	Auramine
Black	Nigrosine
Orange	Chrysoidine
Brown	Bismark Brown

Oil Soluble Dyes

Red	Azo Oil Red
Yellow	Azo Oil Yellow
Orange	Azo Oil Orange
Black	Oil Black
Blue	Alizarin Oil Blue
Violet	Alizarin Oil Violet
Green	Oil Green

When using dyes to color preparations always dissolve them first and determine by trial the amount of the solution needed to get the right tint.

TABLES

Weights and Measures

Troy Weight

24 grains = 1 pwt.
20 pwts. = 1 ounce
12 ounces = 1 pound

Apothecaries' Weight

20 grains = 1 scruple
3 scruples = 1 dram
8 drams = 1 ounce
12 ounces = 1 pound

The ounce and pound are the same as in Troy Weight.

Avoirdupois Weight

27 11/32 grains = 1 dram
16 drams = 1 ounce
16 ounces = 1 pound
2000 lbs. = 1 short ton
2240 lbs. = 1 long ton

Dry Measure

2 pints = 1 quart
8 quarts = 1 peck
4 pecks = 1 bushel
36 bushels = 1 chaldron

Liquid Measure

4 gills = 1 pint
2 pints = 1 quart
4 quarts = 1 gallon
31½ gals. = 1 barrel
2 barrels = 1 hogshead
1 teaspoonful = ⅙ oz.
1 tablespoonful = ½ oz.
16 fluid oz. = 1 pint

Circular Measure

60 seconds = 1 minute
60 minutes = 1 degree
360 degrees = 1 circle

Long Measure

12 inches = 1 foot
3 feet = 1 yard
5½ yards = 1 rod
5280 feet = 1 stat. mile
320 rods = 1 stat. mile

Square Measure

144 sq. in. = 1 sq. ft.
9 sq. ft. = 1 sq. yard
30¼ sq. yds. = 1 sq. rod
43,560 sq. ft. = 1 acre
40 sq. rods = 1 rood
4 roods = 1 acre
640 acres = 1 sq. mile

Metric Equivalents

Length

1 inch = 2.54 centimeters
1 foot = 0.305 meter
1 yard = 0.914 meter
1 mile = 1.609 kilometers
1 centimeter = 0.394 in.
1 meter = 3.281 ft.
1 meter = 1.094 yd.
1 kilometer = 0.621 mile

Capacity

1 U. S. fluid oz. = 29.573 milliliters
1 U. S. liquid qt. = 0.946 liter
1 U. S. dry qt. = 1.101 liters
1 U. S. gallon = 3.785 liters
1 U. S. bushel = 0.3524 hectoliter
1 cu. in. = 16.4 cu. centimeters
1 milliliter = 0.034 U. S. fluid ounce
1 liter = 1.057 U. S. liquid qt.
1 liter = 0.908 U. S. dry qt.
1 liter = 0.264 U. S. gallon
1 hectoliter = 2.838 U. S. bu.
1 cu. centimeter = .061 cu. in.
1 liter = 1000 milliliters or 100 cu. c.

Weight

1 grain = 0.065 gram
1 apoth. scruple = 1.296 grams
1 av. oz. = 28.350 grams
1 troy oz. = 31.103 grams
1 av. lb. = 0.454 kilogram
1 troy lb. = 0.373 kilogram
1 gram = 15.432 grains
1 gram = 0.772 apoth. scruple
1 gram = 0.035 av. oz.
1 gram = 0.032 troy oz.
1 kilogram = 2.205 av. lbs.
1 kilogram = 2.679 troy lbs.

Approximate pH Values

The following tables give approximate pH values for a number of substances such as acids, bases, foods, biological fluids, etc. All values are rounded off to the nearest tenth and are based on measurements made at 25° C.

pH Values of Acids

Hydrochloric, N	0.1
Hydrochloric, 0.1N	1.1
Hydrochloric, 0.01N	2.0
Sulphuric, N	0.3
Sulphuric, 0.1N	1.2
Sulphuric, 0.01N	2.1
Orthophosphoric, 0.1N	1.5
Sulphurous, 0.1N	1.5
Oxalic, 0.1N	1.6
Tartaric, 0.1N	2.2
Malic, 0.1N	2.2
Citric, 0.1N	2.2
Formic, 0.1N	2.3
Lactic, 0.1N	2.4
Acetic, N	2.4
Acetic, 0.1N	2.9
Acetic, 0.01N	3.4
Benzoic, 0.1N	3.1
Alum, 0.1N	3.2
Carbonic (saturated)	3.8
Hydrogen Sulphide, 0.1N	4.1
Arsenious (saturated)	5.0
Hydrocyanic, 0.1N	5.1
Boric, 0.1N	5.2

pH Values of Bases

Sodium Hydroxide, N	14.0
Sodium Hydroxide, 0.1N	13.0
Sodium Hydroxide, 0.01N	12.0
Potassium Hydroxide, N	14.0
Potassium Hydroxide, 0.1N	13.0
Potassium Hydroxide, 0.01N	12.0
Lime (saturated)	12.4
Sodium Metasilicate, 0.1N	12.6
Trisodium Phosphate, 0.1N	12.0
Sodium Carbonate, 0.1N	11.6
Ammonia, N	11.6
Ammonia, 0.1N	11.1
Ammonia, 0.01N	10.6
Potassium Cyanide, 0.1N	11.0
Magnesia (saturated)	10.5
Sodium Sesquicarbonate, 0.1N	10.1
Ferrous Hydroxide (saturated)	9.5
Calcium Carbonate (saturated)	9.4
Borax, 0.1N	9.2
Sodium Bicarbonate, 0.1N	8.4

pH Values of Foods

Apples	2.9–3.3
Apricots	3.6–4.0
Asparagus	5.4–5.8
Bananas	4.5–4.7
Beans	5.0–6.0
Beers	4.0–5.0
Beets	4.9–5.5
Blackberries	3.2–3.6
Bread, white	5.0–6.0
Butter	6.1–6.4
Cabbage	5.2–5.4
Carrots	4.9–5.3
Cheese	4.8–6.4
Cherries	3.2–4.0
Cider	2.9–3.3
Corn	6.0–6.5
Crackers	6.5–8.5
Dates	6.2–6.4
Eggs, fresh white	7.6–8.0
Flour, wheat	5.5–6.5
Gooseberries	2.8–3.0
Grapefruit	3.0–3.3
Grapes	3.5–4.5
Hominy (rye)	6.8–8.0
Jams, fruit	3.5–4.0
Jellies, fruit	2.8–3.4
Lemons	2.2–2.4
Limes	1.8–2.0
Maple Syrup	6.5–7.0
Milk, cows	6.3–6.6
Olives	3.6–3.8
Oranges	3.0–4.0
Oysters	6.1–6.6
Peaches	3.4–3.6
Pears	3.6–4.0
Peas	5.8–6.4
Pickles, dill	3.2–3.6
Pickles, sour	3.0–3.4
Pimento	4.6–5.2
Plums	2.8–3.0
Potatoes	5.6–6.0
Pumpkin	4.8–5.2
Raspberries	3.2–3.6
Rhubarb	3.1–3.2
Salmon	6.1–6.3
Sauerkraut	3.4–3.6
Shrimp	6.8–7.0
Soft Drinks	2.0–4.0
Spinach	5.1–5.7
Squash	5.0–5.4
Strawberries	3.0–3.5
Sweet Potatoes	5.3–5.6
Tomatoes	4.0–4.4
Tuna	5.9–6.1
Turnips	5.2–5.6
Vinegar	2.4–3.4
Water, drinking	6.5–8.0
Wines	2.8–3.8

pH Values of Biologic Materials

Blood, plasma, human	7.3–7.5
Spinal Fluid, human	7.3–7.5
Blood, whole, dog	6.9–7.2
Saliva, human	6.5–7.5
Gastric Contents, human	1.0–3.0
Duodenal Contents, human	4.8–8.2
Feces, human	4.6–8.4
Urine, human	4.8–8.4
Milk, human	6.6–7.6
Bile, human	6.8–7.0

CONVERSION OF THERMOMETER READINGS

F°	C°	F°	C°	F°	C°	F°	C°	F°	C°	F°	C°
—40	—40.00	30	—1.11	80	26.67	250	121.11	500	260.00	900	482.22
—38	—38.89	31	—0.56	81	27.22	255	123.89	505	262.78	910	487.78
—36	—37.78	32	0.00	82	27.78	260	126.67	510	265.56	920	493.33
—34	—36.67	33	0.56	83	28.33	265	129.44	515	268.33	930	498.89
—32	—35.56	34	1.11	84	28.89	270	132.22	520	271.11	940	504.44
—30	—34.44	35	1.67	85	29.44	275	135.00	525	273.89	950	510.00
—28	—33.33	36	2.22	86	30.00	280	137.78	530	276.67	960	515.56
—26	—32.22	37	2.78	87	30.56	285	140.55	535	279.44	970	521.11
—24	—31.11	38	3.33	88	31.11	290	143.33	540	282.22	980	526.67
—22	—30.00	39	3.89	89	31.67	295	146.11	545	285.00	990	532.22
—20	—28.89	40	4.44	90	32.22	300	148.89	550	287.78	1000	537.78
—18	—27.78	41	5.00	91	32.78	305	151.67	555	290.55	1050	565.56
—16	—26.67	42	5.56	92	33.33	310	154.44	560	293.33	1100	593.33
—14	—25.56	43	6.11	93	33.89	315	157.22	565	296.11	1150	621.11
—12	—24.44	44	6.67	94	39.44	320	160.00	570	298.89	1200	648.89
—10	—23.33	45	7.22	95	35.00	325	162.78	575	301.67	1250	676.67
— 8	—22.22	46	7.78	96	35.56	330	165.56	580	304.44	1300	704.44
— 6	—21.11	47	8.33	97	36.11	335	168.33	585	307.22	1350	732.22
— 4	—20.00	48	8.89	98	36.67	340	171.11	590	310.00	1400	760.00
— 2	—18.89	49	9.44	99	37.22	345	173.89	595	312.78	1450	787.78
0	—17.78	50	10.00	100	37.78	350	176.67	600	315.56	1500	815.56
1	—17.22	51	10.56	105	40.55	355	179.44	610	321.11	1550	843.33
2	—16.67	52	11.11	110	43.33	360	182.22	620	326.67	1600	871.11
3	—16.11	53	11.67	115	46.11	365	185.00	630	332.22	1650	898.89
4	—15.56	54	12.22	120	48.89	370	187.78	640	337.78	1700	926.67
5	—15.00	55	12.78	125	51.67	375	190.55	650	343.33	1750	954.44
6	—14.44	56	13.33	130	54.44	380	193.33	660	348.89	1800	982.22
7	—13.89	57	13.89	135	57.22	385	196.11	670	354.44	1850	1010.00
8	—13.33	58	14.44	140	60.00	390	198.89	680	360.00	1900	1037.78
9	—12.78	59	15.00	145	62.78	395	201.67	690	365.56	1950	1065.56
10	—12.22	60	15.56	150	65.56	400	204.44	700	371.11	2000	1093.33
11	—11.67	61	16.11	155	68.33	405	207.22	710	376.67	2050	1121.11
12	—11.11	62	16.67	160	71.11	410	210.00	720	382.22	2100	1148.89
13	—10.56	63	17.22	165	73.89	415	212.78	730	387.78	2150	1176.67
14	—10.00	64	17.78	170	76.67	420	215.56	740	393.33	2200	1204.44
15	— 9.44	65	18.33	175	79.44	425	218.33	750	398.89	2250	1232.22
16	— 8.89	66	18.89	180	82.22	430	221.11	760	404.44	2300	1260.00
17	— 8.33	67	19.44	185	85.00	435	223.89	770	410.00	2350	1287.78
18	— 7.78	68	20.00	190	87.78	440	226.67	780	415.56	2400	1315.56
19	— 7.22	69	20.56	195	90.55	445	229.44	790	421.11	2450	1343.33
20	— 6.67	70	21.11	200	93.33	450	232.22	800	426.67	2500	1371.11
21	— 6.11	71	21.67	205	96.11	455	235.00	810	432.22	2550	1398.89
22	— 5.56	72	22.22	210	98.89	460	237.78	820	437.78	2600	1426.67
23	— 5.00	73	22.78	215	101.67	465	240.55	830	443.33	2650	1454.44
24	— 4.44	74	23.33	220	104.44	470	243.33	840	448.89	2700	1482.22
25	— 3.89	75	23.89	225	107.22	475	246.11	850	454.44	2750	1510.00
26	— 3.33	76	24.44	230	110.00	480	248.89	860	460.00	2800	1537.78
27	— 2.78	77	25.00	235	112.78	485	251.67	870	465.56	2850	1565.56
28	— 2.22	78	25.56	240	115.56	490	254.44	880	471.11	2900	1593.33
29	— 1.67	79	26.11	245	118.33	495	257.22	890	476.67	2950	1621.11

ALCOHOL PROOF AND PERCENTAGE TABLE

U. S. Proof at 60° F.	*Per Cent Alcohol by Volume at 60° F.*	*Per Cent Alcohol by weight*
0	0.0	0.00
1	0.5	—
2	1.0	0.80
3	1.5	—
4	2.0	1.59
5	2.5	—
6	3.0	2.39
7	3.5	—
8	4.0	3.19
9	4.5	—
10	5.0	4.00
11	5.5	—
12	6.0	4.80
13	6.5	—
14	7.0	5.61
15	7.5	—
16	8.0	6.42
17	8.5	—
18	9.0	7.23
19	9.5	—
20	10.0	8.05
21	10.5	—
22	11.0	8.86
23	11.5	—
24	12.0	9.68
25	12.5	—
26	13.0	10.50
27	13.5	—
28	14.0	11.32
29	14.5	—
30	15.0	12.14
31	15.5	—
32	16.0	12.96
33	16.5	—
34	17.0	13.79
35	17.5	—
36	18.0	14.61
37	18.5	—
38	19.0	15.44
39	19.5	—
40	20.0	16.27
41	20.5	—
42	21.0	17.10
43	21.5	—
44	22.0	17.93
45	22.5	—
46	23.0	18.77
47	23.5	—
48	24.0	19.60
49	24.5	—
50	25.0	20.44
51	25.5	—
52	26.0	21.28
53	26.5	—
54	27.0	22.13
55	27.5	—
56	28.0	22.97
57	28.5	—
58	29.0	23.82
59	29.5	—
60	30.0	24.67
61	30.5	—
62	31.0	25.52
63	31.5	—
64	32.0	26.38
65	32.5	—
66	33.0	27.24
67	33.5	—
68	34.0	28.10
69	34.5	—
70	35.0	28.97
71	35.5	—
72	36.0	29.84
73	36.5	—
74	37.0	30.72
75	37.5	—
76	38.0	31.60
77	38.5	—
78	39.0	32.48
79	39.5	—
80	40.0	33.36
81	40.5	—
82	41.0	34.25
83	41.5	—
84	42.0	35.15
85	42.5	—
86	43.0	36.05
87	43.5	—
88	44.0	36.96
89	44.5	—
90	45.0	37.86
91	45.5	—
92	46.0	38.78
93	46.5	—
94	47.0	39.70
95	47.5	—
96	48.0	40.62
97	48.5	—
98	49.0	41.55
99	49.5	—
100	50.0	42.49
101	50.5	—
102	51.0	43.43
103	51.5	—
104	52.0	44.37
105	52.5	—
106	53.0	45.33
107	53.5	—
108	54.0	46.28
109	54.5	—
110	55.0	47.24
111	55.5	—
112	56.0	48.21
113	56.5	—
114	57.0	49.19
115	57.5	—

U. S. Proof at 60° F.	*Per Cent Alcohol by Volume at 60° F.*	*Per Cent Alcohol by weight*
116	58.0	50.17
117	58.5	——
118	59.0	51.15
119	59.5	——
120	60.0	52.15
121	60.5	——
122	61.0	53.15
123	61.5	——
124	62.0	54.15
125	62.5	——
126	63.0	55.16
127	63.5	——
128	64.0	56.18
129	64.5	——
130	65.0	57.21
131	65.5	——
132	66.0	58.24
133	66.5	——
134	67.0	59.28
135	67.5	——
136	68.0	60.32
137	68.5	——
138	69.0	61.38
139	69.5	——
140	70.0	62.44
141	70.5	——
142	71.0	63.51
143	71.5	——
144	72.0	64.59
145	72.5	——
146	73.0	65.67
147	73.5	——
148	74.0	66.77
149	74.5	——
150	75.0	67.87
151	75.5	——
152	76.0	68.92
153	76.5	——
154	77.0	70.10
155	77.5	——
156	78.0	71.23
157	78.5	——
158	79.0	72.38
159	79.5	——
160	80.0	73.53
161	80.5	——
162	81.0	74.69
163	81.5	——
164	82.0	75.86
165	82.5	——
166	83.0	77.04
167	83.5	——
168	84.0	78.23
169	84.5	——
170	85.0	79.44
171	85.5	——
172	86.0	80.62
173	86.5	——
174	87.0	81.90
175	87.5	——
176	88.0	83.14
177	88.5	——
178	89.0	84.41
179	89.5	——
180	90.0	85.69
181	90.5	——
182	91.0	86.99
183	91.5	——
184	92.0	88.31
185	92.5	——
186	93.0	89.65
187	93.5	——
188	94.0	91.02
189	94.5	——
190	95.0	92.42
191	95.5	——
192	96.0	93.85
193	96.5	——
194	97.0	95.32
195	97.5	——
196	98.0	96.82
197	98.5	——
198	99.0	98.38
199	99.5	——
200	100.0	100.00

Buffer Systems

The following table gives some common buffer systems and the approximate pH of maximum buffer capacity. The zone of effective buffer action will vary with concentration but the general average will be ± 1.0 pH from the value given, for concentrations approximately 0.1 molar.

Buffer system	pH
Glycocoll - Sodium Chloride - Hydrochloric Acid	2.0
Potassium Acid Phthalate-Hydrochloric Acid	2.8
Primary Potassium Citrate	3.7
Acetic Acid-Sodium Acetate	4.6
Potassium Acid Phthalate-Sodium Hydroxide	5.0
Secondary Sodium Citrate	5.0
Carbonic Acid-Bicarbonate	6.5
Primary Phosphate-Secondary Phosphate	6.8
Primary Phosphate-Sodium Hydroxide	6.8
Boric Acid-Borax	8.5
Borax	9.2
Boric Acid-Sodium Hydroxide	9.2
Bicarbonate-Carbonate	10.2
Secondary Phosphate-Sodium Hydroxide	11.5

Courtesy of W. A. Taylor & Company

COMMON NAMES OF CHEMICAL PRODUCTS

A

Common Name	Chemical Name
Acacia Gum	Gum Arabic
Acetate of Lime	Calcium Acetate
Acetic Ether	Ethyl Acetate
Acetin	Glyceryl Monoacetate
Acetyl Salicylic Acid	Aspirin
Acetylene Tetrachloride	Tetrachlorethane
Adeps Lanae	Lanolin
Alcohol	Ethyl Alcohol
Alumina	Aluminum Oxide
Aluminum Potassium Sulphate	Alum
Ammonia, Aqua	Ammonium Hydroxide
Aniline	Aniline Oil
Animal Charcoal	Bone Black
Aqua fortis	Nitric Acid
Argols	Crude Cream of Tartar
Arsenic, red	Arsenic Disulphide
Asphaltum	Mineral Pitch

B

Common Name	Chemical Name
Baking Soda	Sodium Bicarbonate
Banana Oil	Amyl Acetate
Barytes	Barium Sulphate, Natural
Benzene	Benzol
Benzine	Petroleum
Black Boy Gum	Accroides Gum
Black Lead	Graphite
Blanc Fixe	Barium Sulphate, Artificial
Bleaching Powder	Calcium Hypochlorite
Blue Stone Blue Vitriol	Copper Sulphate
Boiled Oil	Boiled Linseed Oil
Bone Black	Animal Charcoal
Boracic Acid	Boric Acid
Borax	Sodium Borate
Brazil Wax	Carnauba Wax
Brimstone	Sulphur
British Gum	Dextrin
Bromo "Acid"	Tetrabrom Fluorescein
Burnt Sugar Coloring	Caramel Color
Butanol	Butyl Alcohol
Butter Color	Annatto
Butter of Antimony	Antimony Chloride
Butyric Ether	Ethyl Butyrate

C

Common Name	Chemical Name
Calcium Phosphate, Acid	Calcium Phosphate, Monobasic
Calomel	Mercurous Chloride
Caoutchouc	India Rubber
Capsicum	Red Pepper

Carbolic Acid	Phenol
Carragheen	Irish Moss
Catechu	Cutch
Caustic Potash	Potassium Hydroxide
Caustic Soda	Sodium Hydroxide
Ceresin Wax	Ozokerite and Paraffin Mixture
Chalk	Calcium Carbonate
China Clay	Kaolin
China Wood Oil	Tung Oil
Chinese Wax	Insect Wax
Chloride of Lime	Calcium Hypochlorite
Cholestrin	Cholesterol
Chrome Green	Chromium Oxide
Cinnabar	Mercuric Sulphide
Citronella Oil	Verbena Oil
Cognac Oil	Oenanthic Ether
Colloidal Clay	Bentonite
Collodion	Nitrocellulose "solution"
Cologne Spirits	Ethyl Alcohol (pure)
Colophony	Rosin Pine Resin
Columbian Spirits	Methyl Alcohol (pure)
Colza Oil	Rape Seed Oil
Copper Aceto Arsenite	Paris Green
Copper Arsenite	Scheele's Green
Corn Sugar	Dextrose
Corn Syrup	Glucose
Corrosive Sublimate	Mercuric Chloride
Corumdum	Aluminum Oxide
Cream of Tartar	Potassium Bitartrate
Cresol	Cresylic Acid
Crude Oil	Petroleum (crude)
Cyanamid	Calcium Cyanamide

D

Dead Oil	Creosote Oil
Decalin	Decahydronaphthalene
Degras	Wool Grease
Dope	Pyroxylin "solution"
Dutch Liquid	Ethylene Chloride

E

Earth, Infusorial	Earth, Diatomaceous
Egg Oil	Egg Yolk
Elaterite	Mineral Rubber
Epsom Salts	Magnesium Sulphate
Ether	Ethyl Ether
Ethyl Nitrite	Nitrous Ether

F

Fir, Balsam	Canada Balsam
Flaxseed	Linseed
Flea-seed	Psyllium
Fluorspar	Calcium Fluoride
Fool's Gold	Iron Pyrites
Formalin	Formaldehyde (40% solution)
French Chalk	Talc
Fuchsine	Magenta
Fusel Oil	Amyl Alcohol (fermentation amyl alcohol)

G

Galena.............................Lead Sulphide
Glance Pitch.......................Manjak
Glass, Water.......................Sodium Silicate
Glauber's Salt.....................Sodium Sulphate
Glycerin...........................Glycerol
Glycol.............................Ethylene Glycol
Graphite...........................Plumbago
Green Soap.........................Soft Soap
Green Vitriol......................Ferrous Sulphate
Ground Nut Oil (Arachi's Oil)..........Peanut oil
Gum Lac............................Shellac
Gun Cotton.........................Nitro-Cellulose
Gypsum.............................Calcium Sulphate

H

Heavy Spar.........................Barium Sulphate
Hematite...........................Iron Oxide
Hexamine...........................Hexamethylenetetramine
Hydrochloric Acid ....Muriatic acid
Hydrosylphite (hydrosulfite)...........Sodium Hydrosulphite

I

Ichthyol...........................“Ammonium Sulfo Ichthyolate”
Indene.............................Para-cumarone
Indian Gum.........................Karaya, Gum
Isinglass, Japanese................Agar Agar
Italian Red........................Iron Oxide (red)
Ivory Black........................Bone Black

K

Kauri Gum..........................Copal, Gum
Kieselguhr.........................{Tripoli / Diatomaceous Earth}

L

Lanum..............................Lanolin
Lead Chromate......................Chrome Yellow
Lead Sulfate, Basic................Whitelead, Sublimed
Lemon, Salts of....................Potassium Binoxalate
Licorice...........................Glycyrrhiza
Ligroin, Light.....................Petroleum Ether
Lime...............................Calcium Oxide
Lime, Slaked.......................Calcium Hydroxide
Limestone..........................Calcium Carbonate
Litharge...........................Lead Monoxide
Liver of Sulphur...................Potassium Sulphide
Lunar Caustic......................Silver Nitrate
Lye................................Sodium Hydroxide

M

Magnesium, Calcined................Magnesium Oxide
Magnesium Silicate.................Talcum
Maize Oil..........................Corn Oil
Malt Sugar.........................Maltose
Metol..............................Methyl-para-aminophenol Sulphate

Microcosmic Salt........................Sodium Ammonium Phosphate
Milk Sugar..........................Lactose
Mineral Pitch........................Asphalt
Minium..............................Lead Oxide (red)
Mirbane Oil..........................Nitrobenzol
Muriatic Acid........................Hydrochloric Acid
Myrtle Wax..........................Bayberry Wax

N

Naphtha, Solvent....................Coal Tar Naphtha
Naples Yellow.......................Lead Antimonate
Nickel Salts, Double................Nickel Ammonium Sulphate
Nickel Salts, Single................Nickel Sulphate
Niter...............................Potassium Nitrate
Niter Cake..........................Sodium Bisulphate
Nitrocellulose (soluble cotton)..........Pyroxylin

O

Oleic Acid..........................Red Oil
Olein...............................Glyceryl Tri-oleate (natural)
Oleum...............................Sulphuric Acid (fuming)
Olive Oil...........................Sweet Oil
Orange Mineral......................Orange Red Lead Oxide
Orpiment............................Arsenous Sulphide (yellow)

P

Paraffin Oil........................{Mineral Oil / Petrolatum, Liquid}
Paris White.........................Whiting
Pearl Ash...........................Potassium Carbonate
Petrol..............................Gasoline
Petrolatum..........................Petroleum Jelly
Plaster of Paris....................Calcium Sulphate plus 1 mol. water
Potassium Bicarbonate...............Salaterus
Prussian Blue.......................Ferric Ferrocyanide
Prussiate of Potash, Red............Potassium Ferricyanide
Prussiate of Potash, Yellow.........Potassium Ferrocyanide
Prussic Acid........................Hydrocyanic Acid
Pyramidon...........................Amidopyrine
Pyrethrum...........................Insect Flowers (powdered)
Pyroligneous Acid...................Wood Vinegar

Q

Quicklime...........................Calcium Oxide
Quicksilver.........................Mercury

R

Red Oxide...........................Ferric Oxide, Red
Rochelle Salt.......................Potassium Sodium Tartrate
Rottenstone.........................Tripoli

S

Saccharine..........................Glucoside
Sal Ammoniac........................Ammonium Chloride
Sal Soda............................Sodium Carbonate, Hydrated

Salad Oil....................Cottonseed Oil
Salt....................Sodium Chloride
Salt Cake....................Sodium Sulphate (by-product)
Saltpeter....................Potassium Nitrate
Scale Wax....................Paraffin Wax (low melting)
Silica....................Silicon Dioxide
Sod Oil....................Degras
Soda Ash....................Sodium Carbonate, Anhydrous
Sodium Bisulphite....................Sodium Acid Sulphate
Sodium Phosphate, Dibasic....................Disodium Phosphate
Sodium Phosphate, Monobasic....................Monosodium Phosphate
Sodium Phosphate, Tribasic....................Trisodium Phosphate
Sodium Thiosulphate....................Hypo
Sperm Oil....................Whale Oil
Spirits of Turpentine....................Turpentine
Stannous Chloride....................Tin Crystals
Stearin....................Tristearin
Storax....................Styrax
Sucrose....................{Cane Sugar / Beet Sugar}
Sugar of Lead....................Lead Acetate
Sulfonated Castor Oil....................Turkey Red Oil
Sulphur Olive Oil....................Olive Oil Foots
Sulphuric Acid....................Oil of Vitriol
Sulphuric Ether....................Ether

T

TNT....................Trinitrotoluene
Tartar Emetic....................Antimony Potassium Tartrate
Tetralin....................Tetrahydro Naphthalene
Theobroma Oil....................Cacao Butter
Titanium Dioxide....................Titanium Oxide
Toluene....................Toluol
Triacetin....................Glycerol Triacetate
Trinitrophenol....................Picric Acid

V

Verdigris....................Copper Acetate, Basic
Vermilion....................Mercuric Sulphide, Red

W

Whale Oil....................Train Oil
White Arsenic....................Arsenic Trioxide
White Bole....................Kaolin
White Lead....................Lead Carbonate, Basic
White Metal....................Babbitt Metal
White Wax....................Beeswax (bleached)
Whiting....................Chalk, Refined
Wintergreen Oil, Synthetic....................Methyl Salicylate
Wood Alcohol....................Methyl Alcohol

Y

Yacca Gum....................Accroides Gum

Z

Zinc White....................Zinc Oxide
Zinc Yellow....................Potassium Zinc Chromate
Zinc Sulphate....................Salts of Vitriol

TUBE SIZE AND CAPACITY CHART FOR COMMONLY USED PRODUCTS

Product	*Fluid Capacity*	*Tube Size*	*Tube Material*	*Tube Opening*	*Market*
Dental Creams	3½ dram 1½ oz. 2 oz.	⅝x3½ 1x4½ 1⅛x5	Tin " "	Round or Ribbon	10¢ store Regular Regular
Shaving Creams	1 oz. 2½ oz. 4 oz.	⅞x4 1¼x5 1⅜x6½	Tin " "	Round " "	10¢ store Regular Regular
Toilet Creams	1½ oz. 2 oz.	1x4½ 1⅛x5	Tin "	Round "	Regular Regular
Ladies' Handbag Size	1½ dram 2¾ dram	½x2 ⅝x2½	Tin "	Round "	Regular Regular
Ointments	1 oz.	⅞x4	Tin	Round	Regular
Medical Jellies	2 oz. 3¼ oz.	1x5½ 1¼x6	Tin "	Round "	Regular Regular
Fish Paste	2 oz.	1⅛x5	Tin	Ribbon	Regular
Food Products	1¼ oz. 2 oz.	1x4 1x5½	Tin "	Round or Ribbon	Regular Regular
Tinting Colors	6 dram	¾x4	Tin or Lead	Round	Regular
Oil Colors	1¾ oz.	1x5	Tin	Round	Regular
Metal Polish	3¼ oz.	1¼x6	Lead	Round	Regular
Shoe Polish	1 oz. 2½ oz.	⅞x4 1¼x5	Tin or Lead "	Round "	10¢ store Regular
Cements	1½ oz.	1x4½	Tin	Screw Eye	Regular
Glues	2 oz.	1x5½	Lead	Round or Screw Eye	Regular
Pastes	2 oz.	1x5½	Lead	Round or Ribbon	Regular
Greases	5½ oz.	1½x7	Lead	Round	Regular

REFERENCES CONSULTED

American Druggist
American Perfumer
British Soap Manufacturer
British Jol. of Dental Science
Chemical Formulary Vols. I, II & III
Chemiker-Zeitung
Chemist & Druggist
Der Parfumer
Drug & Cosmetic Industry
Drug Trade News
Druggists' Circular
Jol. of Amer. Dental Ass'n.
Jol. of Amer. Medical Ass'n.
Jol. of Amer. Pharmaceutical Ass'n.
Les Materies Grasses
Manufacturing Chemist
Parfum, Moderne
Perfumery & Essential Oil Record
Pharmaceutica, Acta Helva
Pharmaceutical Journal
Practical Every Day Chemistry
Pharm. Monatshefte
Pharm. Zeitung
Seifenseider Zeitung
Soap
Soap Gazette & Perfumer
Soap, Perfumery & Cosmetics

WHERE TO BUY RAW MATERIALS

This section will be of great value to the cosmetic manufacturer as it lists manufacturers and wholesale agents for most raw materials required. It should be borne in mind, however, that these concerns may not be equipped to sell small quantities. Most materials and laboratory supplies, in small quantities, can be obtained most quickly from your druggist. What is unobtainable there may be usually obtained from any of the following:

Supply Houses (Raw Materials & Laboratory Supplies)

Howe & French .... Boston, Mass.
Kemkit Chemical Corp. .... Brooklyn, N. Y.
B. Preiser Co., Inc. .... Charleston, W. Va.
A. Daigger & Co. .... Chicago, Ill.
Greene Bros. Inc. .... Dallas, Texas
Frank W. Kerr Co. .... Detroit, Mich.
Mine & Smelter Supply Co. .... El Paso, Texas
K. C. Laboratory Supply Co. .... Kansas City, Mo.
Marshall Dill .... Los Angeles, Calif.
Roemer Drug Co. .... Milwaukee, Wis.
Cuthbert Co. .... Minneapolis, Minn.
Central Chemical Co. .... Newark, N. J.
Lewis Chemicals Inc. .... New York, N. Y.
R. F. Revson Co. .... New York, N. Y.
W. J. Gilmore Drug Co. .... Pittsburgh, Pa.
Phipps & Bird Inc. .... Richmond, Va.
Will Corp. .... Rochester, N. Y.
Marshall Dill .... San Francisco, Calif.
Scientific Supplies Co. .... Seattle, Wash.
Refinery Supply Co. .... Tulsa, Okla.

Since there are thousands of different synthetics (aromatics), perfume bases, essential oils etc., it may be necessary to deal with a number of sources, if many different and rarer ingredients are used.

Where to Buy Specialty Raw Materials in Foreign Countries

Argentina, Buenos Aires—W. H. Goetz
Calle Sarandi 315
Australia, Adelaide—Robert Bryce & Co., Pty., Ltd.
27 Chesser St.
———, Melbourne—Robert Bryce & Co., Pty., Ltd.
526–32 Little Bourke Street
———, Sydney—Robert Bryce & Co., Pty., Ltd.
414 Kent Street
Canada, Montreal—Chemicals, Ltd.
384 St. Paul St., W.
———, Montreal, P.Q.—R. E. Loane
512 McGill St.

———, Toronto 2—CANADA COLORS & CHEMICALS, Ltd.
1090 King St., W.
———, Vancouver, B.C.—SHANAHAN'S, Ltd.
Ft. of Campbell Ave.
CUBA, Havana—J. M. SIERRA
Aquiar 73, Dpt. 710, Apartado 363
ENGLAND, London—REX CAMPBELL & Co., Ltd.
7, Idol Lane, Eastcheap E.C.3
FRANCE, Paris—MINERAIS, ALLIAGES, PRODUITS CHIMIQUES
22, Ave. De La Grande-Armee (17E)
MEXICO, Saltillo, Coah—A. C. GARCIA
Apartado 168
NEW ZEALAND, Wellington—ROBERT BRYCE & Co., Pty., Ltd.
19 Lower Tory Street
PALESTINE, Tel-Aviv—E. HUPPERT
Box 1159, 10 Melchettstr.
So. AFRICA, Johannesburg—PHILIP ELZAS & Co.
23 Olga Bldgs., 121 President St.

MANUFACTURERS AND AGENTS FOR LARGE QUANTITIES OF RAW MATERIALS

Supplier †

† The numbers given below refer to the suppliers given at the end of this section.

If a compound name is not found in one place it should be looked up under the second name, e.g., gum acacia if not found under gum will be found under acacia.

Raw Material *

* Note—It is inadvisable to list the thousands of aromatic materials (perfuming oils and chemicals) used in small quantities. If unable to find such a material in this list communicate with an essential oil or synthetic supplier.

Absorption Bases....70, 71
Acacia, Gum....see Gum Arabic
Acetanilide....49, 51
Acetic Acid....14, 63
Acetone....42, 28
Acetone Oil....73A
"Acimul"....70
Adeps Lanae....see Lanolin
Adipic Acid....51
Agar (Agar-Agar)....116, 50A
Albumin....50A, 151
Alcohol....161
Alcohol, Sulphated or Sulfonated Fatty....51, 70
Aldehydes....55, 69
Alkalies....98, 157A
Alkaloids....96, 100
Alkanet....116, 115A
Alloxan....79B, 127A
Almond Meal....2A
Almond Oil....95, 158A
Alum....6, 73
Aluminum Powder....2A, 49C
Aluminum Acetate....6, 63
Aluminum Aceto Tartrate....127A
Aluminum Chloride....80, 101
Aluminum Palmitate....77, 100A
Aluminum Stearate....58A, 100A
Ambergris....96A, 48
Aminophenylglycine....52
Aminostearin....70
Ammonia....16, 63
Ammoniated Mercury....110C, 119A
Ammonium Carbonate....104A, 173
Ammonium Linoleate....70
Ammonium Stearate Anhydrous....70
Amyl Acetate....88, 110B
Amyl Alcohol....58, 139
Amyl Butyrate....110B, 58
Amyl Salicylate....162, 55
Anilin Dyes....70, 122
"Aquaresin"....70
Arachis Oil....see Peanut Oil
Aromatics,....see Synthetics
Arrow Root....102A, 116
Astringent Powder....70
Balsams....95, 110B
Barium Sulphide....14, 63
Barks....115A, 81
Beef Marrow....11A, 172A
Beeswax....91A, 172
"Bentonite"....5, 185
Benzaldehyde....98, 79A
"Benzocaine"....138A
Benzoic, Acid....138A, 29A
Benzoin....81, 116

Benzoinated Lard....98A, 81
Bergamot Oil....94A, 60
Betanaphthol....51, 105
Betanaphthol Disulphonate....127A
Bismuth Salts....110C, 119A
Bolus, white....56, 171
Boracic Acid....see Boric Acid
Borax....113A, 150
Boric Acid....113A, 150
Bromo "Acid"....110D, 70
"Butanol"....see Butyl Alcohol
Butyl Acetate....88, 184
Butyl Alcohol....28, 42
Butyl Stearate....42, 88
Cacao Butter....see Cocoa Butter
Calamine....14, 110C
Calcium Carbonate....171, 173
Calcium Phosphate....101, 166
Calcium Sulphate....63, 101
Calcium Sulphide....14, 63
"Calgon"....see Sodium Metaphosphate
Calomel....110C, 119A
Camphor....49A, 98A
Carbamide....see Urea
"Carbitol"....28
Carbolic Acid....see Phenol
Carbon Black....19, 74
Carbon, Decolorizing....45, 133
Carmine....56, 88A
Carnauba Wax....129A, 83
Carob Bean Powder see Locust Bean Gum
Castile Soap....see Soap
Castor Oil....14A, 145
Castor Oil, Sulphonated ....see Sulphonated Oils
Caustic Potash....see Potash, Caustic
Caustic Soda....see Soda, Caustic
"Cellosolve"....28
"Cellosolve" Acetate....28
Celluloid Scrap....81A, 186
"Ceraflux"....70
Ceresin Wax....20A, 78A
"Cetamin"....70
Cetyl Alcohol....69, 142B
Chalk....see Calcium Carbonate
Charcoal....56, 19
Cherry Kernel Oil....49A, 95
Chloral Hydrate....101, 110C
Chlorbutanol....162
Chloroform....96, 100
Chlorophyll....4A, 119
Chlorthymol....100
Cholesterin....119, 172A
Cholesterol....see Cholesterin
Cinnabar....56
Citral....138, 165
Citric Acid....119A, 14
Citronella Oil....43A, 49B
Clay....173, 5
Cobalt Nitrate....77, 63
Cocoa Butter....127A, 81B
Coconut Butter....182, 145
Coconut Oil....170, 187
Cod Liver Oil....49B, 129B
Colloidal Clay....see Clay
Collodion....see Nitro Cellulose
Colors, Insoluble Dry....84A, 56
Colors, Soluble....84A
Corn Syrup....44, 145A
Cresol (Cresylic Acid)....16, 101
Damar....6, 156A
Deramin....70
Derris....115A, 116
Dextrin....102A, 151
Diacetone Alcohol....42, 101
Dibutylphthalate....87, 184
Diethylene Glycol....28
Diethylene Glycol Stearate....70
Diethyl Phthalate....161, 184
Diglycol Laurate....70
Diglycol Stearate....70
Dyestuffs....56
Egg Oil....83, 74B
Emulsifying Agents....70, 101
"Emulsone B"....70
Eosin....88A, 9
Epsom Salts....49, 63
Erythrosine....110D, 127A
Essences....94A, 95
Essential Oils....see Oils
Ester Gum....17, 115
Ethyl Acetate....161, 184
Ethylaminobenzoate....59
Ethyl Lactate....6, 161
Ethylene Diamine....28
Ethylene Glycol....28
Eucalyptol....120A, 158A
Extracts, Fluid & Solid....138B, 110E
Fatty Acids....174, 187
Flaxseed....145, 10
Flea Seed....see Psyllium Seed
Flower Waters....158A, 96A
Fluid Extracts....98A, 110E
Fluorescein....122, 56
Formaldehyde....79A, 51
Formalin....see Formaldehyde
Fuller's Earth....133, 171
Galagum....70
Gelatin....11A, 50A
Glaubers Salt....see Sodium Sulphate
Glucose....see Corn Syrup
Glycerin....39, 91B
Glycerin Substitutes....70, 111
Glyceryl Mono Stearate....70, 71
Glyceryl Oleate....70
Glyceryl Monoricinoleate....70
Glyceryl Tristearate....70
Glycol Bori-Borate....70
Glycomine....70
"Glycomel"....70
Glycopon....70
Glycosterin....70
"Glyco Wax A"....70
Gum Arabic (Acacia)....58B, 156A

Gum Benzoin....................115A, 81
Gum Karaya....................51A, 58B
Gum, Locust Bean............51A, 58B
Gum Tragacanth....................83
Gum "Tragacol"..............70, 58B
Hamamelis.............see Witch Hazel
Harcol...........................70
Henna.......................81, 116
Herbs.......................see Barks
Hexamethylenetetramine......79A, 110C
Hormones..................11A, 172A
Hydrazine Hydrochloride..........4, 52
Hydrogen Peroxide...............96, 51
Hydrogenated Oils & Fats
...............see Coconut Butter
Hydroxyphenylglycine...............52
"Icthyol"......................96, 100
Infusorial Earth................133, 85
Irish Moss....................83, 115A
Iodine........................96, 100
Isocholesterin............see Cholesterin
"Isohol"..........................70
Isopropyl Alcohol..............147, 184
Japan Wax....................83, 129B
Kaolin, Colloidal..............96, 127A
Kerosene, Deodorized..........143, 141
Lactic Acid......................9A, 73
Lakes, Color.....................9, 88A
Lampblack......................19, 81C
Lanolin.......................19A, 119
Lard.......................see Tallow
Latex...............see Rubber Latex
Lecithin.....................6B, 172A
"Lemenone"........................70
Locust Bean Gum.............58B, 83
Lycopodium..................115A, 116
Magnesium Carbonate.........73A, 173
Magnesium Stearate...........58A, 121
Maleic Acid...................101, 105
Magnesium Sulphate....see Epsom Salts
Menthol.....................129B, 110C
Menthyl Salicylate............59, 127A
Mercuric Chloride..........110C, 119A
"Mercurochrome"..................81D
Methyl Alcohol (Methanol).......28, 42
Methyl Ethyl Ketone...........28, 73A
Methyl Salicylate...............79A, 49
Mercury Compounds........175A, 110C
Methyl Cellulose....................2
Methyl "Parasept"..................79A
Methyl Parahydroxy Benzoate......79A
"Moldex"..........................70
Naphthalene.....................16, 25
Nickel Nitrate....................77, 63
Nipagin...........................71
Nitrocellulose....................79, 51
Nitrophenylglycine.................52
Ochre.........................56, 127A
Oils, Essential................95, 120A
" , Fish.....................49B, 98A
" , Mineral....................78A, 141
" , Vegetable................157B, 187
Oleic Acid.......................32, 91B
Olein...........................32, 91B
Olive Oil........................95, 170
Ondulum...........................70
Oxy-Cholesterin..........see Cholesterin
Oxy-Quinolin Sulphate.............145B
Ozokerite....................87A, 151A
Pancreatin...................11A, 172A
Parachol...........................70
Paraffin Oil............see Oil, Mineral
Paraffin Wax....................12, 141
Para-aminophenol.................25, 52
Parachlormetaxylenol...............101
Paradichlorbenzol.................80, 51
Parahydroxybenzoic Acid or
Esters.......................70, 127A
Para-phenylenediamine.........25, 165A
Peanut Oil......................170, 187
Pearl Essence....................31, 99A
Pectin.......................170A, 25A
Peppermint Oil..............110A, 112A
Perfume Bases.................43A, 56B
Permosalt..........................70
Peroxide of Hydrogen
............see Hydrogen Peroxide
Petrolatum......................12, 141
Petroleum Jelly..........see Petrolatum
Phenol...........................16, 49
Phenylenediamine...................52
Pigments.........................19, 56
Phosphoric Acid.................63, 101
Picric Acid.......................51, 83
Pilocarpine Hydrochloride.....110C, 79B
Pine Oil..........................67, 79
Polycol............................70
Polyglycols...............see Polychol
Potash, Caustic................157A, 83
Potassium Carbonate............83, 188
Potassium Chlorate..............83, 63
Potassium Nitrate................63, 83
Potassium Silicate.................120
Preservatives.....................70, 49
Propyl "Parasept"..................79A
Propyl Parahydroxy Benzoate.......79A
Propylene Glycol...................28
Psyllium Seed.................115A, 116
Pumice..........................83, 171
Pyrethrum....................115A, 116
Pyroxylin............see Nitrocellulose
Quillaja Bark..............see Saponin
Quince Seed....................81, 115A
Quinine Compounds..........100, 110C
Red Oil..........................32, 45A
Resorcin (Resorcinol)..........63, 110C
Ricinoleic Acid.................14A, 187
Rose Water......................94A, 95
Rosin.............................67, 79
Rosin Oil..........................107
Rubber Latex....................108, 127
Saccharin.......................79A, 101
Salicylic Acid....................49, 101
Sal Soda..........see Sodium Carbonate